Beating Lyme Disease: Living the Good Life In Spite of Lyme

David A. Jernigan, B.S., D.C.

SP

Somerleyton Press
Wichita, Kansas, USA

Copyright ©2008 Dr. David A. Jernigan, B.S., D.C.

All rights Reserved. No part of this book may be used or reproduced, stored in a retrieval system, or transmitted by any means, electronic, mechanical, photocopying, recording, or otherwise, without written permission from the author.

ISBN 978-0-9674623-3-2

For information:

SP

Somerleyton Press
545 North Woodlawn
Wichita, Kansas 67208 USA

Edited by Katy Penner
Cover Design and Book Layout ©2008 by Katy Penner

Manufactured in the United States of America

In Memory

In memory of my cousin, Dr. Chris Harazda, O.M.D., Lic. Acc., poet, teacher, shakuhachi player using the Japanese kotchiku flute, philosopher, friend to all who met him.

Dedication

Dedicated to those doctors in the trenches who struggle to achieve lasting results in their Lyme patients; who fight a politically incorrect illness; who through sweat and tears fight stealth microbes; who struggle without any medical and insurance company agreement; who bravely reach beyond their conventional training for the betterment of their patients.

This book is also dedicated to my patients, and the patients of other Lyme-literate doctors, who, in desperation at times, stick with us while we continue to learn how to deal with this most dastardly of illnesses.

Acknowledgements

I would like to recognize the following with special thanks.

Julie Taylor and family, who started me on this journey, fed me my first information about Lyme Disease, and who patiently stayed with me as I struggled to put the pieces together that ultimately led to the development of Borrelogen™.

Dr. Milton Dowty, D.C., my friend and mentor, and founder of Chiro-Plus Kinesiology; who set my foundation on a higher mountain; and who taught me CPK, a tool which led me to the development of Bio-Resonance Scanning™.

Dr. John Brimhall, D.C., whose intellect, wisdom and passion to teach doctors to become healers is unparalleled, whose love for God-designed healing through the latest technology inspires me to be a better doctor and a better person.

My heart cannot express the profound appreciation I feel for the many hours of work by my editor, Katy Penner, to ensure that this book is edited and formatted in such a way that it is easy and enjoyable to read. I am eternally grateful for her loyalty and love in persevering through my idiosyncrasies to help bring forth a quality product.

Special thanks to Michele Menzel, a great healer in her own right, who read the early release copy of this book and grasped the book in its entirety, better than I did myself, and helped rearrange the topics so that the protocol and information is easier to read by those suffering from Lyme Disease.

Disclaimer

This book is intended as an educational tool and guide for doctors and patients seeking alternative methods for addressing the human body suffering from Lyme Disease. All of the therapies and recommendations are designed to facilitate the restoration of the structure and function of the body's tissues rather than "treating disease." The recommendations, therapies, and methods described in this book are for the most part alternative, which, by definition, have not been investigated and/or approved by any government or regulatory agency. Accordingly, it is recommended that one consult with their healthcare professional before using any therapy. Pregnant women are especially advised to consult with their healthcare professional before using any therapy.

Your health is important. Ultimately you must realize it is your body, and it is your decision how to address any illness. You, the reader, must take full responsibility for your health and how you use this book.

The publisher and the author expressly disclaim responsibility for any adverse effects resulting from your use of the information that is contained in this book. Check with your healthcare professional before starting any of the dietary supplements and therapies in this book.

Various chapters in this book describe the clinical practice of the author as it exists at the time of publishing.

Contents

Introduction i

Section 1: Understanding Lyme Disease
1. The "New" Great Imitator 3
2. What is Lyme Disease? 15
3. "Fiber Optic" Communication of Microbes 25
4. What Factors Lead to Illness From Microbes? 45
5. Borrelia burgdorferi & Mycoplasmal Infections 59
6. Beating Lyme Disease is More Than Killing Bacteria 63
7. Body Circuits and Circuit Healing 71
8. Illuminated Physiology and Medical Uses of Light..........89

Section 2: Detoxification
9. Why Detoxify if I Have Lyme Disease? 113
10. Lyme Toxins and a Toxic World...119
    Bacterial Toxins 120
    FACT Scoring 123
    Lyme Leaky Brain Syndrome (LLBS) 127
    Worsening of Symptoms 130
    Ammonia 135
    ALS & Lyme Ammonia 137
    Parkinson's & Lyme Ammonia 138
    Environmental Toxins 138
    Skin Toxins 142
    New Invention: Nanoderm Lotion 143
    Detoxification in Pregnancy and Breastfeeding 145
    The First-Timer's Response.. 147

Section 3: The Perfect-7 Treatment and Detox Protocol™
11. The Perfect-7 Treatment and Detox Protocol™ Summarized .153
    Includes introduction to following sections of Expanded Perfect-7 Steps

---

Perfect-7 Protocol Steps by Section:

Step 1: Restore the Body's Regulation of Microbes
12. Borrelogen™, Lymogen™, Microbojen™ 163

Step 2: Detoxify Lyme Toxins
13. Neuro-Antitox II Formulas™..173
14. Dr. Jernigan's Detox Coffee, Detox Tea, and Detox Cocoa 177
15. Dry Skin Brushing 181

16. Infrared Sauna 183
17. Dr. Joseph's Colon Cleanse™ 189
18. Hydrogen Peroxide/Epsom Salt Detox Bath.............. 195
19. Dr. Jernigan's Mustard Foot Bath™............................ 201
    Hot/Cold Contrast Mustard Foot Bath............................202
20. Strengthening/Nutritive Bath 203
21. Master Longevity Body Cleanse.................................. 207
22. Liver and Gallbladder Flush 215

Step 3: Break Up Bacterial Biofilms and Inflammation
23. TPP Protease® 221
24. Beyond Chelation-Improved® 225

Step 4: Support the Bio-Energetic Fields of the Body
25. Essential Oils Protocol 229
26. Electromagnetic Pollution and BioPro® Products 233
27. Lyme and Low Body Temperature 237
28. Causes of Low Body Temperature 249
29. The Warmth Organization of the Body 267

Step 5: Address all Structural Interferences
30. Doctors of Chiropractic 275
31. What to Expect with Biological Medicine 281
    Cases from the Hansa Center...285

Step 6: Align Lifestyle to Optimize Health
32. A Better Way to "Fight" Infectious Disease: Balanced Living . 301
33. Redesigning Your Life to Overcome Illness 307
34. 50 Thoughts to Live On 315
35. Diet and Nutrition... 319
36. "No Brainer" Things to Do... 327

Step 7: Identify and Address Emotional Triggers
37. German New Medicine™: Revelations Concerning Symptoms 333
    Includes Article by Caroline Markolin, Ph.D.: Reading the Brain...................336
38. Childhood Stress and Lyme Disease 341
39. Adult Stress and Lyme Disease 349
40. Miasms: Predisposition to Illness 353

Section 4: Remedy Suggestions and Emotional Conflicts
41. Remedy Suggestions and Emotional Conflicts for Specific Symptoms.. 361

Section 5: Advanced Techniques for Doctors
42. Advanced Techniques for Doctors of Lyme Patients 399
43. Two-Person Energy Balancing For Stress Resolution................. 407
44. ST-8 Lymphatic Drainage Therapy 415
45. IonCleanse Detoxification.. 419
46. Valve Corrections for Colon Problems 423

Section 6: Advanced Diagnostic Considerations
47. Computerized Regulation Thermography (CRT) 427
48. Lyme Disease Meets Biological Dentistry 433

Appendix A: Dealing with the Alcohol in Remedies 437
Appendix B: The Secret to Proper Tick Removal 445
Appendix C: Lemon Wheel Throat Wrap 449
Appendix D: Iodine Stain Test 451
Appendix E: Recommended Reading 455
Appendix F: Internet Resources 457
Appendix G: Research on Borrelogen™ 459
Appendix H: Other Jernigan Nutraceutical products 465

Glossary 471
Product Ordering 475
Index 477

Introduction

My Story

Through the years, thousands of people have come to my clinic, thousands more have read my books, and yet very few ever knew the health adversities I have personally experienced in my life. So few knew of these challenges I have faced because, after years of working on restoring my own body, mind, and spirit, I am blessed to enjoy virtually perfect health almost all the time now. The health problems I have weathered have been like signposts guiding me towards not only greater health, but also to greater maturity on all levels.

I grew up mostly healthy and doing hard work. In my late teens I cleared land, cutting trees for a housing development, and sometimes putting medium-sized trees under my arm and dragging them to a pile. Older men would shake their heads and say, "You really shouldn't do that to your back." But what did I care? At 6'7" tall, it felt good to be strong. Within a year, my back began to have periods of paralyzing pain.

I didn't know "what I wanted to be when I grew up," so I just did what sounded like fun until it wasn't fun anymore. All my fun involved very strenuous jobs. I worked on seven different riverboats on the Mississippi River, and I worked on oil rigs as a roustabout in the Gulf of Mexico for over a year; that is when my back really first gave me a wake-up call. I was flown by helicopter to a hospital, unable to stand or walk. It was to be the first of three times in my life where I didn't know whether I would ever walk again. The last time, while in the U.S. Air Force, the doctors thought I had broken a bone in my back.

I smoked cigarettes throughout those 11 years "just socially." I would not smoke in my house or car, and never when I was dating someone. I sometimes went weeks without a cigarette, so I never thought I was addicted...until I really tried to quit! In the midst of severe life stress, I began to develop difficult respiratory infections that ultimately led to two bouts of severe pneumonia, and doctors literally saved me at the brink of death.

I spent thirty days in a military hospital after a grueling surgery to remove benign tumors along my spine. This was followed by thirty days of drugs (morphine) to quell the post-surgical pain. It was 90 days after being released from the hospital before I could work out, which was made more difficult by the 45 pounds I gained in the previous three months of immobilization.

In the late 1990's, Lyme Disease entered my life with chronic fatigue, brain fog, cognitive dysfunctions, joint pain, muscle pains and twitching, and the most disturbing symptoms – heart arrhythmias and palpitations. Fresh in my mind is the memory of lying in bed at night and feeling my heart seem to make huge rolling movements inside my chest. It would beat hard and erratic and then stop completely! I would reach up and feel the carotid artery in my neck and see if it really wasn't beating—it wasn't--and then it would race and flip around again. At one point, after facing many nights of wondering if this night I would die, I decided dying was not the worst thing that could happen. Not that I wanted to die, but after facing the possibility night after night, it just didn't hold the fear it once did.

Other family members tested positive for having Lyme spirochetes as well, and one was so sick that he could barely get out of bed for months because of the severe pain and neuropathies. Later on, my oldest daughter's legs became paralyzed from West Nile virus in her spine, thankfully to be ultimately miraculously healed! Do I understand some of what you are going through? Yes! Do I know you can gain greater health than you had before? Yes!

Sharing Health

In 1995, I founded a healing center dedicated to helping the medical "lost causes" of the world, including myself and my family. The present-day clinic is not just for "lost causes," but it is also for those who just want help to realize optimal coherence in the body, mind, and spirit.

It has been years since any major symptom has been a problem for me and my family, and health and happiness now flourish. As each of you can attest to, the journey to health can feel life-long, but it is beyond worthwhile in the realizations and maturity gained along the way!

I have been blessed to treat over 4000 people, with good to great results, using the principles discussed in this book. Over 80% of our patients come to us from out of the state or out of the country. We have treated everyone from day-old babies to centurions, Olympic hopefuls to people in comas. We have facilitated the health of people all over the world, from restoring the ability to walk in a young woman in England, to fighting malaria in Ghana, Africa. Our success has been due to our focus, indeed our specialization, of restoring the integrity of the body, mind, and spirit. We worked to develop new medicines with new modes of action to really restore lives, restore the quality of lives, to give hope, and to facilitate the personal and spiritual growth of all who come to us.

I KNOW it is possible to be restored from any malady. I am living proof, as is my daughter, and as are so many other now-healthy people I have met while on my own personal journey. I have had many teachers, facilitators, and guides that have appeared in Divine synchronicity to my willingness to learn. I give thanks to God and to each of them all for the health, knowledge, and wisdom I now enjoy on all levels of my being.

As I have told so many of my patients, "We are co-mentors upon this journey." True healing and existence is a team effort.

My desire is to see you liberated from the fear of Lyme Disease. I want you to replace the fear with a heart-knowingness that all you need will be provided as you walk in a perpetual state of confidence and love, and as you seek to only use treatments and lifestyle choices that help restore the perfect design and function of your body, mind, and spirit. (More on this in my book *Everyday Miracles by God's Design*.)

It might amaze many of you that I have never read one chapter or any part of any other book on Lyme Disease! The reason is that I value what I call "Original Arrangements of Thought." I have almost given up on the idea of "Original Thought" since I find that so many of my "Original Thoughts" have been thought before. I am a product of the U.S. Public School system of education, and therefore I was programmed to simply take in written information as truth and be able to regurgitate it on a test. In this book, I want to share with you what I have learned in applied knowledge, without bias to the thoughts and ideas of someone else on the topic.

I also want you to know that there is more than one right path to optimum health. This book is what it is -- it is not the end-all dissertation on Lyme Disease or the only way by any means! I hear good results are being achieved from the knowledge of several books on *natural* approaches to Lyme Disease. My recommendation is to find the book or protocol that seems to resonate best with you, and to follow it as closely as possible until it is evident whether it is going to work for you or not. If it doesn't work for you, take what you have learned from the first process and find another protocol that can aid in your forward progress.

People have often asked me if the protocol listed in this book is the same as what we do in my clinic. The answer is no.

Introduction

This book is an effort to provide you with a general protocol that will hopefully empower you enough to heal yourself. Our clinic strives to teach, coach, facilitate, and apply carefully orchestrated therapies and treatments, all tailored to your incredible uniqueness and determined by careful observation and examination. This all pivots around the amazing technology of Bio-Resonance Scanning™ and the philosophy of Circuit Healing™.

As you read this book, you will begin to realize that I devalue the role of the microbes in the ultimate disease process, compared to 99% of Lyme doctors. Dealing with the microbes does matter, but not to the degree you might think.

You will see herein, there are many myths in the "scientific art of medicine." Sincerity is no guarantee of truth. I tell you this because so often doctors state the "facts" as though they were written in stone. The only problem is the "stones" often get replaced with new stones. Each is promoted as the sincere truth. Although I am very sincere in what I am telling you in this book, it is just my truth, based upon the best science and research I have found.

I really appreciate what T. Harv Eker states in his motivational seminars and books:

> "Don't believe a word I say. Why would I say that? Because I can only speak from my own experience. None of the concepts and insights I share are inherently true or false, right or wrong. They simply reflect my own results, and the amazing results I've seen in the lives of thousands and thousands of my students. Having said that, however, I believe that if you use the principles I'm teaching you, you will totally transform your life. Study these principles like your life depended on it. Then try the principles out for yourself. Whatever works, keep doing. Whatever doesn't you're welcome to throw away."[1]

Biological Medicine Philosophy

This book is intended to present a natural protocol for people suffering from Lyme Disease, based on a relatively new philosophy within what is generically termed Alternative Medicine. This new philosophy is called Biological Medicine. Biological Medicine recognizes that all aspects of the body, mind, and spirit must be addressed and brought into optimal integrity before lasting health can be achieved.

Unlike other body/mind/spirit philosophies of the healing arts, American Biological Medicine is unique in that it is able to utilize the highly scientific, adjunctive diagnostic and treatment technique, Bio-Resonance Scanning™ (BRS), as well as conventional tests and the ancient healing arts of observation and intuition, to rapidly and accurately determine where interferences exist within the body, mind, or spirit. BRS helps to greatly diminish the educated "guesswork" of doctoring. BRS can be used to flow dynamically, in real-time, from interference-diagnostics to treatment selection and its correct application. (The scientific explanation of Bio-Resonance Scanning is addressed later in Chapter 8.)

The reason it is important to discuss Biological Medicine and Bio-Resonance Scanning™ here is so that the content of this book can be appreciated as not promoting another "cookbook" solution to healing from Lyme Disease. Cookbook healing means that, once diagnosed, the patient is put on a standard "recipe" that is supposed to heal everyone. The reality is that as different as each of us look from one another on the outside, we are all just as unique on the inside. For instance, it is now known that the supposed benefits of taking aspirin daily for the heart only works for about one third of people. Two thirds of the people taking aspirin for this purpose are getting no benefit because their body digests aspirin differently than the one third. (The natural supplement Nattokinase, a systemic proteolytic enzyme, works better than aspirin and is effective in over 95% of people.)

Introduction

The reality of medicine and healing is that the world's most astute and celebrated physicians cannot heal even the simplest paper cut, much less a complex illness such as Lyme Disease. Also, giving the body allopathic (symptom-based) prescription medicines or allopathically-oriented natural remedies that do not work synergistically with the body, but seek instead to bomb the bacteria or suppress a symptom, might as well be black magic! These medicines create only the illusion of health. The reality underneath the illusion is that the illness is still there, evidenced by the fact that if you remove the medicine, all the symptoms return. Roughly 80% of western medicine simply enables you to die faster without feeling it.

If the physician cannot actually heal anything, and forcing the body into drug-induced illusions of health does not heal anything, then the focus of all health-related efforts must be to identify everything interfering with the optimal function and integrity of the body and then provide the body with the corrective/restorative treatments that will work to *enable the body to heal itself.*

Ultimately, healing is achieved by facilitating the body, mind, and spirit with:

- Corrective information.
- Restoring the transmission and reception of bio-information.
- Providing the building blocks needed to restore optimal function and integrity.
- The removal of structural, chemical, stress-related, and electromagnetic interferences to the normal structure and function of the body.
- Replacing "disease mentality, and negative thought and emotional patterns with sustained, powerful DNA transforming thoughts and emotional patterns.
- Restoring the integrity within the interdependent and interconnected body, mind, and spirit.

It is a myth that you will be truly well when your doctor can kill all of the bacteria. Later chapters will reveal how some of the bacteria always survive every form of treatment and also explain what is required by you and your health care team to achieve the disappearance of any symptom and any disease.

A companion to this book is my new book, *Everyday Miracles by God's Design*. The *Everyday Miracles* book teaches powerful DNA-changing processes and truths that will supercharge the body while the remedies and therapies listed in this book are doing their work. It is a book written to empower you to take charge of your life and health, and to finally be liberated from needing any doctor ever again. *Everyday Miracles* is not a book filled with stories of miraculous events. It is written after seeing thousands of people appear at my clinic, seeming to believe that they were only responsible for 1) Showing up for their appointments, and 2) Taking their remedies/medicines.

I have written the *Everyday Miracles* book to teach people how they are ultimately in control of the healing process – and how to live a life filled with miracles of health, miracles of wealth, and miracles of joy.

Beating Lyme Disease is written for lay people and physicians who desire to learn some of the healing options that I have used to facilitate healing in over 4000 people suffering from virtually every imaginable symptom. The remedies, therapies, and treatments mentioned have been applied in literally tens of thousands of office visits at our clinic.

One can easily pick up literature about a myriad of vitamins, minerals, botanical medicines, glandulars, homeopathic remedies, enzymes, and colloidal metals and minerals, all promising to "cure" what ails you. I see patients from all over the world who have been everywhere and tried everything (and many have the bags and sometimes suitcases full of medicines and remedies to prove it!). You may have Lyme Disease, but when it is chronic, the infection is well-entrenched, and the only way to route it is to change the environment of body so that it is no longer enabling the overgrowth of certain microbes.

Complex cases often require more than just pills and natural remedies for the body to balance and heal itself. Often required are hands-on treatments with a doctor and many types of therapeutic devices, such as Frequency-Modulated Low-Level Lasers, Infrared Saunas, ST-8 Lymphatic Machines, Fascia-Release therapies, Colymed™ hydrotherapy, and many other clinical techniques and technologies. Health strategy is all about using the correct tool for the job. Often too much is being expected from the pills, IV therapies, and other medications – many times we have seen that no combination of medicines will unlock the chronically ill body without these other modalities.

You must deal with all the areas of the body that are weak and out of balance. The cookbook method of conventional treatment is to simply take a rotating, seemingly never-ending cocktail of various antibiotics. The reality is that even intravenous antibiotics will often only kill 85% of the bacteria at their very best, leaving 15% alive and now antibiotic-resistant.[2] In the long term, the body is not enhanced or improved in any way with antibiotics. The short-term gains of antibiotics blind many people to their insidious long-term adverse effects. Now before you throw this book down because of my "anti-antibiotic" stance, please know that it is not because I believe that antibiotics don't kill bacteria, it is just that I believe more strongly in the body's ability to heal in a more optimum manner if given the less harmful natural support it needs.

Just because popular opinion sustains the opinion, it is not necessarily true that prescription and/or natural antibiotics are the ultimate answer.

Someday the practice of forcing the body into drug-induced illusions of health will hopefully be viewed as just as barbaric as not washing hands. The reality is that no microbe can replicate out of control in a healthy body. The body's own blood component albumen is six times better as a bacteriostatic (blocks bacteria from reproducing) than penicillin! Its ability to control and stop the overgrowth of bacteria vanishes when the body becomes imbalanced. Restoring balance in the body, mind, and spirit also restores the albumen's ability to stop the bacteria from continuing to thrive. Albumen is just one, and by no means is the primary, mechanism the body has to control microbes! The body has many different mechanisms like albumen to regulate microbes if given a chance.

The protocol presented in this book revolves around frequency-matched remedies and the principles of Circuit Healing™ and American Biological Medicine. Circuit Healing™ and American Biological Medicine are, in my opinion, the most pure and advanced healing methods and philosophies available today.

Health in a bottle is a myth!

Most people with Lyme Disease have already used many antibiotics with limited success or may be intolerant and allergic to them.

This is the fourth revision of this book. Each new edition is more refined as greater understanding is realized. Each book has been written because my heart goes out to so many people suffering using prescription or natural antibiotics. These people erroneously believed, "If my doctor can kill these bacteria, then I will be well." "Health in a bottle" is a myth.

Optimum health is the product of living with the highest degree of integrity within the body, mind, and spirit. Optimum health is also the ability of the body, mind, and spirit to adapt correctly to any changes in its internal and external environment.

Healing is the product of guiding and facilitating the restoration of integrity through thoughtfully applied physical treatments, natural medicines, therapies, and through teaching and coaching the whole person back to optimum integrity within the mind, emotions, and spirit.

Preface to this edition of *Beating Lyme Disease*

The first two editions of the book were called *Surviving Lyme Disease; Using Alternative Medicine*. The only reason I wrote this first book was because so many people were trying to use Borrelogen™ like an antibiotic, taking a few bottles and expecting to be "cured." Readers of these first two editions responded by saying they wanted to do more than just survive. Thus was born the third edition, *Beating Lyme Disease; Using Alternative Medicine and God-Designed Living*.

Feedback from some doctors was that they couldn't get some people to read the book because it had the word "God" in the title. The principles of "God-Designed Living" are the life issues revolving around understanding what I feel are universal laws, meaning things which are true no matter who you are or what your religious orientation. No matter how powerful and clever the combination of medicines, if you don't play by the universal laws, you can never really win. This information is vitally important because if you do not know the very definite rules that must be followed to learn how to live in maximum quality of existence, you will be a slave to drugs and remedies forever.

These topics of universal laws are now covered in my book *Everyday Miracles by God's Design*, which deals with the latest research I have found regarding what, other than taking medicines and doing therapies, is truly necessary to completely heal. For those who want to know only about Lyme Disease without the mention of God, this edition will focus solely on that topic. Others wanting to gain a more complete picture of health, happiness, and beyond can read the *Everyday Miracles by God's Design* book in addition to this book.

This edition of the *Beating Lyme Disease* book is subtitled *Living the Good Life In Spite of Lyme* because advances in creating more powerful microscopes and in laboratory diagnostics reveal that our bodies are a "soup" of microbes which are held in synergistic form and function only when the optimal integrity of the body, mind, and spirit is maintained. (Synergy = both microbes and you live in harmony, both receiving benefits from the relationship.) You most definitely can "live the good life in spite of Lyme microbes" by enabling the body to naturally bring down the population of potentially problematic microbes and by restoring the integrity of the body, mind, and spirit.

The concepts and protocol presented in this book are the result of ongoing research of doctors around the world to find and/or develop better "informational" remedies and therapies. The healing protocol in this book is called the *Perfect-7 Treatment and Detox Protocol*. You will find that the Treatment Protocol and the Detox Protocol are identical. This is because the idea that one can treat without detoxifying the body, or detoxify without dealing with the primary source of the toxins (the microbes) is a flawed idea.

Although we have trained doctors in the practice of American Biological Medicine, most doctors are classically trained and many of the concepts presented in this book will seem foreign. It is my hope that more doctors, as well as patients, will become interested upon reading this and be liberated from the "germ theory" and "drug mentality" that is so pervasive in today's clinics and hospitals.

I pray that you prosper and find good health all the days of your life.

Dr. David A. Jernigan

[1] Eker, T. Harv, *Secrets of the Millionaire Mind: Mastering the Inner Game of Wealth*, 2005. Harper/Collins, New York.
[2] Martinez J, Baquero F. 2000. Mutation frequencies and antibiotic resistance. Antimicrob. Agents Chemother. 44:1771-1777, Coates A, Dormancy and Low Growth States in Microbial Disease. 2003. Cambridge University Press.

Section 1
Understanding Lyme Disease

1
~

The NEW Great Imitator

Quick Facts About Lyme Disease

- Lyme Disease is initiated by a spiral-shaped bacteria (spirochete) called Borrelia burgdorferi, but the actual disease always involves loss of the body's control of several different "co-infections" of virtually every microbial class, i.e., viral, mycoplasmal, fungal, parasitic.
- Toxins from the bacteria are actually the primary cause of all of your symptoms!
- Lifelong optimal health can be achieved even if every single Lyme spirochete in your body has not been killed.
- It is well recognized that the best natural or pharmaceutical antibiotics can at best only kill 85% of the target bacteria in the body.
- Antibiotics may do more harm than good. Antibiotics can activate bacteriophages (viruses) that infect the Lyme spirochetes and insert their toxin-generating genes into the bacterial chromosomes. These viruses can turn basically harmless bacterium into killers through

this genetic sequencing of toxins by causing the bacteria to produce greater amounts of neurotoxins (nervous system poisons).
- The allopathic philosophy of medicine (antibiotics, etc.) often predisposes one to Post-Lyme Syndrome (PLS).
- After prolonged illness a person would not likely be symptom-free or truly healthy even if it were possible to kill every spirochete, because restoring health requires more than killing the bacteria.
- It is possible to have Lyme spirochetes and yet <u>never</u> manifest any symptoms.
- The unique symptoms experienced by an individual are from the microbes revealing a person's weakest, and therefore most vulnerable, areas in the body.
- High-powered microscopes have revealed that our bodies are a soup of innumerable and greatly unrecognized microbes. There are 20 times more microbes than cells in your body. Another way of saying this is that 90% of the cells in your body are microbes.
- A Herxheimer reaction (herx) is a sign of a <u>poor</u> treatment plan and is unnecessary. A herx greatly increases the toxic load on the body; at its worst it can kill an illness-weakened patient outright. A herx can temporarily or permanently disable the body, mind, and spirit.
- The sustained restoration of the optimal function and integrity of the body, mind, and spirit will naturally resolve any infection.
- No microbe can replicate at will or unchecked in a healthy body.
- A component in your blood called albumin is six times stronger than penicillin as a bacteriostatic (preventing microbial replication).

- Until the patient's body can maintain microbial balance without the help of medications, the patient will never reach the point of not needing the medications.
- Some of the best research facility laboratories report that they have rarely found any person's blood to be completely clear of spirochetes, even after every type of long-term natural or pharmaceutical intervention.
- Tick bites are <u>not</u> the only way to get Lyme Disease.
- Less than half the people diagnosed with Lyme Disease ever have a bulls-eye rash.

The "New" Great Imitator

The new "Great Imitator," Lyme Disease, is increasingly being confirmed in cases of misdiagnosed chronic illnesses. It is said to be the "great imitator" because its symptoms are so diverse that it can mimic 200 illnesses.[3] This fact, and the fact that there have been no good laboratory tests available to positively confirm Lyme Disease, has led to the polarization of the medical and scientific community on the topic of Lyme. I have seen people in my clinic who have seen many specialists and been subjected to as many as 700 different tests without conclusive results. These patients were usually labeled "Atypical Lupus," "Atypical ALS," "Atypical MS," or some other symptom-based diagnosis. When I checked the person (using Bio-Resonance Scanning™, which will be explained later) for frequencies of Lyme bacteria, I often found it positive in both the blood and urine. Upon returning to their other doctors with the news, many times the doctors told the patient, "We don't know what you have, but it isn't Lyme Disease!" Even when faced with positive Lyme tests, and even in the face of symptoms that are known to be possible in Lyme Disease, as Dr. Ed Masters, M.D., presented at the 1999 International Conference on Lyme Disease, and even in the face of overwhelming evidence he so eloquently demonstrated, Lyme Disease is apparently a "politically incorrect" illness. Dr. Masters presented many photographs of the classic bull's-eye rash on his patients, a picture of the tick, the lab report verifying that the tick did indeed have the Lyme spirochetes in its stomach, the blood and urine lab tests of the patient that were positive, and the list of symptoms that are commonly found in Lyme Disease patients. When he took his evidence to the Health Department of his state to ask them to warn the public to take precautions when doing outdoor activities, it is reported that the officials there said something like, "With all due respect Dr. Masters, if we had Lyme Disease in our state, more doctors would be finding it."

Apparently ticks that attach to geese and other waterfowl in Connecticut fall off as the birds cross the state line, thus preventing the spread of infected ticks to every other state in the country. What?? This idea that Lyme could only exist in one part of our interconnected country is ridiculous. Actually, Lyme Disease experts such as Dr. Ray Stricker now acknowledge the impact potential of migratory birds in the now-worldwide spread of Borrelia burgdorferi.[4] Another of my favorites is when I hear that only one type of tick is classically recognized as carrying Lyme spirochetes. Some seem to believe that any other blood-sucking insect that drinks the blood of an infected deer mysteriously filters out the Lyme spirochete. This idea is also not based on facts.

Some Lyme researchers have estimated that mosquitoes, deer flies, black flies, horse flies, and fleas have and could potentially transmit Lyme bacteria. Mosquitoes, fleas and lice may also carry Borrelia.[5] It only makes sense that Lyme could be transmitted by just about any blood-sucking insect, especially when the Centers for Disease Control in Atlanta estimate that every 1/20th of a second, someone contracts a mosquito-borne illness, and every 20 seconds someone dies from one. Until recently, the lab tests could only detect the "shadow" or the "possibility" that your body has seen the Lyme bacteria, *Borrelia burgdorferi*, via serum antibody tests. Serum antibody testing, such as the Lyme Western Blot IgG/IgM, in reality does not confirm the actual presence of the

Lyme bacteria. The presence of the Lyme-specific antibody seen in a Lyme Western Blot can arguably show that your body has simply "seen" this type of bacteria before, but it does not necessarily have an active infection. If you had Strep throat, your doctor could perform a throat culture and definitively confirm the presence of the actual Strep bacteria. The doctor could also test and find that the white blood cell count and neutrophils were elevated, further confirming the strep bacterial infection. The *Borrelia burgdorferi* is a type of bacteria which can elude your body's immune system; therefore, the lab tests often show no elevated white blood cells, or neutrophils. Your body's immune system apparently often cannot see these bacteria, leading some of the world's Lyme researchers to label the bacteria as a "Stealth Pathogen."[6] You can see why so many otherwise-intelligent doctors have a difficult time acknowledging Lyme Disease as a possible diagnosis for their patients. The training that most doctors receive dictates that one must confirm facts with laboratory tests. If it does not show up on lab testing, if the patient does not fit the profile, or (the greatest ignorance of all) if the patient is not in the Connecticut area, then most doctors absolutely will not consider Lyme as a possible answer.

Thankfully, recent advances in laboratory testing have improved the detection of the actual microbe that causes Lyme. Newer, FDA-approved Lyme PCR testing detects the genetic structure of Lyme in whole blood serum or cerebral spinal fluid.

Keep in mind that NO bacteria or virus can replicate out of control in a healthy body! Therefore, just testing positive with any test method does **not** mean you will definitely develop any symptoms--ever!

You are only as strong (and as resistant to infectious disease) as your weakest link in your body, mind, and/or spirit.

If you have many weak tissues and organ systems, then you may manifest many of the symptoms on the following pages (This listing is certainly not all of the potential symptoms).

---

[3] Blanc, Frederic. Med Mal Infect, 2007.
[4] Stricker, Ray. York 2004 LDA Conference.
[5] Agric Environ Med, 2002; 9: 257–9.
[6] Mattman, L., *Cell Wall Deficient Forms: Stealth Pathogens, Third Edition* CRC; October 26, 2000.

Section 1: Understanding Lyme Disease

Lyme Disease Symptoms

	Symptom	Borrelia burgdorferi	Babesia (babesiosis)	Bartonella henselae	Ehrlichia (Ehrlichiosis)	Mycoplasma Fermentans Incognitus	Check Your Symptoms
1	Abdominal pain		✓	✓			
2	Air hunger		✓				
3	Anemia		✓	✓	✓		
4	Anorexia				✓		
5	Anxiety	✓		✓		✓	
6	Back stiffness	✓	✓	✓			
7	Bites from infected ticks				✓		
8	Bladder dysfunction	✓					
9	Burning or stabbing sensations	✓					
10	Cardiac impairment	✓					
11	Change in bowel function	✓					
12	Chills		✓	✓	✓		
13	Chest pain	✓					
14	Confusion	✓			✓	✓	
15	Cough	✓	✓		✓		
16	Depression	✓	✓			✓	
17	Diarrhea		✓		✓		
18	Difficulty thinking	✓			✓	✓	
19	Difficulty with concentration and reading	✓				✓	
20	Difficulty with speech, writing	✓					

Lyme Disease Symptoms Continued…

		Borrelia burgdorferi	Babesia (babesiosis)	Bartonella henselae	Ehrlichia (Ehrlichiosis)	Mycoplasma Fermentans Incognitus	Check Your Symptoms
21	Difficulty finding words; name blocking	✓					
22	Disorientation: getting lost, going to wrong places	✓					
23	Disturbed sleep: too much, too little, fractionated, early awakening	✓		✓		✓	
24	Ears/Hearing: buzzing, ringing, ear pain, sound sensitivity	✓		✓			
25	Emotional lability	✓	✓			✓	
26	Encephalopathy	✓	✓	✓			
27	Endocarditis	✓		✓			
28	Exaggerated symptoms or worse hangover	✓					
29	Eyes/Vision: double, blurry, increased floaters, light sensitivity	✓					
30	Facial paralysis (Bell's palsy)	✓					
31	Fatigue, tiredness, poor stamina	✓	✓	✓	✓	✓	
32	Fevers		✓	✓		✓	
33	Forgetfulness	✓					
34	Gastrointestinal problems	✓			✓		
35	Headache	✓	✓	✓	✓	✓	
36	Heart block	✓					
37	Heart murmur	✓					
38	Heart palpitations	✓					

Section 1: Understanding Lyme Disease

Lyme Disease Symptoms Continued…

#	Symptom	Borrelia burgdorferi	Babesia (babesiosis)	Bartonella henselae	Ehrlichia (Ehrlichiosis)	Mycoplasma Fermentans Incognitus	Check Your Symptoms
39	Heart valve prolapse	✓					
40	Hemolysis		✓	✓			
41	Hepatomegaly (enlarged liver)		✓	✓			
42	Imbalance without true vertigo	✓	✓				
43	Immune deficiency	✓		✓			
44	Increased motion sickness	✓					
45	Insomnia	✓		✓		✓	
46	Irritability	✓				✓	
47	Irritable bladder	✓					
48	Jaundice			✓			
49	Joint stiffness	✓	✓			✓	
50	Joint pain or swelling	✓	✓	✓		✓	
51	Leukopenia, persistent				✓		
52	Light headedness	✓					
53	Liver enzymes elevated			✓	✓		
54	Lymph nodes swollen			✓		✓	
55	Malaise (generalized ill feeling)	✓	✓	✓	✓	✓	
56	Mood swings	✓				✓	
57	Muscle pain or cramps	✓	✓	✓	✓	✓	
58	Myalgias	✓	✓	✓	✓	✓	
59	Myocarditis	✓		✓			

Lyme Disease Symptoms Continued…

#	Symptom	Borrelia burgdorferi	Babesia (babesiosis)	Bartonella henselae	Ehrlichia (Ehrlichiosis)	Mycoplasma Fermentans Incognitus	Check Your Symptoms
60	Nausea, vomiting		✓		✓		
61	Neck creaks & cracks	✓					
62	Neck stiffness, pain	✓	✓				
63	Night sweats	✓	✓			✓	
64	Numbness	✓				✓	
65	Papular or angiomatous rash			✓			
66	Paralysis	✓					
67	Pelvic pain	✓					
68	Poor appetite	✓	✓				
69	Poor attention/concentration	✓				✓	
70	Poor balance	✓				✓	
71	Poor short-term memory	✓				✓	
72	Problem absorbing new information	✓					
73	Pulse skips	✓					
74	Rib soreness	✓					
75	Rigors				✓		
76	Seizures (rarely)			✓			
77	Sexual dysfunction or loss of libido	✓					
78	Shaking chills		✓				
79	Shooting pains	✓					
80	Shortness of breath	✓	✓	✓			
81	Skin hypersensitivity	✓					

Section 1: Understanding Lyme Disease

Lyme Disease Symptoms Continued…

#	Symptom	Borrelia burgdorferi	Babesia (babesiosis)	Bartonella henselae	Ehrlichia (Ehrlichiosis)	Mycoplasma Fermentans Incognitus	Check Your Symptoms
82	Somnolence			✓		✓	
83	Sore throat	✓		✓			
84	Splenomegaly		✓	✓			
85	Swollen glands/lymph nodes	✓		✓		✓	
86	Testicular pain	✓					
87	Thrombocytopenia				✓		
88	Tingling	✓				✓	
89	Tibia pain, severe			✓			
90	Tremor	✓		✓			
91	Twitching of the face or other muscles	✓		✓			
92	Unavoidable need to sit or lay down	✓					
93	Unexplained breast pain	✓					
94	Unexplained fevers, sweats, chills or flushing	✓	✓				
95	Unexplained hair loss	✓					
96	Unexplained menstrual irregularity	✓					
97	Unexplained milk production	✓					
98	Unexplained weight loss / gain	✓					
99	Urine dark or with blood		✓				
100	Upset Stomach or abdominal pain	✓		✓			
101	Vertigo	✓					

Lyme Disease Symptoms Continued...

		Borrelia burgdorferi	Babesia (babesiosis)	Bartonella henselae	Ehrlichia (Ehrlichiosis)	Mycoplasma Fermentans Incognitus	Check Your Symptoms
102	Weakness	✓	✓			✓	
103	Weight loss	✓	✓	✓		✓	
104	Wooziness	✓					

2

~

What is Lyme Disease?

In the United States, what ultimately came to be known as Lyme Disease started in the city of Lyme, Connecticut, in early 1975 with an epidemic of "juvenile rheumatoid arthritis." By 1982, Dr. William Burgdorfer, M.D., identified the cause of an illness sweeping the area as a spiral-shaped bacterium (spirochete), ultimately named *Borrelia burgdorferi*.

Of course, this type of bacteria has been with us throughout history. Historical records document what is now called Lyme Disease as far back as 1882 in Europe. The classic presentation was a tick bite and bulls-eye rash with joint pain and neurological symptoms. For years, it was thought to be confined to a few northeastern states, but as time passed it became apparent that surrounding states were also reporting the infection at an alarming rate. Research now confirms that Lyme disease is rampant throughout much of the United States and Europe.[7]

In the 2008 Open Eye Pictures movie *Under Our Skin; The Untold Story of Lyme*, an important quote stands out, "The Centers for Disease Control admits that more than 200,000 people may acquire Lyme Disease each year, a number greater than AIDS, West Nile Virus, and Avian Flu combined."

Many people with confirmed infection never remember being bitten by a tick. Some of my patients have told me that they have <u>never</u> personally even seen a tick in their lives. It was once thought that one must have the bulls-eye rash in order to have Lyme Disease, but it is now known that only about 30% of individuals bitten by a Lyme-infected tick even develop a bulls-eye rash, so having no rash does not rule out Lyme Disease.[8,9]

Lyme spirochetes may lay dormant for weeks or years after initial infection. This dormancy is due to the fact that no bacteria or virus can replicate (reproduce) at will in a healthy body. This will be discussed in detail later. For now, understand that the Lyme spirochetes may lay dormant in a healthy body until the individual experiences a stress on the body that weakens the body's control mechanisms, thereby allowing the spirochetes to replicate and spread out of control.

Deer are considered one of the primary carriers of Lyme bacteria, but in fact no animal has been found immune to infection. Even dogs, cats, and farm animals have often been found infected with Lyme Disease. It is this author's belief that a large percentage of all domesticated livestock are already infected.

The fact that Lyme spirochetes have been cultured from virtually every body fluid in cows, including whole blood, colostrum and fresh milk, with no conferred immunity, makes one question the safety of such products. A report of research conducted with the School of Veterinary Medicine, University of Wisconsin, stated, "Because spirochetes (Borrelia burgdorferi) could be isolated from blood, synovial fluid, colostrum, and urine, these animals (cows and horses) could be important in providing an infected blood meal for ticks and bringing B. burgdorferi in direct contact with humans."[10]

Being a vegetarian never sounded so good! At the very least, avoiding undercooked meat seems prudent.

There is practically no better immune-boosting dietary supplement on the market than the fractionated colostrums.

Colostrum is the initial mother's milk, high in immune system-stimulating factors, that is only produced for a few days after delivering a baby. Whole cow colostrum is dehydrated into a powder which is sold as an immune system booster for human consumption. However, screening needs to be performed on each batch of whole colostrums to ensure there are no Lyme spirochetes present. Keep in mind that a cow only produces a limited quantity of colostrum, and after freeze-drying it, there is little powdered colostrum produced. This means many cows are needed to produce the hundreds of thousands of capsules to supply the public demand. Using more cows means a greater risk of being infected and contaminating the entire lot of colostrum.

While there is no evidence of Lyme infection from taking an infected colostrum product, I don't recommend risking it. I have had patients who only started manifesting symptoms of Lyme Disease after starting to use colostrum products. These patients were told by the company who produced the colostrum product that the new symptoms were their immune systems coming online and fighting microbes. This is also a plausible possibility.

My favorite colostrum products are the immune-stimulating *fractionated* colostrums, such as Transfer Factors, and not whole colostrums, unless the batches have been screened by an independent laboratory.

Infection

The first step in the life cycle of a Lyme-infected tick is to attach to, and thereby infect, a deer. The ticks fall off and each have hundreds of baby ticks, all of which will be infected from birth with Lyme spirochetes. The baby ticks can be smaller than the head of a pin. These hundreds of baby ticks climb onto blades of grass, working their way up to the tip of the blade. From there, the tick holds onto the blade of grass with a few legs and spreads its other legs wide to catch onto animals, birds, or people passing by. The tick burrows its head through the skin and injects stomach fluid and anesthetizing chemicals so that you don't feel it breaking the skin. This injection of fluids transmits the bacteria into your body. This is one way to get infected.

Another might be that the deer is bitten by a tick, the tick falls off, has babies, and the babies attach to a goose which is infected. The goose migrates all over the country, where the ticks fall off and later infect other animals and people. Of course, our local ticks and mosquitoes could bite the infected goose, resulting in an eventual plague of Lyme Disease as those ticks and mosquitoes later bite other animals and people in the area. The truth of this scenario is evident today in the United States as the West Nile Virus is being identified in a growing number of states, due to the migration of infected crows. The infected crows are bitten by local mosquitoes. These mosquitoes go on to bite and infect people in the area.

I am not trying to scare anyone, although caution is warranted. My goal is to help patients and their physicians wake up to the very real possibility of Lyme Disease in their communities. Until the proper diagnosis is determined, the proper treatment cannot be applied. And when Lyme Disease looks like so many other illnesses, one may be getting the absolute wrong treatment. For example, steroid medicines, such as prednisone, are contraindicated in Lyme Disease but often used in treatment of other illnesses.

Many cases of Multiple Sclerosis (MS) and ALS are misdiagnosed and are actually what some call "Neuro-borreliosis." Recent research by Dr. Lida Mattman, Ph.D., et al., which is due to be published soon, has identified another strain of Borrelia spirochete to be found in every case of MS, as well as a different strain in cases of ALS. This would explain the improvement often seen in treating these illnesses as Lyme Disease. Both of these newly-found strains react, as we can see on blood tests, to Lyme Borrelia antibody, which is why so many of these cases are called Lyme Disease. They are, in fact, different species of Borrelia. The good thing is that these strains will often respond to the same treatments as the classic *Borrelia burgdorferi* of Lyme Disease.

Improvement following correct treatment also confirms the diagnosis. Compare this to typical MS treatments, which only work to slow down the progression of the illness. (By the way, if you have MS, ask any doctor what causes it – you will have difficulty getting a straight answer.) Why not a Borrelia type of cause?

Patients must understand that every doctor can only go as far as they have been taught. If they are taught that Lyme is only in Connecticut and the surrounding states, they will not even consider Lyme or look for it in diagnoses.

The nice thing about the correct diagnosis of Lyme Disease is that it is treatable, with a hope of permanent recovery. I have seen and heard many people who have taken their positive Lyme lab tests to their M.D. It is quite common for the doctor to say, even in the absence of any other positive identifying lab work, "I don't know what you've got, but its not Lyme Disease." I don't understand this! It seems that some doctors would rather diagnose people with what I call a "non-diagnosis" -- Unilateral Cephalgia, Fibromyalgia, Chronic Fatigue Syndrome, or atypical this or that. These are not a diagnosis! All the doctor is doing is turning what you told him into Latin or simply describing your symptoms. A good diagnosis should name the cause of the symptom. These other "non-diagnoses" are just fine if all you plan for treatment is providing unending symptomatic relief. Unilateral cephalgia in the example above is really nothing more than the doctor translating what the patient said into Latin, "pain on one side of your head." With this diagnosis, a doctor can do no more than prescribe pain killers, which do nothing to treat the <u>cause</u> of the pain.

Opponents of the diagnosis of Lyme Disease (even with positive lab tests, there are many who deny its diagnosis for some political or other reason) outside of New England are afraid that one may arrive at the incorrect diagnosis of Lyme Disease. This is mainly because the exact cause of the supposed autoimmune diseases is not known in most cases, and there seems to be fear that patients would be not receiving their traditional symptomatic treatments to slow the illness.

There is a compelling book, *Lab 257: The Disturbing Story of the Government's Secret Germ Laboratory*, which takes place at Plum Island in the Long Island Sound off the coast of Connecticut. This book reveals what may be the cause of the resistance to the diagnosis of Lyme Disease. This book suggests that Borrelia burgdorferi may indeed be a "Genetically Modified Organism" -- a manmade bug! Read the book and draw your own conclusions.

I am not saying we should treat every autoimmune disease as if it were Lyme. However, in the absence of any labs identifying the *cause* of your condition, and if you get a positive blood or urine test for Lyme Disease *and* improve upon correct treatment, I say it confirms the diagnosis of Lyme. Most treatments for autoimmune diseases seek only to mask the symptoms or slow down the progression of the disease.

Pleomorphism of Lyme Spirochetes

The ability of bacteria to change shape, pleomorphism, has been greatly debated since the discovery of bacteria. I am definitely in the camp that believes bacteria do indeed morph in response to changes in their environment. However, whether bacteria can morph or not matters very little in the scheme of the ultimate patient treatment philosophy and frequency-matched remedies presented in this book. In the end, no matter what we call it or how we describe it, dealing with illness always comes down to how we are going to correct what has gone wrong in the human organism, since we are not treating bacteria but people. Understanding the potential for pleomorphism is important in understanding why it is not necessary to completely annihilate every Lyme microbe in order to achieve lasting and permanent health.

Dr. Lida Mattman, Ph.D., the author of three university textbooks on the scientific validation of pleomorphism, presents convincing research substantiating that Borrelia burgdorferi (Bb) are *pleomorphic* organisms.[11] A pleomorphic organism takes on a different shape at different life stages or in reaction to changes in its environment. A butterfly is said to be pleomorphic because it changes from a caterpillar to a cocoon to a butterfly. The Lyme bacteria are known to be pleomorphic. The different pleomorphic stages of Borrelia burgdorferi are unclear, but research suggests that it can definitely exist as *cell-walled bacterium or cell-wall deficient bacterium*, depending on its lifecycle. Again, each stage of the cycle is relatively "stealth," or basically invisible to the immune system.

A cell wall is requisite in order for the spirochete Borrelia burgdorferi to achieve its spiral shape. Some antibiotics act by disrupting the mechanisms in the cell wall of the Bb in order to kill the bacteria. It is suspected that the long-term antibiotic attack on the cell walls can cause the spirochete to revert into a *"cell-wall deficient"* form as a survival mechanism. The problem is that the Bb can revert back and forth between the classic spiral shape and the cell wall deficient shapes. To complicate matters more, the Bb can exist simultaneously as both forms. Dr. Lida Mattman, Ph.D., a leading researcher in L-Form bacteria, has found that it is common to see three Lyme spirochetes for every seven Lyme L-Forms in a blood specimen. Also, it is not uncommon to see only L-Forms with no spirochetes to be found.[12]

The cell wall-deficient form is synonymously called *L-Forms* and *spheroplasts*. Many different bacteria and fungi can achieve this form. For unification purposes, scientists now refer to the cell wall deficient stage as L-Forms.[13]

It may sound strange that any organism can exist at all without a cell wall. This term can be a little deceiving in that there is a membrane where there formerly was a cell wall.

Without its cell wall, the Bb cannot hold its characteristic spiral shape. It has been speculated that Lyme-infected ticks can also harbor the L-Form of Bb, which may explain why not every infected person develops a bulls-eye rash or tests positive on initial blood tests.

Indications are that the Bb can be forced into remission for weeks to years with long-term aggressive use of antibiotics. During this remission, there are usually no detectable Bb spirochetes, and titers go down to undetectable levels. The Bb could possibly be latent in its L-Form during this stage.[14] Apparently when the conditions in the body are right, the latent L-Form infection reverts back to the spirochete form, the symptoms return, and the titers go up, leaving the patient to wonder if they were bitten again by an infected tick.

Not only does the spirochete change from a cell-walled bacterium to an L-form bacterium, but it is also possible for each life stage to exist independently from the other stage.[15] Recent research has shown that laboratory animals injected with dead fragments of the classic spirochetal Borrelia burgdorferi contracted Lyme Disease.[16] This is significant because bacteria do not replicate themselves from eggs, but from fission. Therefore, a possible explanation might be that the undetected cell wall-*deficient* life stage actually was responsible for these laboratory-induced infections.

Bacterial pleomorphism is not unique to the Lyme bacteria. Treponema palladums, also a spirochete, and the bacteria known to cause Syphilis, are also widely known to prefer different shapes depending on where they are found in the body.[17]

Recently, scientists unlocked the genetic sequencing of the Bb bacteria and found that 50% of its genetic makeup is identical to that of the Syphilis bacteria.[18] Due to the homeopathic law of *similars,* or "like cures like," doctors should consider a single dose, or a few doses, of the homeopathic miasm remedy Syphilinum 200c. Miasms are the tendencies and predisposition to certain physical and psychological problems, either acquired or inherited due to illness or suppressive treatments.[19] Upon reading the homeopathic Materia Medica reference book, one will see a great many similar symptoms of the chronic Lyme patient that may be corrected by this one homeopathic remedy.

The ability to change shape is thought to be the reason why the Lyme bacteria, once well established in the body, are able to survive even after long-term antibiotic therapies. It is possible that the Lyme bacteria flip-flop between several shapes to escape the antibiotics. People who receive antibiotic treatment soon after infection often recover completely, since the organism has not had time to "dig-in" and cycle into the other pleomorphic shapes. The fact that most antibiotics only address the cell-walled spirochetal bacterial stage may also explain why many people under antibiotic therapy feel improvement while on the antibiotics, only to relapse soon after discontinuing the antibiotics. The antibiotics may kill some of the spirochetal phase, but ultimately the bacteria get smart and shift to shapes that are resistant to the antibiotic, and these shapes may not be as pathological or cause as many symptoms.

One of the "stealth" or cloaking mechanisms of these bacteria is to "attach to or invade human cortical neuronal cells," say researchers at the National Center for Infectious Diseases in Colorado, part of the U.S. Centers for Disease Control and Prevention (CDC). This makes the bacteria difficult to detect and kill by the immune system.[20]

An analogy of the use of antibiotics as the sole treatment of Lyme Disease might be seen in the following example. If you have termites eating their way through the wood of your house, you can call an exterminator to come to your home and kill the termites. By killing the termites, you have eliminated any worsening of the problem; however, you have done nothing to correct the myriad of tunnels through the woodwork of your house. To make matters worse, you now have a very toxic chemical insecticide in your home.

Those placing their faith in antibiotics to "cure" them of *chronic* Lyme Disease will, in most cases, be disappointed. Drug therapies such as antibiotics address only the offending bacteria in certain stages but do nothing to heal the body as a whole.

---

[7] Barbour, Alan G. Fall and rise of Lyme Disease and other *Ixodes* tick-borne infections in North America and Europe, *Bntish Medical Bulletin* 1998,54 (No 3).

[8] Stricker, .R.B et al: Lyme Disease without erythema migrans: cause for concern? *Am J Med* 2003; 115:72.

[9] Centers for Disease Control and Prevention (CDC). Lyme Disease – USA, 2001–2002. *Morb Mortal Wkly Rep* 2004;53(17):365–369.

[10] Burgess, E.C, Borrelia burgdorferi infection in Wisconsin horses and cows. Ann N Y Acad Sci 1988;539:235-43.

[11] Mattman L, 1992 *Cell Wall Deficient Forms, Stealth Pathogens*, 2nd Ed.

[12] Mattman 1992

[13] Mattman 1992

[14] Infection, 1996; 24: 218–26.

[15] Mattman L, 1999 Per telephone conversation with Dr. Lida Mattman Ph.D., July.

[16] Cotran, Kumar, Robbins, *Robbins Pathological Basis of Disease*. 4th Edition.

[17] Cotran et al.

[18] Mattman 1992

[19] Murphy R. *Lotus Materia Medica*, Lotus Star Academy Publishing.

[20] Microbes Infect, 2006; 8: 2832–40).

3

~

"Fiber Optic" Communications of Microbes

In every epidemic, there are those who walk through it unscathed. This immunity goes beyond simply having a healthy immune system. While strengthening the body's immune system with supplements like thymus gland, mushroom extracts, and antioxidants is a good idea, these interventions will likely not be enough to deal with rapidly progressing, highly virulent microbes. The following outlines a new and better understanding of how the body naturally controls the overgrowth of microbes.

<u>There are 20 times more microbes than cells in your body!</u> Another way of saying this is that "90% of the cells within us are not ours but microbes."[21] So for someone to say, "I've gotten an infection" is quite an understatement! You are a walking, talking "infection" if we want to hold on to the definition of infection as the presence of a microbe! As you will see here and begin to appreciate, it is not a war of "us against them;" instead, we *are* them and they *are* us! Even in Lyme Disease, the bacteria and other associated microbes cannot in and of themselves cause disease in an individual who is in

optimum coherence and integrity within the body, mind, and spirit. This fact is manifest in the thousands and tens of thousands of individuals who are "carriers" of the Borrelia burgdorferi but have no apparent symptoms.

Bacterial species function as a collective unit. Every bacterium is part of the collective thought matrix of the entire microbial society. A microbial "collective consciousness" accurately describes bacteria, viruses, parasites, and fungi functioning as a complete community inside the human body. This community has a food chain of producers, consumers, and decomposers. They are all fighting and striving to survive, and they all need each other in order to survive. Any attack on the bacterial collective may hurt them, but they immediately use their collective intelligence to adapt, repair, regenerate, change tactics, and survive.

To give your body a pharmaceutical or natural antibiotic is like dropping a bomb on the microbial collective; it may hurt, but the microbes work together to adapt. It is a "war" within your body -- only because we have declared it so, by attacking the "bad guys" but also by attacking virtually all that we as humans are – the proverbial microbial soup!

When there is a microbial overgrowth, we must recognize it for what it truly indicates. It indicates that you are suffering from a breakdown of coherence between the body, mind, and spirit! Recognizing this is important in order to regain the quality of health you desire. All therapeutic efforts must be applied in all haste to restore the body's ability to adapt correctly to changes within its internal and external environment.[22] This is accomplished by thoughtfully applied natural treatments and therapies that are not harmful in any way to the human organism. These treatments and therapies should work with the goal of correcting the loss of integrity, and therefore correcting the function within the physical body, the mind, and the spirit.

Correcting the body, mind, and spirit in this way will reset the body's holographic blueprint, which will resolve the microbial overgrowth and eliminate every symptom. We will discuss the body's holographic blueprint in detail later in Chapter 8's article, "Illuminated Physiology and the Medical Uses of Light."

The following is an excerpt from one of my next books, *Infectious Perceptions: Living and Healing in a World of Designer Microbes*:

> Why go into all this explanation? Because the reality is that it truly is not a war of "us against them." We are them and they are us, living in synergy. When the body shifts from its normal healthy integrity the microbes work to help us correct the problem. The reality is that the human body is not dumb as it may seem when it is suffering from apparent infections. Virtually every occurrence of fever, chills, and achiness of an infection is during the Healing Phase of the event. How we respond from a treatment perspective during this symptomatic phase will dictate the ultimate outcome. It will determine if the infection persists and maims or kills you, or if the point of the entire "infectious process" is able to complete its task, thereby restoring order and health. It is important that you understand that no matter the illness, you can overcome it by restoring the proper rhythm and balance of every aspect of life and of the body. It is also just as important to realize that illness can be avoided by maintaining the same, all the time.
>
> It is easy to see why we have come to this "war mentality" regarding microbes. With 50% of cancer patients dying from secondary infections, it appears that the bacteria are the bad guys. The reality is that the microbial challenges (often Staph or mycobacterium) seen

in cancer are actually now recognized to be the "clean up crew" to assist in eliminating the abnormal cells.[23] More damage is caused by chemotherapy and radiation, and the cancer is cyclically placed in the "Active Phase" through repeated triggering of emotional conflicts that instigated the cancer in the first place. As this continues, the microbes insistently push to decompose the ever-increasing abnormal cells of the cancer to complete the natural healing of the body, instead of progressing through the Healing Phase.

It is vitally important, now more than ever, that you be finally delivered from the erroneous mindset, "If my doctor can kill this bacteria or virus, then I will be well." You will be well when your tissues are no longer a dysfunctional environment that has lost its integrity through unresolved conflicts within the body, mind, and spirit.

It is said that in Chess, the game is often lost within the first few moves. If you start the game with the same predictable moves, you will likely see a consistent and predictable outcome. This is also true in the "game" of illness. If every doctor reacts to illness with the same basic move, then every step of the unsuccessful outcome can be microscopically analyzed and tested. But in the end, the game is lost, and millions of people die or are debilitated needlessly from the infection.

If virtually the entire world accepts this model of treatment, and all the researchers work from this model, then it isn't that the data they uncover is wrong. It may be found that "The microbial proteins may actually damage components of the immune system within this system of treatment," but it is possibly simply describing the inner workings of the flawed process that has been irrevocably altered from the natural order of things through the "first few moves."

To research a person who has been treated for all their life with antibiotics, who was never allowed to fight their own fights, nor even allowed to generate a functional fever, deferring instead to "better health through chemistry," and to study the person who is in an active infectious disease process is to extract data from a flawed database. The data extracted is from a body which has been interfered with from virtually every avenue possible.[24]

One might read this and say that it is well and good if you don't have "truly dangerous" bacteria involved. Let's look at some compelling research to demonstrate the flaw in this mindset. Tests on volunteers revealed that, when given Cholera bacteria, it required extremely high concentrations at 10^8 to 10^{11} organisms before any one of the volunteers became sick with the disease. Interestingly, the amount needed to cause disease dropped by half if they neutralized the volunteer's stomach acid.[25] We see here that abnormal changes in the body increase the chance of developing a disease even from a potentially very deadly microbe. Need more convincing? Other research has shown that only one out of 100 receptive poliovirus infected individuals will actually develop polio, the disease![26] As you see, the microbe is almost the last determining factor in contracting a disease.

In the previous edition of this book, I stated that I had developed a theory of intermicrobial communication as a method of microbial growth and survival in the human body.

We now know that this is a fact, not a theory. Research has determined that all living tissue, whether the body's tissues or foreign microbes, are made up of unique molecular liquid-crystalline structures.[27] We refer to the human body as the crystalline matrix, which conducts bio-information via light referred to as biophotons. Photons are the energy packets of light. The liquid-crystalline structures within the crystalline matrix, including Lyme spirochetes and the other co-infecting microbes, are capable of creating and transmitting laser-like bio-photons for the purpose of communication between tissues, molecules within the body, and even transmitting great, almost limitless distances to the outside world.

Much of our understanding of how chemical molecules, such as hormones, function is now being recognized as a matter of proximity (transmitting their hormonal information via light and vibrations through the crystalline matrix with the body) rather than actual physical contact of the hormone in the classic "lock and key" explanation we have used for years. In fact, research reported by James Oschman, PhD., in his book, *Energy Medicine: The Scientific Basis*, states that even the frequencies emitted by a person having an allergic reaction can trigger a spontaneous reaction in another allergy-prone person.[28] It is <u>all</u> vibration!

Everything in the universe is simply our perception of vibrations. Light, sound, tastes, the chair you are sitting in, the shirt you are wearing, the apple you ate today, the thought you think -- all are just vibrations. Another way of talking about vibrations is to call them frequencies. Let's carry this a little further so that you can really grasp what a very important role your mind, emotions, and spirit play in promoting health or sickness. If you have a glass of deadly poison, it is poisonous to you because its vibration or frequency is so disruptive to the frequencies of your body. In the same way, your thoughts are also frequencies. Negative, fearful thinking creates absolutely poisonous frequencies! Thoughts of love and joy are like Miracle Grow is to plants and produce nutritious, healing frequencies. I am not playing with words here; these are true physical concepts.

If you see your body and life as if it is an apple tree, and the fruit appears small and unhealthy, would you say the fruit was determined by what you could see above the ground or by what was unseen – the roots? Of course, the roots determine the integrity of the fruit. Could you run lab tests on the fruit and find that it was low in some nutrient? Certainly, but the correction for what is wrong with the fruit will ultimately require you to deal with the roots.

In this scenario, all of your symptoms are the fruit and simply reflect the problems in your body's root system. What are your roots? They are the mind (your thoughts), your emotions (energy in motion), and your spirit. These three absolutely determine your physical fruit! If you desire to understand the integrity of your root system, then look at the fruits. The fatigue, the knee pain, the nerve and brain problems are the result of problems in the mind, emotions, and spirit. It is all vibration and either produces health or illness. Correct the roots, and your fruit will reflect the vibrational changes. All of the chemistry of your body, the entire crystalline matrix, and indeed the entire universe, shifts dynamically to root changes at virtually the speed of light!

You cannot pour Miracle Grow plant food on the roots and follow that with poison and expect to get anything but a sick plant with poor fruit! In the same way, you cannot live juggling fear and negativity with loving and joyful thoughts and expect anything but negative symptoms and illness.

It is through the unique vibrations of the molecular structure of hormones, and indeed any pathology (including microbes), that gives it its own unique electromagnetic signature, often called a molecular signature. Understanding this concept, one can begin to see how a radio station can also be likened to this communication link on a much larger scale. If the electrons of the radio station transmitter are oscillating at the same frequency as the setting on your radio, you can receive all of the songs and information embedded within the signal. The communications between the transmitter (radio station) and the receiver (your radio) is known as co-resonance. All other radio stations in the area would be operating at a different frequency and would therefore not interfere with your ability to hear the selected radio station.

On a microscopic scale, because of their unique molecular structure and oscillatory frequency, microbes can transmit and tune in to each other across great distances within the human body via coherent laser-like biophotonic emissions. Embedded within these microbial transmissions is the information needed by other microbes, "tuned" into the same frequency, about how they need to mutate in order to survive against an antibiotic, how to work together to change the host environment (your body) to one more conducive to their overall population, or to transmit just about any type of communication.[29] Millions of microbes can be communicating in this manner with signal velocities estimated at upwards of the speed of light. Does this seem incredible? I can use my cell phone and carry on a virtually instantaneous conversation with someone on the other side of the earth. Often we accept this technology without thinking about how truly amazing it is! Why then is it any more or less believable that microbes are "tuning in" to each other within the body?

Just like the radio station example, by nature these microbial communications would not be restricted or impaired by illness-weakened human tissue. In fact, microbes most likely interface with the body's own crystalline matrix in order to communicate. It is also likely, that this bacterial communication is cut off, making it impossible to communicate microbe-to-microbe, when health is restored in the human.

The first time a prescription antibiotic is introduced into the body, it is like a surprise attack, and there is not time for the first bacteria to adapt. As these bacteria die, the message is sent out via bacterial transmission of bio-photons and/or electromagnetic signals, like a distress call to all the rest of the microbes that were not affected by the antibiotic. This communication is what they need in order to mutate, thereby becoming antibiotic-resistant. "Microfibers, including DNA within microbes, and cytoskeleton polymers, can function as biological antennae..." for receiving these intermicrobial communications.[30] We now know for certain that the bacteria can mutate around the antibiotic sometimes within 20 minutes of taking the first dose.

If there were no communication between microbes as the antibiotic worked its way through the body, it would be a surprise to each individual microbe and would effectively kill every microbe! It is the arrogance of mankind that insists we are the only intelligent life on the planet.

In other words, it is believed that bacteria, viruses and other microbes can and do communicate with each other through their unique molecular crystalline matrix, and are transmitting and receiving vibrational resonance, laser-like coherent signals from each other. This communication is made possible by sending signals through the human body's own cellular matrix.[31]

This molecular crystalline matrix concept is found in all living tissue, i.e. bone, muscle, tendon, ligament, all of which operate and respond in cooperation in order to adapt the body to the ever-changing surrounding environment. We usually think of crystals as hard faceted minerals; however, all living tissue is indeed composed of long, thin, pliable molecules that are soft and flexible, which are considered "liquid crystals."
[32,33]

Several scientific studies have identified that, along with the microbes of the body, the molecules of the body also interact with each other via crystalline vibrational coherent fields. Within this type of crystalline matrix, bio-information/communication signals move through the tissues of the body at an astonishing rate, potentially up to half the speed of light or more. Understand that when there is an overgrowth of foreign microbes, their molecular crystalline vibrational fields are integrated and imbedded within the matrix of the human body.[34,35]

Now we turn to foreign microbes. With only a few foreign infectious microbes in the body's matrix, those microbes such as Borrelia burgdorferi or Cholera would normally not be a component of the "20 times more microbes than cells in your body" crowd. The foreign microbes will be held in check forever by the energetic aspects of the *healthy* human body. These infectious microbes may have little impact on the human and never develop into a disease. However, in an illness-weakened human, a few infectious microbes can multiply unimpeded. They now have a voice and can influence the form and function of the human, even influencing the mind and emotions, via their cooperative crystalline communication network. This can be seen as a computer virus overwriting the body's software in order to create a more hospitable environment for the bacterial collective.

Microbes need the human body to have a certain temperature in order to communicate efficiently. Too hot will mean their biophoton communications will overshoot their target, and too cold will cause their signals to be too weak to communicate.[36] However, a colder than normal human body may, at times, be exactly what some types of foreign infectious microbes need to communicate efficiently. This may be why people with severe chronic Lyme Disease tend to have a low core temperature. Therefore, it is likely that one of the first things microbes work together to achieve in a new host is an optimizing of the host's temperature to suit their needs. Later you will read more regarding the importance of treatments for re-establishing a normal body temperature distribution throughout the body (see Chapter 27**Error! Reference source not found.**, Lyme and Low Body Temperature).

If we assign this form of intelligence to microbes, one begins to wonder at the toxins these microbes produce, most of which are neurotoxins functioning to impair the body's nervous system and organ systems from setting up energetic antimicrobial growth-restricting fields.

Following this same line of thought, one can see why so many infections disturb heart function. The heart is now known to be primarily an electromagnetic generator for the entire body, generating 1,000 times more electricity than the brain and nervous system.[37] The electromagnetic energy from the heart is carried very well by the saline-rich blood through 50,000 miles of blood vessels. Without the heart-generator, organ function, body chemistry/metabolism, and core temperature plummet. How better to weaken the human body's energetic "force fields" than by weakening its power generator?[38,39]

The following explanation of cellular cascade and amplification by James Oschman, Ph.D., may provide the scientific rationale for how microbes can work to alter the human organism physically, mentally, and emotionally to promote a more hospitable environment:

> "A single antigen (microbe), hormone, pheromone, growth factor, or smell or taste or neurotransmitter molecule, or single photon of electromagnetic energy, can produce a cascade of intracellular signals that initiate, accelerate, or inhibit biological processes. This is possible because of enormous amplification – a single molecular event at the cell surface can trigger a huge influx of calcium ions, each of which can activate an enzyme. The enzymes, in turn, act as catalysts, greatly accelerating biochemical processes. The enzymes are not consumed by these reactions, and can therefore act repeatedly. Some of the reactions are sensitive to electromagnetic fields, some are not, and others have not yet been tested. Some frequencies enhance calcium entry, others diminish it. Steps in the cascade involving free radical formation

are likely targets of magnetic fields. Some of the products of the cascade are returned back to the cell surface and into the surrounding extracellular space. Molecular events within cells set up electronic, photonic, and electromechanical waves (phonons) that propagate as solitons through the cellular and extracellular matrix. These feedbacks enable cells and tissues to form a functionally organized society. **The cells whisper to each other in a faint and private language. They can 'tune into' each other over long ranges.**"[40]

This crystalline matrix theory could also help explain psychological abnormalities individuals experience that seem to be unique to each type of microbial infection. Doctors all over the world will attest to the fact that various types of infections seem to cause the infected person to be more prone to certain emotional patterns, such as depression, irritability, anxiety and frustration, as well as food cravings. Anyone suffering from Candida (yeast) overgrowth can attest to the almost-unreasonable craving they have for sugar, which just happens to be yeast's favorite food. In light of the molecular crystalline nature of microbes, along with their potential to use your own tissues to control their environment, your thoughts or cravings may not be "your thoughts" at all, but they may in fact be a superimposed thought pattern induced by the collective influence of microbes.

Microbial intercommunication is likely the reason why certain microbes seem to work in cooperation, such as the Borrelia burgdorferi of Lyme Disease working synergistically with Babesia microti, Ehrlichia, Bartonella, and various viruses such as the Human Herpes virus-6, Cytomegalovirus, and Epstein-Barr virus.

It appears that many people accumulate several strains of herpes viruses and other microbes, which may interfere with normal body function, as discussed in Chapter 10 (Lyme Toxins and a Toxic World). However, it seems that when Lyme bacteria come on the scene, they quickly assume a leadership position within the *susceptible* or weak human body. Lyme bacteria seem to organize the other microbes into a collective effort to work together to master their environment – your body.

All species of the world strive for survival. All attempt to control their environment or adapt to their environment in order to survive. Bacteria are no different. They work to change your body to suit their unique survival needs. However, no bacteria can overpower or alter a *healthy* body. They cannot get a foothold and replicate in large enough numbers to "have a voice" and alter the internal environment of the healthy human body. A healthy human body sets up energetic interference fields within the body to control the growth mechanisms of disease-causing microbes. It is only when the body's own crystalline matrix becomes impaired that infection can set in. Understanding this can help doctors recognize infections such as Strep throat as a weakness or breakdown of the throat's electro-energetic crystalline matrix. This may be due to emotional distress, physical stress, or other causes, but it is definitely not due to the invasion of Strep bacteria, which are now known to be present in everyone's throat. **How does this theory of "intermicrobial communication" change the way we treat people with infectious disease?**

Using the knowledge of the crystalline-matrix network of the human body and how microbes communicate, I developed a technique called Bio-Resonance Scanning™ (BRS) to tap into this biophotonic communication network of the human body. (See further detailed scientific information about BRS in Chapter 8.) Using BRS, I was able to create a completely new class of unique, highly-effective, frequency matched, botanical formulas (Virogen™, Paragen™, Yeast Ease™, Borrelogen™, Pomifetrin™, Microbojen™) to enhance and support the body's control mechanisms against microbial overgrowth. A good way to look at these unique remedies is to see the microbial overgrowth as having caused a "computer virus" of sorts. The computer virus doesn't kill you directly; it only tampers with certain aspects or programs in the operating software of your body. These targeted remedies create the inverse frequencies in the body that enable the body to rewrite, or overwrite and delete, the microbial computer virus program. Other treatments and therapies are then necessary to facilitate the actual repair and restoration of the damaged tissues. As the integrity of the entire matrix of body, mind, and spirit is restored, health follows.

Recall that in every epidemic there are those people that walk through it unharmed. They likely had the microbe in their body, but they never manifested the microbial disease. The microbial overgrowth is held in check by the energetic aspects of their crystalline matrix. These frequency-matched formulas enhance this same energetic aspect of "immunity" that is missing in the people who have developed the infectious disease or those who are susceptible to catching it.

To continue in computer language, these formulas are frequency-matched to "overwrite" the microbial matrix and facilitate one's ability to restore the mind, emotion, and spirit "roots," rebooting the original body programming "fruits." Each formula's complex molecular crystalline array matches those frequencies that the healthy human body uses to prevent specific types of microbes from being able to communicate and replicate, while simultaneously guiding the body back to healthy coherence. In essence, the desire in any infectious disease is that the treatments will help bring down the number of microbes and restore the body's ability to control the microbe's livelihood.

These formulas target the proper structure and function of the body rather than targeting the virus or microbe. In my opinion, this is the most pure form of intervention developed to date, in that it works *with* God's optimal design of the human body. Antibiotics and high-power drug interventions figuratively take a sledgehammer to God's perfect design.

Of course, the printed research on these high-power drugs is overwhelming in the scientist's optimism regarding their drug's effect on the microbes; however, they leave the sledgehammer side-effects to the small print section of the article.

I am always amazed at the anger that comments like these about antibiotics rouse in some people when even the conventional medical establishment admits that they are running out of antibiotics that will work. Not only does the medical establishment desire to abandon the present antibiotic model, but the major push in the pharmaceutical research world is also working to create better ways to deal with bacteria from avenues other than antibiotics.[41]

Keep in mind, sincerity is no guarantee of truth. Your doctor may still sincerely believe antibiotics are the best. I too am very sincere in what I say; however it is the truth as I see it, based on the best research and intuition we have to date.

All doctors and scientists attempt to explain the exact mechanism of illness based upon their area of expertise. Each describes illness from their unique perspective. It is like the story of the three blind men describing an elephant -- one at the trunk, one at the side, and one at the rear. Each may be absolutely correct in how they perceive the elephant, but each is simply describing the elephant from their perspective. So, while one scientist may focus on the microscopic, molecular, and morphological properties of the microbe, others may focus on the autonomic changes in the body, and others may focus on the effect of antibiotic "cocktails." Still others may focus primarily on the electromagnetic properties. You see, doctors and scientists may all be correct in their assumptions but completely erroneous in their treatment rationales.

Often there seems to be the assumption that the human body is dumb and needs drugs to help kill microbes. The truth is that the human body is highly intelligent and

simply needs support. I heard one of the best examples of this truth while attending a lecture by Dr. Thomas Rau, M.D., of the world-famous Paracelsus Klinik in Switzerland. He gave an example of the need to recognize the body's intelligence in a story about a dog that had swallowed a bone too large to pass through the stomach into the small intestines. The dog's normal stomach acid was unable to digest the bone; therefore a stomach cancer began to grow. The stomach cancer created so much acid that the bone finally dissolved and passed on through. Once the bone passed out of the stomach, the tumor rapidly disappeared – without treatment. Apparently the cancerous tumor served a purpose, but most doctors' mentality and training is to diagnose the cancer and remove it, either by surgery or chemotherapy, which is really just a chemical scalpel.

In the same way, doctors should not give pharmaceutical drugs which basically tell the body, "Step aside! I'll kill these bacteria for you!" Instead, doctors should learn to facilitate the body's own natural ability to regain control over the bacteria. To do this, the doctor must use frequency-matched nutraceuticals that enhance the energy already being created by the body to bring the bacteria under control, in combination with other natural treatments and therapies *that work to optimize perfect design and function of the body*.

The doctor must facilitate the body's ability to heal itself by removing anything that is interfering with its ability to heal. Potential interferences are many; therefore efforts must be made to remove anything and everything that ideally should not be there. This can be improved by detoxifying the body of heavy metals and organic toxins like pesticides, herbicides, and petroleum-based toxins that jam up the machinery and crystalline matrix of the body. Scars can be primary sources of interference due to the fact that scars act as a dam to the flow of electrical information passing through the meridian system, the pathways of acupuncture. Cold laser therapy can help reconnect these electro-energetic pathways through the scar thereby restoring the body's ability to communicate with itself unimpeded. These are but a few examples of many ways your doctor should be working with the body to help facilitate healing on every office visit.

At the same time, the doctor should be providing the information and building blocks needed by the body to repair the molecular matrix. This must occur in order to restore the body's healthy environment, making it non-conducive to microbial overgrowth.

Treatments and therapies should be applied with the goal of providing the body with the information it needs to heal itself. This is what the *Perfect-7 Treatment and Detox Protocol* is designed to do.

High-power prescription drugs are designed to provide you the illusion of health only. Does anyone really believe that aspirin is truly "fixing" the cause of your headache? The disturbance in your body is still there, but you can't feel it anymore. When your doctor gives you a medication for high blood pressure, does he ever say "Take this medicine for six months and then you should be well and be able to stop taking it"? No, he says you must take the medicine until the day you die or until it quits working, because the medicine is not truly fixing anything. The underlying disturbance in your body's matrix remains untouched. The drug simply creates the illusion of a healthy nervous system or organ system.

Antibiotics used in chronic infections also create the illusion of health; you may feel a little or a lot better while taking them, but they damage the body's healthy crystalline matrix further and simply push the microbes into a different shape. That is why if you stop taking the antibiotics, the infection often returns within weeks to months, leading one to wonder if they were re-infected or if it is the same infection returning that never truly went away.

Many people defend their conventional medical doctor because he/she "also uses vitamins along with the antibiotics."

It is great to incorporate vitamins, but vitamins are not enough to effect permanent change and long-term restoration of true health. Remember, to give your body an antibiotic or vitamin is like dropping a bomb on the microbial collective; it may hurt their population, but they work together to adapt.

Of course, none of this new understanding of microbes does away with the scientific facts of following good hygiene and using sanitary precautions. History is full of epidemics that killed millions of people and were caused by microbes due to unclean scalpels, unwashed hands, and contaminated food. This research helps us understand how to get control of microbes now that we know that antibiotics are not the "silver bullet – cure-all" we originally thought they would be.

This book outlines many issues that must be addressed to provide the body with the information, energy, and building blocks needed to facilitate the body's natural ability to heal itself and stay healthy.

This is not the all-inclusive compendium of treatment possibilities or even everything I do in my clinic, as the reader would get lost in all of the nuances of being a doctor. You will see that we are not just another doctor trying to sell you vitamins and supplements. As a matter of fact, a person can substitute many great remedies and supplements into each step of the Perfect-7 Treatment and Detox Protocol. This protocol is simply a template for all to use. I am presenting what I feel works best, based upon the latest research and my clinical experience. Doctors using these methods are not able to restore every patient to perfect health again, but we are definitely helping the majority and extending longevity.

I get calls from people from all over the world wanting to know if they can take my frequency-matched formulas and follow our protocols while taking antibiotics. The answer is yes, you can, but hopefully you see antibiotics and aggressive drug therapies are unnecessary and harmful in most cases.

[21] Glausiusz, Josie. Your Body is a Planet, Discover, 2007.
[22] Cloos, W. The Living Earth, London: Lanthorn Press 1977.
[23] Hamer, G. Summary of the New Medicine 3rd Edition, 2000.
[24] Jernigan, David A. *Infectious Perceptions: Living and Healing in a World of Designer Microbes.* To be released at a future date.
[25] Hornick, W., et al. Bulletin of the Academy of Medicine, 47 1971 p. 1181.
[26] Joppich, G. Lehrbuch der kinderheilkunde, Stuttgart 1975.
[27] Oschman, JL. 2001. *Living Crystals.* Energy Medicine, The Scientific Basis.
[28] Oschman, JL. 2001. Energy Medicine, The Scientific Basis.
[29] Popp, FA, Gu Q, Li K, (1992). Recent Advances in Biophoton Research and its Applications. Singapore: *World Scientific Recent Advances in Biophoton Research and its Applications.* Singapore: World Scientific
[30] Jenson, GS, 2002 Lecture Dec. Second annual conference on applied neurobiology; Treating Lyme and Co-infections.
[31] Vogel, R., Submuth, R., 1998. *Bioelectrochemistry and Bioenergetics*, 45, 93-101.
[32] Oschman 2001.
[33] Bouligand, Y. 1978 *Liquid crystals and their analogs in biological systems.* In: Liebert L (ed) Liquid crystals. Solid State Physics, Supplement 14:259-294.
[34] Allen, HC. Cross PC, 1963. Molecular Vib-rotors. John Wiley, New York.
[35] Smith, CW.1994. Biological effects of weak electromagnetic fields. In: Ho MW, Popp F.A, Warnke U (eds) Bioelectrodynamics and biocommunication. World Scientific, Singapore, Ch 3, pp 81-107.
[36] Slawinski, J., and Popp, F., 1987 J. Pl. Physiol., 130, 111-123.
[37] Oschman, J. *Energy Medicine: The Scientific Basis.* 2000
[38] Marinelli, R., van der Furst, Zee, H., McGinn, A., Marinelli, W., 1995, *The heart is not a pump: a refutation of the pressure propulsion premise of heart function.* Temple University Frontier Perspectives 5:15-24.
[39] Schwenk, T. 1996. *Sensitive Chaos*, Rudolf Steiner Press pp 90-93.
[40] Oschman 2001.
[41] Lewis, R., *The Rise of Antibiotic-Resistant Infections.* FDA Consumer magazine. September 1995.

4

~

What Factors Lead to Illness From Microbes?

I have been asked by doctors at conferences where I was teaching, "Why is Lyme Disease so prevalent, and why now? The answer is somewhat simple. In developed countries, mankind is moving away from the "inflammatory" diseases of the 19th and 20th centuries and towards the "cold and sclerotic" diseases. What has changed? We have! We have spent generations chasing "Better Health through Chemistry," a slogan of one of the pharmaceutical drug companies. Now we are dealing with the consequences of all the covering up of illness with illusionary medicine. Not only is our physical body over-cooling, but the complexity of mental, emotional, and spiritual life is shifting in huge leaps as more information floods in on the Information Highway. All of these rapid changes lead to becoming more out of balance, in turn leading to the "evolutionary" susceptibility to Lyme Disease.

Dr. Otto Wolf quotes the ecological research (The study of the environmental causes of disease) of Charles Elton who found that "diseases appear only after populations have already begun to decline."[42] Otto Wolf, M.D., goes on to state that "diseases are therefore not primary agents of evolution, but rather only indicators of a developmentally changed situation which they help to intensify or complete."[43]

We have all heard the saying, "A chain is only as strong as its weakest link." This is true in every aspect of the human body. I am talking about balance and living in integrity throughout the interconnectedness of your body, mind, and spirit. Any area of your life that is out of healthy rhythm and balance becomes a weak point. The body's healthy crystalline matrix, discussed in the previous chapter, is compromised by its inability to adapt rapidly enough to prolonged imbalance and irritation, making it vulnerable to the overgrowth of microbes.

Weak links in a person's life can often be identified by where the focus of infection is located in the body. For instance, viruses much prefer nerve tissue, while bacteria prefer blood and metabolic tissues. Nerve tissues can become susceptible to viral infection from mental, emotional, or otherwise sensory overload. Bacterial challenges often may be the result of nutritional deficiencies, toxin overload, weather extremes that weaken tissue resistance, and physical injuries such as cuts and abrasions. If your body is out of it optimum coherence and integrity, then no medication will ever truly return you to the quality of life you seek. In the human body, all treatments and therapies should seek to change the environment inside the body back to one that is inhospitable for microbial overgrowth.

The factors that may lead to microbial illness through the upsetting of the body's healthy integrity are numerous. The following is by no means complete:
- Fear, by any of its names
- Imbalanced body pH (too acidic or too alkaline)
- Prolonged or acute exposure to weather extremes
- Loss of the predominantly negative polarity of the tissues of the body
- Lowered core body temperature
- Prolonged personal suppression from people in your environment

Section 1: Understanding Lyme Disease

- Prolonged negative emotions
- Inherited predispositions and constitutional weaknesses
- Overuse of antibiotics, steroids, and other prescription medicines
- Vaccinations/immunizations
- Prolonged biomechanical stress
- Infection activated through auto-suggestion - usually the news media
- Dietary imbalances/Food maladaptive syndrome
- Tissue toxin overload
- Poor function of the organs of elimination, i.e., colon, urinary tract, lungs, skin.
- Geopathic stress
- Overwork
- Over/under sleeping
- Excessive prolonged stress
- Spiritual distress
- Electromagnetic pollution
- Mental overexertion
- Depression/emotional imbalance
- Poor hygiene
- Lack of creative stimulation
- Loss of connection to the world around you
- Loss of direction and purpose
- Lost love and affection
- Hate/unforgiveness

Basically, any influence that leads to an over- or under-stimulation, or an inability of the body to adapt correctly to changes of its internal or external environment, can adversely alter your receptivity to infection. Lyme spirochetes may lay dormant in the body for years, only to erupt into a major problem when the environment changes within the body.

The type of symptoms and the areas affected are determined by the factors involved. Sometimes several of the above-listed factors are involved in creating the illness. The point is that an effective treatment strategy must include therapies that will correct any and all factors leading to the receptivity.

Most people have taken antibiotics at some point in life. Once the symptoms are gone, most people don't give them another thought. Yet the best antibiotic in the world only kills about 85% of the bacteria at the very most. **Remember, some bacteria have already mutated or changed shape within the first 20 minutes of interacting with the antibiotics!** Taking more of the antibiotic, prolonging the treatment period, or switching from a pill form to intravenous won't matter.

Research reported by Ricki Lewis, Ph.D., states, "According to a report in the April 28, 1994, New England Journal of Medicine, researchers have identified bacteria in patient samples that resist all currently available antibiotic drugs."[44] Lewis also quotes one of the world's top experts on antibiotics as saying "Whenever antibiotics are used, there is selective pressure for resistance to occur. It builds upon itself. More and more organisms develop resistance to more and more drugs," says Joe Cranston, Ph.D., director of the department of drug policy and standards at the American Medical Association in Chicago.[45]

Historically, if you have a case of Strep throat or an ear infection, your medical doctor would prescribe an antibiotic for 7-10 days, and if you were diagnosed with Lyme Disease, your doctor would give an antibiotic for 6 weeks. The reality is that with Strep throat and ear infections, the illness would be over in 7-10 days even if you don't treat with antibiotics. The same thinking was applied for the standard medical protocol of six weeks of antibiotics for Lyme Disease -- surely the body could take over again within that time frame. Unfortunately, the body often cannot take over again after the discontinuation of antibiotics.

When you balance all aspects of your body and life, and your healthcare team has restored the integrity of the environment within your body using Circuit Healing and American Biological Medicine, the bacteria will be brought to a greatly reduced and symbiotic condition, and the symptoms will disappear, never to return as long as you stay in balance.

Antibiotics undoubtedly have saved lives and suffering in early stage, early-diagnosed Lyme. At times antibiotics may seem to have been used with some success in some chronic cases. It is more likely in these "success cases" that these people made meaningful changes in their lives during the ordeal that resulted in the cure. These meaningful changes might be new reconciliations in the mind (returning to a condition of love/peace/joy, thoughts of deliberate creation and intention), in their emotions (forgiveness, releasing fear and negative energy, redirecting more energy towards living and acting in a more loving condition to themselves and those around them), and lifestyle (improving diet, detoxing, exercising, getting natural therapies and treatments).

I personally have had five family members test positive for Lyme, one severely affected. My own children have tested positive on several occasions. I have treated over two thousand people who tested positive to Lyme, either through resonance, blood, and/or urine testing. I have seen and heard the horror stories of patients at the hands of doctors who tell many that because their basic conventional blood tests didn't find anything wrong, the person is basically a psychiatric case -- it's all in the head. I have had many women tell me that they feel like they must go to the doctor with no makeup on and in wrinkled clothes because they look too good to feel as bad as they are telling the doctor, especially when blood tests are negative. It reminds me of a tombstone I read about with the inscription, "I told you I was sick!"

Lyme Disease is a difficult proposition for anyone, but it should make sense to all that in the world of the future one will hopefully only feel *better* from medical treatments. In the world of today, the severe Herxheimer reactions or toxic effects of the strong antibiotics often create more problems than they fix.

There will always be those who insist that antibiotics, and lots of them, are the only way to address chronic Lyme. I have just not seen this to be true. I was at a recent Lyme conference with about 50 medical doctors in attendance; every doctor there acknowledged that antibiotics provided only limited relief at best. I was pleased to see that these brave few MDs are seeking new, more natural alternatives for helping their Lyme patients! So for those of you out there with no hope, here is real hope: a small but growing number of health professionals not only acknowledging the widespread existence of Lyme, but also seeking more effective and *natural* methods of treating people with Lyme.

Lyme Disease is serious, and just like there are very few Lyme-literate medical doctors, there are also very few doctors who practice natural medicine that are Lyme-literate. It is my hope that this book will help both types of doctors, as well as every person suffering with Lyme. Much of what I have learned about Lyme and healing has been from my patients. You can help plant seeds in your doctors' minds by taking them this book or suggesting gently that they might like to read it.

Realities of Antibiotics

It may seem that I am anti-antibiotics, but the reality is that there is a time and a place where they can be beneficial for some people. I appreciate the way the renowned German medical doctor Otto Wolf, M.D. says the following about antibiotics:

> "Summing up, we may state that antibiotics negatively influence the organism's healing reactions, and are thus the opposite of a true remedy. That is not to say that they cannot save

lives, but the same must be said here as was said about insulin: it can undoubtedly save and lengthen life, but does not heal diabetes, since it is only substitution therapy. To the extent that bacteria are only a symptom of the underlying disease, antibiotics act only symptomatically...The use of antibiotics should therefore not be a first therapeutic step, but rather should be reserved for situations in which the organism is overtaxed...The objection that "antibiotics should be used in every serious case" completely misses the point; it demonstrates a lack of understanding regarding illness, healing, and the principles of effective therapy. 'Serious cases' will generally not arise if the organism's own meaningful reactions are recognized and stimulated from the beginning and the organism is thereby guided through the disease...The use of antibiotics can be compared to throwing a life ring to someone who has fallen into the water. Although even the best swimmer can find himself in a situation where a lifesaver is required, it is still better to teach people to swim than it is to rely on such devices. By no means is the lifesaver the "true" remedy to the problem of deaths by drowning."[46]

Antibiotics are definitely not a solution I recommend if avoiding them is at all possible, due in part to their increasingly poor results in the long run, and primarily due to the many very real direct and unavoidable adverse effects on the integrity of the body, not to mention their potential for side effects and allergic reactions.

I am amazed at how many people already know they are allergic to at least one class of antibiotic. The problem I have seen repeatedly is that a worsening of symptoms is expected by many doctors as an indication to them that the medicine is working -- the proverbial "herx." But how does one know when it is a true adverse reaction to the drug instead of a bacteria die off? Many, if not most, people we have tested were allergic to the antibiotics they were using. Keep in mind that it doesn't mean that the antibiotic isn't killing bacteria, but many are experiencing adverse symptoms that have nothing to do with a herx. Just so this point is understood, in the same manner, every single asthma sufferer I have tested has been allergic to their inhaler, and the inhaler tested as a toxic substance to the body, but it still worked for them as a bronchial dilator. These people got the relief they needed from their inhalers but were suffering in other ways due to the allergic and toxic effects on other parts of their body.

It might be a surprise to you to know that the leading type of drug causing adverse reactions is antibiotics! As reported in the scientifically referenced article, "Death by Medicine" by Gary Null, PhD, et al., the leading cause of death in America is adverse drug reactions. It is reported that approximately 800,000 people die yearly due in large part to adverse reactions and conventional medicine's philosophy of care. Over one million hospital admissions annually in the United States are due to adverse drug reactions.

In one year in the United States alone, over 3 million pounds of pure antibiotics are used on humans! This is enough antibiotics to give every man, woman, and child in the United States <u>10 teaspoons</u> of pure antibiotics every year! Now consider that many Lyme Disease sufferers have been on at least two different antibiotics at a time at an average dosage of 600mg each per day. If one has been on antibiotics at this dosage for one year, a full pound of pure antibiotics has been consumed. How many more pounds of antibiotics will it take? **Especially when research has shown that at times bacteria are known to be able to spontaneously mutate around an antibiotic within the first 20 minutes of taking the first pill!**[47] If the bacteria have already mutated around the antibiotic, taking a higher dosage or switching to an intravenous form of the antibiotic (which is a common tactic), will do little good and will likely only increase the toxic burden and aggravate the biochemistry of the body.

Now consider the almost 25 million pounds of antibiotics fed to livestock for non-therapeutic reasons. In the January 18, 1997, issue of New Scientist, researchers reported a link between farm animals given drugs and antibiotic resistance. Individuals who ingested the meat of these animals were found to be more susceptible to resistant strains of *Salmonella* and *Enterococcus faecalis*.[48] Do you think that maybe eating antibiotic altered beef, pork, and other meats might interfere with your body's ability to adapt correctly when you get bitten by ticks, mosquitoes, and fleas? Remember, the actual microbe is almost the last factor which determines whether you will manifest a disease!

This research shows antibiotics as an unacceptable and "last resort only" solution, since they likely lead to years of dependency. Some doctors and patients feel it is justified due to the relief provided, even though it is, but again, simply a drug-induced illusion of health.

Again, many people are angered over information that shows the negative side of antibiotics. Some of this anger is from having lost loved ones to the ineffectiveness of antibiotics or the perception that not enough antibiotics were given to save their loved one. My goal is not to bring people to anger. I have known true loss, and I feel deeply for those who have lost loved ones. It is because of these losses and the suffering of so many that I work hard to develop new, hopefully better, ideas that will save lives. My real hope is that this book will stimulate some young doctor to surpass anything that has been thought or done to date.

Antibiotics and Post-Lyme Syndrome

No one or two medicines or remedies can address all of the problems associated with a multi-system illness, such as chronic Lyme Disease. Each of the remedies, supplements, treatments, and therapies presented in this book complement each other and have a strong synergistic effect on the entire body. When true healing takes place, as it does when using the philosophy of Biological Medicine (as opposed to allopathic medicine), one not only facilitates the natural decrease in the population of spirochetes, but Post-Lyme Syndrome (PLS), which is common with antibiotic and pharmaceutical medicines, can also be avoided. Lyme Disease is similar to another of history's terrifying neurological infections, Polio, whose allopathic treatment left many to suffer with Post-Polio Syndrome. Both syndromes leave the people who have been declared "cured" with a slowly-progressing condition marked by short to long periods of stability.

The severity of PLS depends on the degree of the weakness and disability an individual had leading up to the infection, as well as the residual weakness and disability left behind by the infection and allopathic treatments.

People who had only minimal symptoms from the Lyme Disease and were treated with antibiotics will most likely experience only mild PLS symptoms. People originally hit hard by Lyme Disease and treated with antibiotics often are left with severe residual physical, mental, and emotional problems, and they may develop more severe cases of PLS with the recurrence of many symptoms and more periods of profound fatigue.

PLS is not necessary and is avoidable when the restoration of coherence and integrity of the body, mind, and spirit is the focus of every treatment and therapy.

One may ask, "Is there a time when antibiotics are okay to use?" My answer is yes. Antibiotics have saved many lives since the advent of penicillin. However, in chronic Lyme Disease, it is the opinion of some conventional doctors that the antibiotics should only be used at the time of the initial diagnosis for approximately four months. **My opinion as a doctor specializing in restoring the optimal integrity of the human organism: I would never recommend antibiotics for acute or chronic Lyme Disease.** I have seen too many people overcome Lyme without antibiotics and without severe Herxheimer reactions. As a doctor, I strive to make no one feel guilty for using antibiotics. Everyone must walk their own health road and make their own choices. When treating someone who is taking antibiotics symptomatically, I simply work to counteract any adverse effects they may be causing, while providing the body with the true corrective care it needs to heal.

The prevalent thought seems to be that the human body is unintelligent and needs our help to fix its problems. The reality is that the world's most astute and celebrated physicians cannot fix even the simplest paper cut, much less a serious illness like Lyme Disease. Most physicians specialize in creating drug-induced illusions of health. The human body is not dumb. The body needs the physician to see his role as a being a facilitator in the process of restoring the body's optimal design so that homeostasis can be reestablished and true health can follow.

The drug companies have teams of people who "police" the internet newsgroups and media to monitor the information getting out about natural products that are working. They keep the latest drug in the forefront of people's minds dangled like a carrot that will lead you to the restoration of the quality of life you desire. It is said that this is the Information Age, and he who controls the information controls the world. Apparently all is fair in the "guerilla marketing." For example, when Borrelogen™ was first announced on internet Lyme newsgroups, it caused a war of words between the people who were trying it and reporting that they were getting better versus the drug company people. You can see this war quite easily in the archives of the internet, preserved for eternity.

People would innocently and joyfully report that they were getting better on Borrelogen, and they were getting hate mail from "well meaning, self-appointed newsgroup drug company police." The guerilla warfare continues with another author's writing about the natural treatment of Lyme. To discredit Borrelogen, he simply posted the same message to multiple newsgroups that said "he had tried Borrelogen and it didn't do much for him" and continued to post this same message for months until anyone typing in a search on Borrelogen had to suffer through his monotonous messages. Shortly after doing this, he produced his own book on Lyme. It seems that morality is for sale in America.

I bring this up because one needs to know what is going on in this Information Age. Drug companies and nutraceutical companies often are only concerned with keeping you a loyal customer of their quality-questionable products. I am first and foremost a doctor. I developed my few products simply because nothing I could find was helping my patients. It could be said that I, too, am simply trying to sell you something. My heart is to help people get well, not in a year or two, as is promoted by doctors following the fad "cookbook" natural protocols, but as quickly as I can help you heal. I am a facilitator and teacher only. I want you to be fully informed of the realities of your choices. I don't want anyone to follow a protocol that keeps them suffering for a year or two with the promise that at the end you will feel better. I know *some* of these protocols are "bad medicine" because so many of the thousands of people who have come to our clinic demonstrate improvements within the first two weeks of care – not a year later! Almost all of these people stated that nothing they had ever tried had even helped them. Most of them had only gotten worse with the conventional and natural medicines they had tried.

I do not share this information to benefit my ego or claim in arrogance that "My way is the only way." I feel it is necessary to help you benefit from my work with thousands of people and understand why I felt it necessary to write such a complex book. As you will notice, this book is more about the process of healing than the products I developed. The Perfect-7 protocol I present later in this book can be implemented using a wide range of different natural products, not just the ones I have formulated.

The treatments, therapies, and products we use have helped many thousands of people over the years, but I want you to know that even if they only get you partially well, this is more than many medicines achieve. I like to think it is like you are running a marathon and I am on the sidelines handing you a refreshing drink that may not get you all the way to the finish line, but at least it will get you that much closer so that someone else can help you the rest of the way.

Remember the true reality is that health in a bottle is a myth! Remedies and medicines, even the formulas I have developed, can be of great benefit in helping restore the body; however, many physical problems require a physical correction either through a knowledgably applied manual correction of the musculoskeletal system or through electro-medical devices. True health requires one to use the correct tool for the job. If you dislocate your finger, there isn't a pill in the world that will correct it.

In Lyme Disease, it is unfortunate that once the diagnosis has been made, every symptom is typically blamed on Lyme and its co-infections, when in reality most people have a myriad of problems that have nothing to do with Lyme but are aggravated and enhanced by it, or vice-versa (other symptoms aggravate and enhance Lyme), and must be addressed using the right tools. Along with the physical body, the mind and the spirit must also be addressed.

[42] Wolf, O. and Husseman, F. The Anthroposophical Approach to Medicine, 1989 Vol 3.
[43] Wolf, O. and Husseman, F. The Anthroposophical Approach to Medicine, 1989 Vol 3.
[44] Lewis, R., *The Rise of Antibiotic-Resistant Infections.* FDA Consumer Magazine September 1995.
[45] Lewis, R., *The Rise of Antibiotic-Resistant Infections.* FDA Consumer Magazine September 1995.
[46] Wolf, O. and Husemann, F. The Anthroposophical Approach to Medicine, Vol 3 1989.
[47] Lewis, R. *The Rise of Antibiotic-Resistant Infections.* 1997.
[48] Bonner, J. *Hooked on Drugs.* New Scientist, 24-27. 1997.

5
~

Borrelia burgdorferi & Mycoplasmal Infections

When the Borrelia burgdorferi are in their L-Form phase, the morphology (appearance) cannot be distinguished from that of Mycoplasma organisms. In fact, there is only one primary difference between the two organisms; mycoplasma by definition cannot generate a cell wall.[49]

For those of you who are unfamiliar with the term mycoplasma, do not feel uneducated. It is only recently that the pathogenic nature of these organisms has come into the forefront of the medical mindset. A mycoplasma is larger than a virus and smaller than bacteria. Mycoplasmas are more closely akin to bacteria than viruses. They are said to be the smallest self-replicating life form.[50] Like Borrelia burgdoferi, the mycoplasma can infect deep tissues and create almost all of the same symptoms as Lyme.[51] A plethora of research has connected mycoplasmal infections to many of today's most prevalent illnesses such as Lyme Disease, Chronic Fatigue Syndrome (CFS), Fibromyalgia Syndrome (FMS), and even the Gulf War Syndrome (GWS).[52]

How does this impact you?

Any person suffering from Lyme knows that it is affecting multiple systems of the body. This fact causes a weakened and susceptible immune system. Sufferers of chronic LD/CFS/FMS/GWS become microbe collectors. The body's resistance to foreign invaders such as mycoplasma is greatly reduced. When considering the effects of having multiple pathogenic infections at the same time, it is no wonder that so many people undergo years of treatment without complete resolution of their symptoms. Each of these microbes is part of a community in your body and are either a producer, consumer, or decomposer. With the knowledge of intermicrobial communication, via their crystalline matrix hotwired into the body's normal crystalline matrix, one can see that they are all working together to survive. Successful treatment can only be realized by addressing the entire body to restore the body's own control mechanisms of all microbes.

It is well recognized that people suffering from Lyme Disease may also have other infections going on at the same time, such as Babesia microti, Ehrlichiosis, viruses (EBV, CMV, and HHV-6), and Candidiasis. To make matters worse, we are now realizing that mycoplasmal infections can be detected in the blood of 60-70% of all LD/CFS/FMS sufferers. According to Dr. Nicholson, Ph.D., "Systemic mycoplasmal infections are a major source of morbidity in CFS, FMS, and Gulf War Illness patients, and they need to be treated with antibiotics...and nutritional support".[53] Of course, antibiotics were anticipated in the development of this biological warfare microbe, so it is unlikely antibiotics are a good treatment.

When considering the fact that the Bb can also revert to a mycoplasma look-alike L-Form when antibiotics are introduced, one can begin to grasp the true difficulties of determining an effective treatment protocol. Do not get disheartened; all of this is treatable! I am simply attempting to educate you so that you can know what you are up against and better understand your enemy. Your body is well-equipped to deal with any microbe if given the proper support (I don't mean antibiotics). Anyone who would tell you otherwise is stuck in a medical model of drug interventions on a statistically sick, dysfunctional, and otherwise imbalanced population.

If you have been treated for Lyme Disease and have reached the point where all of the lab tests indicate that you no longer have any Borrelia burgdorferi, yet you are still feeling very sick, then your doctor needs to do a mycoplasma PCR test on you. Also have him test for the other common co-infections: Babesia microti, Ehrlichia, Human Herpes Virus-6, Epstein - Barr virus, Cytomegalovirus, Adeno-virus, and systemic Candida. If you have never tested positive to having Lyme Disease, definitely get your doctor to test for mycoplasmal infections.

---

[49] Mattman, L., *Cell Wall Deficient Forms*, Stealth Pathogens, 2nd Ed., p 13, 1992.
[50] Popular Science, April 1999.
[51] Donta, S.T., Fibromyalgia, Lyme Disease, and Gulf War Syndrome, 12th International Conference on Lyme Disease, New York, 1999.
[52] Nicolson, G.L., Nasralla, M. Hier, J. and Nicolson, N.L. Mycoplasmal infections in chronic illnesses: Fibromyalgia and Chronic Fatigue Syndromes, Gulf War Illness, HIV-AIDS and Rheumatoid Arthritis. Med. Sentinel 1999.
[53] Nicolson, G.L., The Institute for Molecular Medicine, 1999.

6

~

Beating Lyme Disease is More Than Killing Bacteria

I cannot stress enough the need for your doctor to be addressing all the systems of the body on every visit. The body is totally integrated and should perform like an orchestra, with every organ and tissue keeping rhythm with all the rest of the body. Taking a multi-vitamin/mineral, or even Borrelogen™ only addresses a part of what is required by your body to restore its ability to heal.

If one organ becomes dysfunctional due to illness or trauma, it ceases to move with correct rhythm in relation to the three dimensional movement of the other organs. When this happens, it throws off the natural rhythm of the entire body. Eventually no tissue is able to maintain the proper rhythm. It is inevitable that this chain reaction will occur progressively over time if left uncorrected. Proper rhythm is part of what is necessary to maintain the integrity of the communication throughout the entire human organism.

While it is true that there is usually one offending issue that starts the whole chain-reaction, if left undiagnosed and untreated for very long, the problem will become complicated by the after-effects of the original cause. Weakened tissues lose their natural crystalline-matrix resistance to and control of things such as parasitic infection, toxin overload, dysregulated chemistry, and fungal and microbial infection.

Let us use the example of Lyme Disease. A person gets bitten by an infected tick or mosquito and becomes infected with a few of the bacteria known as Borrelia burgdorferi. The few bacteria migrate through the tissues, making their way to the weakest tissues... muscles, joints, connective tissues, organs, the brain, and/or nerves.

If the body is relatively healthy, there may be enough integrity within the body's crystalline matrix to effectively keep the few bacteria from overpopulating, and therefore no illness may ever manifest as long as you maintain the integrity of the body, mind, and spirit.

If the infection is not detected and treated correctly in order to enable the body to adapt, the body's resistance remains weakened, and the few bacteria find the body a perfect breeding ground. The few become many, and the chain reaction begins. The bacterial toxins wreak havoc on your body. To let you know that there is something wrong, your body responds with a multitude of symptoms arising from those weakest areas.

Like every organism, the Lyme bacteria live a certain life span and then die. This means that even without treatment, you will have a certain number of Borrelia burgdorferi bacteria dying off every few weeks. These dying bacteria end up causing problems since they release toxins upon dying (also known as the cause of a Jarish-Herxheimer reaction). These toxins lodge in the tissues of the body and cause a worsening of the symptoms you feel. Research has shown that there is no direct tissue damage from the spirochetes. The damage to tissues is primarily due to the spirochete toxins which increase the inflammatory and immune responses.[54] Here is where the chain reaction begins to be most pronounced.

To better understand the chain reaction, let us start with a hypothetical example. Suppose the toxins are primarily affecting the elasticity of your muscles. The muscles of your right leg become tight and cramp, with wandering pains. You begin to favor that leg, walking with a limp. You are not designed to walk in this manner, so structural integrity is compromised. Your body's structural components are now exceeding their design limitations. The knee and hip joints begin to swell in response to the strain. The pelvis becomes unlevel, throwing the entire spine into fits as it attempts to compensate for the tilted pelvis. The pelvis and intervertebral discs of the spine become inflamed from the changes in weight distribution, which in turn irritate the spinal nerves. The spinal nerves are important in carrying the brain's messages for helping to regulate every organ's function. With the spinal nerve irritation comes radiating pains in different areas of the body, along with tingling, numbness, and loss of muscular control. The organs begin to reflect the spinal problems and cannot get a clear signal from the brain; therefore the chemistry and hormones become dysregulated. Any area of inflammation and weakness in the tissues, such as the spinal nerves, becomes susceptible to viral and bacterial infection. Some of the latest research by Dr. Gary Young, M.D., N.D., has demonstrated microbial infections in the majority of spinal nerve irritations, such as in sciatica, with the pain radiating from the lower back down the legs.[55]

Every organ is on its own dedicated electrical circuit with at least one set of muscles. When there is a problem anywhere in an organ circuit, it causes the entire circuit to become short-circuited. The damaged organ circuit will only work at about 40% of its normal electrical and functional capacity, though it may not show any changes on blood tests. Most Lyme sufferers can relate to this since most of the blood tests, of all types, reveal nothing of significance even though there are many symptoms.

The "short-circuiting" is one of the body's protective mechanisms. The body will "turn down" the available energy to a damaged area so that you cannot damage it further by exerting 100% energy into an area that needs to be repaired. It is like breaking a bone in the leg; upon breaking the bone, special nerve fibers in the muscles called muscle spindle fibers send a signal to the brain to shut down the muscles. In an instant, the brain shuts down the circuit containing those muscles. Otherwise, having 100% energy in the muscles might allow them to break the bone further.

Decreased energy in one circuit disrupts the rhythm of the other organs, which, over time respond one by one, going into compensation mode, where they attempt to "take up the slack" for the dysfunctional organ circuit; eventually they too manifest complete dysfunction.

By now, you are suffering from profound and chronic fatigue as all the muscles of the body are only able to function at 40% of their intended output and you hurt all over. You have tender spots in the muscles. Your joints take turns aching and hurting. Your brain won't seem to work right because the bacterial toxins cause the blood-brain barrier to become "leaky," allowing large proteins to cross the barrier and cause cerebral allergies and localized swelling, and as a result you can't seem to sleep even though you are completely worn out all day long. It seems like nothing in your body is working correctly. You go to the doctor, who may not believe that Lyme is a problem in your state, but who runs other tests, which are "inconclusive." And the Lyme Disease goes on. Electrical Circuitry of the body will be discussed in more detail in Chapter 7.

Finally, you have found a doctor who determines you have Lyme Disease. "Not a problem," he may say. "Just take this antibiotic, and you should be better in six weeks"." At the end of six weeks he proclaims you cured. The problems are just starting; even if you were one of the lucky ones who felt better while on the antibiotics, once the antibiotics are discontinued your symptoms return. Another more common response is that even during the six weeks of antibiotics you don't feel any better or you feel worse, or at the minimum you feel like you are still not well.

Did the doctor address everything? Does the doctor even have the tools and knowledge necessary to address the structural, chemical, stress-issues, and electromagnetic problems? Usually he has only attempted to addressed the infection. The structural imbalances that have now been there for months or years, and no pill will address them adequately. Even if he recommends vitamins, it is often not enough. How about the organ circuits which didn't magically come back online after the antibiotics? Did he address the opportunistic parasites, yeast, and viruses that found a home in your body while your resistance was down? How about the toxins stored in the tissues?

Friends, can you begin to see how difficult it can be to achieve total wellness after a long fight with something terrible such as Lyme Disease? If your doctor is simply giving you antibiotics with the hope that everything will go back to normal as soon as the bacteria is gone, then you need to find a new doctor, one who will cover all the other areas needing healing -- even if you must go outside of your PPO, HMO, or health insurance company. If your auto insurance won't pay to get your transmission fixed when it breaks down, you would find a way to pay to have it fixed because your car and getting around is a priority to you. Where is your priority regarding your body? You must do whatever it takes to get it fixed.

Addressing the totality of the human body is impossible without a technique like Bio-Resonance Scanning™ or other like electro-dermal screening, Voll-testing, Computerized Regulation Thermography (CRT), or Neural Therapy. All of these techniques have been developed by scientists and doctors in order to eliminate much of the educated guesswork, or "cookbook," doctoring that has dominated the last hundred and fifty years. Without these techniques, doctors are just guessing at what is needed and hoping you won't be allergic to the medicines, as well as hoping the combination of medicines won't conflict or create adverse effects in the body.

Using natural methods to help facilitate the body's ability to bring down the population of the bacteria in Lyme Disease can many times be just part of the fight. You now must restore the integrity of every tissue of your body. This restoring of integrity is sometimes called restoring coherence. *Coherence exists when every aspect of the body, mind, and spirit is able to communicate freely and adapt correctly to changes in the internal and external environment.* This takes time. A general rule of thumb in chronic illness is to expect three months of corrective lifestyle/treatments for every year you have had the problem. This doesn't mean that you won't feel better sooner. It simply means that *feeling good and being healthy are two different things.* When most people are initially diagnosed with cancer or heart disease, they say they have "never felt better" and the doctor just found the problem in a routine examination. So, be patient with the body.

Beating chronic Lyme Disease is much more than killing bacteria. Your body will naturally control the population of spirochetes if coherence is restored. Beating Lyme Disease requires your complete attention and cooperation. You cannot simply take the medicines and hope for the best.

Keep a journal so you can see improvement over long periods of time. Rejoice in small triumphs. Control your thinking -- don't allow yourself to become depressed. Do not talk about the various symptoms, talk about the things that are better. See yourself *half-well instead of half-sick.* Cooperate with the different doctors and therapists who are trying to help you. Don't be lazy in your mind; rejoice and actively participate in the healing of your body. You cannot afford to just take the pills and live a dark, dismal life, waiting for the pills to work. Change your routines. Strive to be vital in rebuilding your body. You are not a victim; you are simply living life like everyone else. All have problems to deal with. You cannot afford to allow yourself to "become an illness;" this just leads to a rapid decline. The illness is not who you are. Become one with God and one with yourself, not one with the illness. Get outside in the sunshine and close to nature, and simplify life so that your priorities are correct. The decisions you make today will determine your tomorrow. Above all, control your thinking --it's the one thing you have total control over. It's your free-will choice to accept or reject the illusions and lies that come to your mind. More information concerning the actual how-to as well as the science behind consciously and purposely creating a new reality of health and prosperity can be read in my companion to this book, *Everyday Miracles by God's Design*. You <u>can</u> reclaim your quality of life, and the journey with a worthy destination is the prize.

---

[54] Coyle PK, 1999 Neurologic Lyme Disease Update, International Conference on Lyme Disease, New York
[55] *Essential Oils Desk Reference* (3rd Edition) Essential Science Publishing, 2004.

7

~

Body Circuits and Circuit Healing

The body is set up on electrical circuits much like your own house. In your house you have a circuit breaker box. Each circuit switch has a label that tells you basically what is on each circuit (i.e., kitchen appliances, refrigerator, kitchen lights). The electrical circuits of the body always have one organ, specific teeth, a specific set of muscles, specific joints, and a specific gland all sharing one circuit.

The human body was created this way because, from an electrical perspective, we have very low electrical energy. The circuitry is necessary because if all of the body got all of the energy all of the time, there would not be enough electrical energy to go around. God made it so that each circuit of the body has its own time of highest energy directed to it for three hours only per day.

In a house, if something on a circuit has a problem, it knocks the entire circuit "offline." If the refrigerator from the above example circuit has a problem, it will cause the toaster oven, and kitchen lights that share that same circuit to not work either. Houses were designed this way so that if anything along the electrical circuits is having a problem, the problem would not get so bad that it would cause a fire.

Similarly, in the human body, if something on a circuit has a problem, it can knock the entire circuit "offline" as well. While we don't have a switch that gets turned off as in your house circuit breaker box, God designed our bodies with secondary "wiring" as a backup system in case you blow out the primary wiring. This secondary wiring will carry only about 40% of the normal amount of energy. This means that if the organ becomes diseased, it will cause the teeth, muscles, joints, and gland on that circuit to also only function at 40% of their normal capacity. God designed the body this way so that if anything along the electrical circuits is having a problem, the problem would not get so bad that the problem quickly worsens out of control.

It has been this author's observation that by the age of 20, most people have blown out all of the body's circuits and are living on secondary wiring. One can live a long life on secondary wiring, even reaching over 100 years of age, but the quality of life is less than half what it should have been if all circuits of the body had been maintained correctly.

Section 1: Understanding Lyme Disease

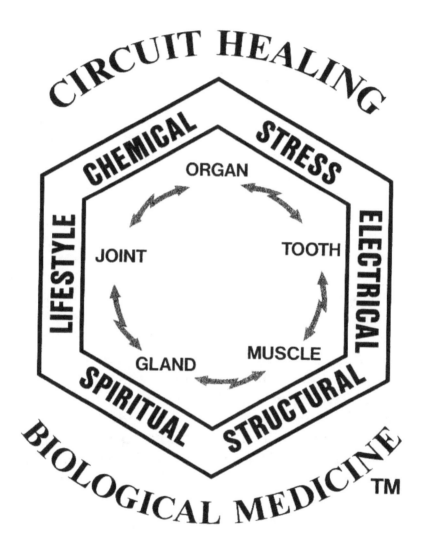

Treating the Body Circuits

The concept of the human body being set up on dedicated, yet interconnected, electromagnetic circuits are not a metaphor. The circuits of the body have been recognized as fact a thousand of years before western scientific thought decided that the microscopic view of the inner workings of the body was more important than the macroscopic (larger) view of the body's circuits.

Conventional medicine truly relies heavily upon a microscopic view of the various body components, blood cells, immune cells, tissues, and fluids. While a doctor cannot throw out medical advancements that have stood the test of time, he must be humble to the realization of where true healing comes from in the first place. Only the human body can heal itself. Doctors do not heal. On the best of days, they can only facilitate the body's own God-designed ability to heal. If you cut yourself, I hope you have a band-aid because I cannot heal that cut. At best, I can provide your body with treatment or remedies to speed the healing.

American Biological Medicine combines the best of the microscopic view with the best macroscopic circuit view of healing. It seeks to find where on the circuit the primary problem is coming from. Finding the primary problem is complicated by the fact that, 85% of the time, where you feel the pain is not where it is coming from. I hope you understand that looking at the body fluids through a microscope may tell you that something is wrong, but it will not tell you from where the primary problem is coming. This is why 88% of all conventional medicine (allopathic medicine) is, by definition treating the symptoms only, as opposed to seeking to correct the cause of the symptoms![56] Conventional medicine could treat the cause if it could identify it. It would only be able to identify it if it would view the body in its entirety, a system of interrelated and interdependent circuits.

The doctor specializing in Biological Medicine is trained to identify where within each circuit the primary problem lies. Once the problem is identified and corrected, the entire circuit goes back to 100% or maximum electrical capacity. Optimal health is achieved and maintained by keeping all of the body circuits functioning as close to 100% as possible.

Circuit Healing and the Swiss Watch

If you were to take the back off of a Swiss watch, you would see an incredibly complex system of gears. The precision that has made these watches famous is created by many gears meshing together. Each of the gears is a separate piece, but each gear is interconnected with the rest of the gears through a complex system to ultimately achieve perfect time keeping.

If you remove or damage one gear, the precision will be lost and the watch completely useless. Not one out of the dozens of gears in a Swiss watch can perform its function if even one part is missing or damaged.

The human body is much more complex than the most intricately designed Swiss watch. However, comparisons can still be made. The circuits of the body can be likened to the various gears in the watch. Each circuit in the body must work in unison with all of the other circuits of the body. The precision of the watch is determined by the perfect timing and rhythm of every single gear. The precision of the body is determined by the perfect function and rhythm of every single circuit.

Imagine, if you will, that the circuits of the body are simply gears that fit together and all have to be turning at the same time in order to function. If all of the gears are stuck, repairing only one of the gears will never get the body functioning correctly. This is the way most medicine is practiced today. The "specialist" type of doctor, such as a doctor specializing in Infectious Disease, attempts to get his "gear" unstuck. He can't tell that the gear is stuck because of something gone wrong in a location far removed from his stuck gear because he is focusing only on his specialty.

Each of the body's circuits is self-contained but interconnected with the other circuits. Problems in one circuit will necessarily create a chain reaction of the other circuits progressively becoming dysfunctional.

The doctor specializing in Biological Medicine is trained to identify where within each circuit the primary problem lies. Once the problem is identified and corrected, the entire circuit goes back to 100% energetic capacity. Optimal health is achieved and maintained by keeping all of the body circuits functioning as close to 100% integrity as possible.

I developed the Circuit Healing chart pictured previously to demonstrate a basic circuit in the body. The outer ring, something I like to call the "Hexagon of Health," represents all of the potential variables that can "blow the circuits" in the body. The doctor specializing in Biological Medicine is trained to address all of these potential problems.

Keep in mind that there can be multiple problems within one circuit. This is more common in severe and chronic conditions. Each problem will need to be addressed before the circuit will come back online.

Individual roles played in Circuit Healing are discussed on the following pages.

The Role of Teeth in Circuit Healing

Certain teeth are on each organ circuit in the body and can therefore cause dysfunction throughout the entire circuit. It must be realized that teeth are alive. They are not bones in your jawbone. Each tooth has up to two miles of micro-dental tubules, small tubes within the tooth, which maintain the nutrient and energetic flow in a healthy tooth.

Conventional dentists are primarily concerned with the appearance of your teeth, repairing cavities, and fighting infection. However, a new type of dentist is emerging -- the Biological Dentist. These dentists recognize that tooth problems will ultimately cause dysfunction in the rest of the circuit.

Keep in mind, that while dental cavities need to be addressed, what I am referring to is the entire tooth mechanism, including not just the tooth, but the gum, and jaw integrity as well.

A bad tooth can cause major problems to arise anywhere within the circuit, such as in the organ or gland that shares its energetic circuit, ultimately causing your untimely and premature death.

Most of the problems in teeth arise from the efforts of dentists, either by placing toxic heavy metals (such as mercury) in the fillings, or by multiple metals in your mouth creating random charges of electrical currents in a battery effect, or through direct toxic waste leaching out of decaying and dead root canals.

In one study in Europe, dental problems were the primary cause of breast cancer in 97% of the cases.[57] As amazing as it may seem, there are at least eight teeth that have direct electrical connections via the body circuits to the mammary glands, and 80% of all breast cancer arises in the mammary glands. Another interesting finding from the same study was that the tumors had up to 80 times more mercury metal than the surrounding healthy tissue. The primary source of mercury (which is 1000x more toxic than lead) in your mouth is from silver/mercury amalgams in your teeth. Experts feel that mercury is leached out of the teeth throughout its entire electrical circuit, potentially ending up in joints, muscles, glands, and organs.[58]

Doctors specializing in Biological Medicine are trained to identify problems anywhere in the body's circuits, even the teeth. If the problem is coming from a tooth, no treatment will work completely until the tooth problem is resolved.

The Role of Joints in Circuit Healing

A joint is where two bones meet. All of the joints of the body share specific electrical circuits with an organ, specific muscles, teeth, and glands. As a part of the circuit, a problem in the joint can and will cause a problem throughout the circuit. This means a problem in a joint can potentially cause a circuit to blow, reducing the available energy in the circuit to about 40% of what it normally should have. Not only does the joint become dysfunctional, but the organ sharing the same circuit will become dysfunctional as well.

Any joint can lead to circuit problems, but the primary joints are the inter-vertebral joints in the spine, pelvis, knees, feet, and the many joints of the skull.

Doctors specializing in Biological Medicine are trained to identify and address joint problems. Problems in joints usually arise from misalignments where the bones are slightly out of normal position, fixations (bones of the joint are stuck and not moving through their correct range of motion), toxic accumulations in the joints (chemical and/or biological poisons have been trapped in the joints), and other joint problems such as bone spurring and degenerative conditions.

Remember, in order to heal completely, every aspect of the body must be functioning as close to 100% as possible. Therefore, it makes sense that the integrity of the joints must be addressed in any type of disease. That is why the adjusting of the spine and other joints of the body by a trained Doctor of Chiropractic is included as a part of Circuit Healing.

No other doctor in the world is as well trained to address the various bio-mechanical problems of the body than a Doctor of Chiropractic. Nor is there a branch of medicine so well-suited to practice Biological Medicine; Chiropractors are now trained almost identically to Medical Doctors, with the exception that Doctors of Chiropractic must work with natural means to facilitate healing. Biological Medicine recognizes the body's interconnectedness and focuses on true healing through natural methods, and it recognizes the body's ability to heal if given the chance.

The Role of Organs in Circuit Healing

I have seen patients who had lifelong perfect teeth until they got very sick, and then their teeth began to exhibit disease. This unfortunate event beautifully demonstrates how absolutely true the concept of body circuits is. As organs malfunction due to disease, the entire circuit is affected; in this case the teeth on the circuit begin to suffer.

Remember, the circuits of the body are electrical pathways that are shared by an organ, a specific set of muscles, glands, teeth, and joints.

Of all of the components in a circuit in the body, the organs are the most critical; major problems arise when organs malfunction, compared to muscles and joints, which cause a progressive problem to arise and result eventually in the disruption of the normal function of the organ.

Imbalance in organs is most often noticed in lab tests but is most often felt in the dysfunction of joints and muscles. If an organ is rigid, stiff, and generally dysfunctional, the muscles and joints on the same circuit will be rigid, stiff, and generally dysfunctional. It really is that easy. The entire circuit will be affected in much the same way.

Doctors specializing in Biological Medicine are trained to recognize and address organ dysfunction from all causes. Organs can malfunction from many different causes: toxic substances, parasites, microbial overgrowth, hormonal, nutritional, and enzymatic imbalances, emotional stress, and electrical circuit problems.

As unfair as it may seem, we are not all born equal. All of us are born with problems that predispose us to organ problems. This is why it is so important to have your children treated using Biological Medicine principles. It will start them on the road to a long and functional life and will benefit every generation to follow. The longer the organ problem has been there, the longer it may take to resolve.

The Role of Symptoms in Circuit Healing

Symptoms are the problems you feel when circuits are not functioning correctly. Pain is a symptom, it is your body's way of saying, "Don't do that, or it will cause more damage." A tumor in a cancer patient is a symptom! (The tumor is not the cause, but the result of dysfunction within the circuits! This is why cutting out the tumor does not cure cancer). Joint swelling, fatigue, neuritis, and depression all are common symptoms in people with Lyme. <u>As a matter of fact, the overgrowth of Lyme microbes is also a symptom!</u> None of these symptoms are the cause but are the result of the underlying incoherence within the body, mind, and spirit. We know this to be indisputably true. If you surgically remove the tumor, the body will generate a new tumor. If you take a pain medication, it will wear off. If you take antibiotics, the bacteria will mutate.

Symptoms are good for alerting us that something is wrong. Symptoms also provide us with a way to learn what not to do that creates pain. Symptoms can also be a way to track your progress while under a treatment program. If you come to Hansa Center, we want to see your symptoms going away, since those are what brought you to us in the first place. However our methods do not work to suppress symptoms.

Doctors specializing in Biological Medicine are trained NOT to treat symptoms. The symptoms will improve, sometimes remarkably fast, when the cause has been addressed.

I can guarantee you that you never have a headache due to a deficiency in Tylenol or aspirin. Taking Tylenol treats the symptoms but does nothing to correct the underlying cause of the headache. You may not feel the pain anymore, but whatever was causing the pain will continue to grow bigger and worse, and eventually the pain medicine will no longer work. Now you are faced with the question of finding a stronger pain medicine or finding a doctor specializing in

Biological Medicine who can finally address the cause. You must trust that the symptoms will go away as the result of your healthcare team facilitating the body's ability healing itself.

A simple blister on your foot may arise from wearing a new pair of shoes. I can "cure" you by convincing you not to wear those shoes. I removed the cause. The blister should not get worse unless you aggravate it while it is healing. No doctor can heal that blister. It will just take time, usually about four weeks for the body to completely heal the skin so that you can't see where it was. In the same way, all healing takes time to be fully manifested. Be patient with your body; the older it is, the longer it may take. And be patient with your team of healthcare professionals, it is not a precise science yet.

The Role of Muscles in Circuit Healing

The muscles are the most obvious way to detect circuit problems. All muscles are controlled electromagnetically. We know this from observing Multiple Sclerosis (MS) and Lou Gherig's Disease (ALS), which damage the electrical pathways, nerves, much like cutting the power cord to your T.V.

No muscle will work without electricity. Muscle problems are very common in Lyme patients. When a circuit in the body is "blown" for whatever reason (problems in the teeth, organ, joint, gland, muscle), the muscle will immediately weaken and stay weak until the cause is addressed. For example, if a tooth is rotten and leaking toxic waste into the circuit, the entire circuit will "blow," reducing the available energy to 40% of normal. When this happens, the muscle will weaken, everytime, and due to its decreased energy, it will also begin to cool in temperature. It will begin to stiffen since it is weak and cold. As it stiffens, it develops a hard knot in its core that is tender to touch. This hardened core is called a trigger point.

The existence of many trigger points is what conventional doctors use to diagnose Fibromyalgia Syndrome (FS). These trigger points are a symptom of multiple organ circuits that are chronically blown. (See also chapters on Lyme and Low Body Temperature for more specifics concerning trigger points and fibromyalgia)

Muscles serve two primary purposes in the body. They move bones, and they move fluids through the body. The joints must have proper muscle control in order for the joint to function without pain. Muscles also provide a pumping mechanism to move toxins out of the tissues and to move nutrients into the tissues.

If there are new or old injuries in the muscles, the effect on the other tissues on the circuit can still be harmful.

Doctors specializing in Biological Medicine are trained to use muscles in testing the integrity of the various organ circuits.

Muscles may need to be addressed directly through the use of myofascial release techniques, Therapeutic Massage, nutritional and homeopathic remedies, essential oils and exercises. However, the muscles reflect the integrity of the entire circuit, so they may not fully release until the rest of the circuit is repaired.

Any healing protocol for chronic Lyme sufferers must recognize the full scope of potential problems in the organ circuits.

The Role of Glands in Circuit Healing

Glands produce hormones. Hormones are chemical messengers to specific organs, which trigger an organ to perform a certain function.

In circuit healing, any time a circuit is "blown," the gland on that circuit will be affected along with each tissue on that circuit (i.e., organ, gland, joint, muscle, tooth).

To say that there is an imbalance in the hormones simply means that there is imbalance in that gland's electrical circuit. Hormones normally are produced or are not produced as dictated by the demands of the body. There are really many types of hormones. Most people are only familiar with estrogen, progesterone, and testosterone because doctors often supplement with those.

Doctors specializing in Biological Medicine are trained to recognize that glands will respond correctly when the circuits have been corrected. Since glands produce hormones that regulate the proper functioning of organs, one can see why this area of the circuits cannot be left out of a successful treatment protocol.

Glands and their hormones can be affected by outside influences, especially the estrogens, which are truly a class of many chemicals with "estrogenic" actions. For example, most petroleum-based cosmetics, shampoos, and personal care products have estrogenic actions on the body. This means that the chemicals from your personal care products are "turning on" or "turning off" the function of some of your estrogen-receptive organs. This normally should only happen when the glands are directed to produce estrogen by the brain.

Your healthcare team will instruct you in ways to avoid substances that may interfere with the glands of the body. After all, how can we get the organs turned back on electrically if the glands are turning them off because of chemical interferences?

[56] Stedman's Medical Dictionary, 27th Edition. accessed October 2007.
[57] Rau T, *Advanced Biological Medicine Training Seminar, Marion Massachusetts*. May 11-13, 2001
[58] Hansen R, The Key to Ultimate Health (Second Edition) Writerservice Pubns (2000)

8

~

Illuminated Physiology and the Medical Uses of Light

The Science and Application of BioResonance Scanning™ and Neurophotonic Therapy™

[This chapter was first published in the peer-reviewed scientific journal *Subtle Energies and Energy Medicine*, Vol. 16, Number 3, Sept. 2006. Written by David A. Jernigan, D.C. and Samantha Joseph, D.C.]

In order to fully appreciate the diagnostic and treatment aspects of light, one must first understand some of the physiology of the light metabolism in the body.

Photons, the energy packets of light, function as a particle or as a wave. The colors that we perceive are simply photons of varying wavelengths. In other words, there are no color pigments in light. Even though a bull is colorblind, the wavelength of what our human brains register as the red color of the bullfighter's cape will still travel through the bull's eyes and through the bull's body to stimulate his adrenal glands, making him angry and charge.

There are two primary functions of the eye. One is to translate light into patterns of electrochemical impulses that are transmitted to the brain. The other function of the eye is to provide an entry point for light to access the crystalline matrix or "fiber optic" network of the body. This light metabolism provides light/photons as stimulatory nutrients and informational packets to every aspect of the body, mind, and spirit.

Based upon our clinical observations, we theorize that light gains access to the crystalline matrix, and ultimately the entire organism, via the eyes, by diverting from the rods and cones into the Müller cells that lie in close proximity. The Müller cells provide direct contact with the living matrix, reaching every aspect of the organism.[59,60] It is this fiber optic-like network, otherwise known as the body's crystalline matrix, upon which we will be focusing. [61, 62, 63]

Research has determined that all living tissues, whether the body's tissues or the molecular structure of microbes, are made up of these unique molecular liquid crystalline structures.[64] These living, pliable, crystalline structures are capable of creating, transmitting and receiving laser-like bio-photons (energy packets of light, generated by the tissues of the body) to communicate between tissues and molecules.[65] While the macroscopic aspects of tissue coherence is discussed herein, it must be understood that non-classical, and non-linear quantum coherence of biophoton transmission through the organism is also relevant.[66] You may think of these two mechanisms, the liquid crystalline matrix and the quantum coherence fields of biophoton transmission, as carrying the bulk of information throughout the body. These biophotons interact with every aspect of the electromagnetic spectrum and travel through the body via the crystalline matrix, seeming to also stimulate spatial optical solitons, which appear to transfer information via quantum coherence fields. (A spatial optical soliton is an extremely stable, solitary, self-guided light wave that transfers a large amount of information in nonlinear media, with a constant velocity and without loss or dispersion of energy or information.)

The fascinating field of nonlinear optics suggests that spatial optical solitons may also derive its movement through the body via a mechanism identified by Fritz-Albert Popp called biophoton sucking.[67,68,69] It is our suggestion that biophotonic sucking is facilitated by electromagnetic-polarization by the collective deoxyribonucleic acid (DNA). DNA is well recognized as an ideal agent in functioning as optical waveguides to facilitate the redirection or distribution of optical information.[70] On the macro-scale the regulation of the electromagnetic-inducing attributes of DNA may be derived from the strongest electromagnetic generator in the body, the heart.[71,72] Compelling research by Rollin McCraty and others documents experimental evidence showing that when our thoughts are held in "heart-focused intention," the coherent electromagnetic and biophotonic emissions of the heart change the conformation of DNA.[73] In other words, what we hold to be true in our heart of hearts creates our reality.

The existence of light within the body is a relatively foreign concept in science and medicine. Many scientists and doctors feel that the use of light-based treatments toward healing is too esoteric. This dissertation by no means covers the wide range of scientific research that has been published in this field. These authors desire to bring well-deserved recognition to the potential of the ongoing research advancing the interpretation of the information encoded in the biophotonic emissions of the body. This promises to advance our knowledge of healing, and indeed life itself, more than the cracking of the human genome since it is potentially the coherent light of the body that regulates genetic expression. [74] As far back as 1976, as well as in more recent validation, research traced the occurrence of tumors back to a definite loss of coherence of the biophoton field.[75,76,77]

The importance of restoring the optimal coherence of light metabolism and the crystalline matrix pathways is that they connect every aspect of the human being to its internal and external environment. On the physical and quantum scale, light enables the body to continually adapt to changes in the environment within and around the body. One doesn't realize it most of the time, but our bodies must constantly adapt to everything that is vibrating around us – the lights in the room, the computer, the music playing in the background, the person or people in the vicinity, the alignment of the planets, whether or not there is a full moon or new moon. Everything vibrates in and around us. There are 60 trillion cells in the human body, all of which must communicate at the speed of light in order to maintain the integrity of the organism.

Imagine the body is constantly morphing or changing shape, literally at the speed of light. The body is changing in reaction to each thought one thinks, the medicines consumed, foods eaten, and in reaction to each and every change in one's internal and external environment—even in reaction to what is held in the heart as truth!

In fact, the body's ability to adapt and transmit information is clocked at less than a hundred-trillionth of a second. To put this speed into perspective, if each trillionth of a second contained the equivalent knowledge gained in one whole second, that second would represent the accumulated knowledge gained over the course of 32 million years! The first law of thermodynamics states that energy can neither be created nor destroyed. It is our belief that each of us has access to the neurophotonic information imprinted in the light energy field which is flowing through the crystalline matrix containing all of the experiences and knowledge of the universe from the beginning of time. This includes the information streaming from the quantum reality of no time, space, or distance. This may explain the hundredth monkey phenomenon[78] and the streaming of extra-sensory knowledge.

The universe may indeed be a progressive learning light hologram.[79] Knowledge may be gained or simply brought to the forefront from the universal hologram, but just as the law of thermodynamics states that energy can never be destroyed, so too no knowledge can be destroyed. The illumination experienced during transfiguration to other dimensions indicates that light is the medium that carries forward in the hologram of all dimensions.

It is the authors' belief that a person's thoughts cause the mind to set up a morphogenetic field, which in turn fuels bio-holographic (coherent light) projections in the heart. These projections use biophotonic (laser-like) coherent emissions to transmit information and control inputs to the DNA, and from the DNA to the entire crystalline matrix to support the thought command. We propose the theory that heart-generated light traveling through the liquid crystalline matrix "optical fibers" of the body can produce "supercontinuum light," thereby maintaining its coherence and resulting in the multi-system-wide effects seen when one biophotonic emission frequency from the heart is sent though the body's crystalline matrix. (Supercontinuum light is coherent light traveling through special optical fibers that can produce or split into multicolored light, enabling light to carry greater amounts of information without loss of coherence or loss of information.) The DNA molecules are known to be photo-receivers and photo-transmitters, and it may be that DNA is where the coherent signal is split into supercontinuum light to produce the "super-bio-hologram" that is the human body.[80] It would seem that thoughts are commands to the heart. The heart then photonically imprints the myriad of DNA throughout the body with the information to make the thought command come true. Thoughts enable the heart to process the sensory information taken in from your environment in order to holographically adapt correctly to environmental changes. Inharmonious thought processing (negative thinking) concerning one's perception of reality or of the internal or external environment may create distortions in the bio-hologram, ultimately resulting in manifest dysfunction in body, mind, and spirit.

The elaborate structure of DNA and its surrounding network of clustered water filaments facilitate the structuring and regulating activity of a coherent field operating within every living thing.[81] DNA emits about 90% of the cellular light (biophotons) and acts as a photonic transmitter, receiver, and storage mechanism for biophotonic or other electromagnetic information.[82,83]

Following Light through the Liquid Crystalline Pathways in the Body

Now with the understanding that the body is a liquid crystalline matrix, the following will review the action of light within the body. "Liquid crystals reflect different wavelengths of light depending on the orientation of its molecules".[84] Based upon this science, we see that when we drive photons of specific frequencies (colors) via the eyes into any molecular structure, be it the liver, heart, or lungs, the tissue will reflect back through the body's crystalline pathways the color frequency unique to its molecular structure.[85,86,87] By this definition of liquid crystals from the mainstream encyclopedia, the liquid crystals of the heart will *conduct* and *reflect* different wavelengths of light (green and red respectively) than the liquid crystals of the liver (yellow and violet). To follow this concept further, if the liquid crystal pathways of the heart are blocked or encounter interference, the stimulation with frequencies of green will result either in no reflection of red (indicating that no stimulation of the tissue is occurring), or some other color frequency may result due to corruption of the crystalline pathways.

The correct structural and energetic alignment, as well as the orientation of the molecules making up the body's crystalline matrix, dictates the integrity of the entire organism. Structural and energetic interferences to the integrity of the matrix are the ultimate source of disease. These interferences include, but are not limited to, scars and surgical interventions, toxins, structural misalignments, inharmonious thoughts, the cellular memory of physical, emotional, and spiritual traumas, and damaged meridians. The alignment and normal functioning of the crystalline matrix also depends upon the temperature of the tissue, so it is important to maintain the optimum core body temperature.[88]

Interferences in the crystalline matrix pathways block the excitation of the end-organ's molecular structure by incoming "colored" light, thereby disrupting the optimal function and regulation of the entire organism. According to Mae Wan Ho, PhD, in her enlightening book, *The Rainbow and the Worm*, any interference in the light metabolism of an organism is going to have local and global effects.

Laser light is called "coherent light photons." Interestingly, the heart and DNA are also said to be transmitting coherent light.[89,90] The really awesome realization of this is that we know lasers, or "coherent light," can rapidly carry a great deal of information and travel long distances without losing signal strength.

For years, maverick physiologists have stated that the ion-transfer mechanism of nerve impulses in the human body are way too slow to account for the huge amount of information transfer that is going on in the body. Desktop computers operate much faster than nerve impulses, yet these computers still cannot compute as fast as humans. It seems that the human physiology and neurology textbooks need to be revised. What was formerly credited with running the body (the central and peripheral nervous system) is just another cog in the wheel, with the crystalline fiber optics network carrying the bulk of the information and maintaining the integrity of the human organism.

The fiber optic networks that are used in the United States for communication purposes can carry "up to three trillion bits of information per second. At that rate, downloading the entire contents of the Library of Congress (over 20 million books), a feat requiring 82 years with a dial-up electronic modem, would take just 48 seconds for a fiber optic modem" (Microsoft® Encarta® Encyclopedia 2003). Interestingly, a single hair-thin fiber optic thread can transmit millions of telephone calls at a time.

Diagnostic Ability of Light

Through the realizations of the crystalline matrix and photonic aspects summarized above, Dr. Jernigan developed a technique that enables the healthcare professional to adjunctively diagnose biophotonic interferences and dynamically treat patient dysfunction with the purpose of restoring optimal coherence of the body, mind, and spirit. This new photonic technique is called Bio-Resonance Scanning™ (BRS). BRS is possibly the first functional method of decoding the information within biophoton emissions. The following is an effort to explain the science which has been extrapolated from the clinical application of BRS.

The ultimate purpose of BRS is to identify specific frequencies of incoherence, from any source, in the tissue (pathology) and identify the corrective remedy or modality that will ultimately restore global coherence in the patient.[91]

An important point is that BRS utilizes a novel understanding of testing the body that does not rely on measuring the body's reactions to frequencies, as in electro-dermal screening devices (a problem since the more degenerative the condition, the less reliable the reactivity of the organism), nor does it rely on meridian testing. Unlike the many computer dermal testing devices which essentially challenge the patient's body with a rapid fire of single frequencies of pathologies, BRS can be used in frequency-sentences to obtain very specific information about the body. An example of a frequency sentence would be to essentially form the following question, "Of all of the different organs and glands that are malfunctioning in any way at any time of the night or day and in any neurological posture, which organ or gland is the worst?"

In cooperation with the inventor and developer of one of the leading electro-dermal screening (EDS) devices, Dr. Jernigan performed an unpublished trial running BRS against the EDS device of that time (1997). BRS performed approximately 22 times faster in determining its findings than the EDS test did. The EDS system required 45 minutes to complete the assessment of the patient and identify the corrective remedies to balance the meridians. BRS required only 2 ½ minutes to achieve the same results which were then verified by the EDS system. The EDS devices are based upon assessment of the body via acupuncture meridians, while BRS evaluates the entire organism globally by performing a dynamic analysis in real-time. Regarding objectivity, in another unpublished research study (Jernigan, Smith, Jernigan, 1997), a tissue slide of breast cancer was placed upon the belly of a patient and the EDS device was unable to detect the pathology. The body was not reacting strongly enough to the frequency emitted by the molecular structure embedded within the tissue sample on the slide. This same slide was hidden by the patient on the body and, using BRS, was correctly and rapidly identified independently by three doctors. Upon review of patient records, additional in-house statistics reveal that BRS diagnostic findings for specific pathologies were confirmed with an 86% accuracy when substatiated by blood tests, x-rays, and MRI's.

BRS utilizes various biological Global Access Points™ (GAPs) to transmit and receive information from remote parts of the body at one access point. BRS can, however, also access localized information from any non-GAP point of the body. It may help to view GAPs with the following example. The administrator of a corporation accesses the mainframe computer through many different terminals connected to all of the centralized information in the mainframe (GAP), while a secretary's access privileges only allow her to view information pertinent to her job (local).

It is these authors' opinion that BRS transmits photoelectrical wavelengths created by the neurophotonic emissions of the doctor's handmodes and thoughts. Handmodes are specific positions made with the physician's fingers. When movement and tension are set up in the tissues, as when the fingers are bent in certain positions, the tension on the fabric or matrix changes the length of the molecular antennae of the myofascial system, and thereby sets up different resonant frequencies.[92]

Another mechanism for generating the handmode frequency is the central nervous system impulse—thought to create and transmit photo-electrical frequencies from the doctor's hand.[93] In these ways, handmodes (frequencies) are capable of harmonically entraining the frequency of a specific pathogen.

The pathogen, whether virus, bacteria, or cancer pathology, has a specific photoelectric frequency signature, based upon its photonic information and molecular structure.

The handmode frequency is believed to be electro-photonically transmitted from the doctor's hand into the patient's body crystalline matrix via the thousands of photoelectrical receptors in the skin.[94] Energy fields held over the skin can have profound biological effects, especially when held over certain active regions of the skin - GAPs.[95] Although GAPs enable the doctor to access total body (global) information from key points on the body, localized and associated information can be accessed from anywhere on the body.[96]

GAPs therefore enable the doctor to identify problems distant to the point of testing.

The most commonly used GAPs are located in four general locations:

    1. Forehead, above and between the brows,

    2. External occipital protuberance (EOP),

3. Anterior heart,
4. Umbilicus.

The crystalline matrix of the patient's body carries or enables the handmode frequency to specifically resonate with the frequency of the pathology in the body and back to a device called a Resonator, the actual photo-electrical-resonance detector.[97, 98, 99]

The Resonator is a belt-worn device with a synthetic polymer membrane. When the Resonator membrane is rubbed by the doctor, an electromagnetic friction occurs as the surface tension of the membrane changes in reaction to the photo-electro-luminescent reflection or radiant transmission from the pathology or pathogen within the patient. This increased surface tension on the Resonator is similar to the *psauoscopy* defined in Dorland's Medical dictionary as "A method of physical examination where the observation of increased friction is experienced when one lightly rubs a finger pad back and forth on the skin over an area of pathology. The finger seems to encounter greater resistance and the skin seems more tense and less supple."[100]

Upon the specific handmode's frequency interaction with the target pathology's molecular frequency, an optical and electrical property (absorption, fluorescence, reflectance, refractive index, etc.) of the pathology's molecular structure undergoes a measurable change. In this way, the modified patho-photo-electrical frequency is guided back through the patient's body crystalline matrix and travels through the body's bioluminescent fields (which have been scientifically documented to surround the body) to the Resonator.

The Resonator membrane is made of a special photo-electrically sensitive, synthetic material. The pathology signal is amplified by the resonator through altering the membrane's surface tension, creating an electromagnetic friction on the membrane that is detectable when the doctor rubs the membrane.

The appropriate forming of the handmode allows the physician to carry out, in real time, specific tests of the target chemical substances. (Deleted reference #14) Diagnostically, BRS enables the physician to create bio-photoelectrical frequencies from the physician's own body to challenge, in real time, the patient's body for an exact frequency match to standardized or otherwise known pathological specimen frequencies. These frequencies are matched either to actual microbes in suspension, or to microbial or tissue pathology frequencies imprinted in vials expressly for the purpose of adjunctive diagnostic techniques.

From a treatment perspective, and as discussed earlier, BRS enables the doctor to sequence photo-electrical "sentences" of frequencies to determine more specific patient information. This type of formatting of frequencies enables one to determine not only the simple presence of pathology, but its degree of priority in the scheme of problems going on in a patient. From the format testing, the physician can determine issues such as the top ten worst organ or gland problems at any time of day or night and in any patient posture. This means that even if the patient's worst organ problem is their heart, and their heart only has problems at three in the morning and only when they lie on their right side, and the patient is in your office at noon, the physician would still be able to detect the three a.m. problem as the patient's worst problem and then proceed to use BRS to determine what exact medicine or treatment is needed to correct the heart problem, be it a structural, chemical, stress-related, electrical, or photonic etiology or correction.

Our theory is that the frequency of the hand mode, and the frequency test pathology, and the frequency of the remedy, are all very close to the same frequency—now perhaps simply reversible—matching the pathology's reverse photonic emission.[101]

Aligning the Crystalline Matrix Pathways with NeuroPhotonic Therapy™

It is amazing that we can facilitate the healing of anyone when we consider the incredible range of things that can cause dysfunction in the body. Regardless of what a doctor calls an illness, in the end it must come down to this: how are we going to restore the integrity of the person as a whole? Forcing the body into drug-induced illusions of health with pharmaceuticals must be relegated to medical museums. Even natural medicine often follows an errant, allopathic mentality, targeting this or that microbe or toxin with the hopes that its eradication will enable the body, mind and spirit to be restored.

The problem has always been how to assess and treat the body as one completely integrated organism, as opposed to the "pieces and parts" reductionist mentality of our training. Through the sequencing of BRS, it is relatively simple to restore the integrity within all of the "organ circuits" of the body. Assessment using electro-dermal scans and kinesiology would at this point reveal "perfect balance" in the body; however, the authors realized that however wonderful and healing this restoration of the organ circuits, it was just balancing the body to the environment of the lighting in the treatment room. After years of practicing in this manner, and enjoying above average success, we realized that if we challenged the newly "balanced" patient with high intensity light of a specific color in their eyes, the entire organism would be thrown into chaos. The challenge of a specific color caused a cascade of biochemical and bioenergetic disturbances, identified via BRS, which affected the organism locally and globally. Every muscle that could be challenged would become weak. The entirety of the patient was shifted adversely by their inability to efficiently process light through the liquid crystalline matrix. To date, the authors have never found anyone who could process light correctly.

This led Dr. Jernigan to develop the treatment technique now called NeuroPhotonic Therapy™ (NPT). Essentially, NPT uses special, variable intensity glasses to challenge the crystalline matrix pathways. Then, using BRS, one can identify the blockages and problems in the matrix and provide the corrective information (using many different frequency treatments, i.e. homeopathy, Solfeggio tuning forks, essential oils, frequency modulated cold-laser, EM field therapy, etc., as determined by BRS) and treatment that results in progressively and near-instantaneous realignment and correction of the pathways. We postulate that the traveling of light through the matrix pathways may be seen as what is known as spatial optical solitons, as discussed in the emerging field of nonlinear optics.

Interestingly, once the pathway's integrity is restored, the previously irritating color will test via BRS as now "highly beneficial" or a "primary" treatment to the body. It is as if the tissues with the greatest affinity to the color used were starved for this frequency stimulation!

By challenging multiple colors and combinations of colors, true restoration of the integrity of the organism as a whole can be achieved. The restoration of the organism's optimal coherence can be monitored and verified by EDS, BRS, applied/clinical kinesiological tests, and in patient subjective improvements. It is likely that as we improve the alignment of the liquid crystalline matrix pathways, there will be increased coherence and the body's fields will get stronger. The key to long-term health and healing is in maintaining the optimal coherence of the body, mind, and spirit over the course of a long enough time frame for the organisms to process through all of the corrective inputs of the treatments. The end result is accelerated healing of the body, mind and spirit, since all three of these are interconnected as part of the one organism.

The reality, it would seem, is that whether a person looks at a red cardinal or a red dress, if they cannot process that color through the crystalline matrix of their body correctly, it will cause global problems. The intensity of the light may dictate the degree of disturbance.

In the quest for ever-greater spiritual enlightenment, we must recognize that the spirit will be hampered in its ability to transcend by incoherence in the body and mind. Bio-Resonance Scanning™ and NeuroPhotonic Therapy™ are appropriately "light-based" technologies that may lead the world closer to a truly holistic approach to facilitating healing and transcendence.

Clinical Example (Names changed to preserve anonymity)

Although an accomplished gymnast as a younger woman, 45-year-old Jennifer Doe's health and vitality took a dramatic turn for the worse. As a young mother of three, she was smitten by Lyme Disease, a bacterial infection transmitted most often by ticks, mosquitoes and other blood-sucking insects. Lyme Disease had stolen years from her life—at its worst, she was wheelchair bound and unable to hold her head upright. MRIs of the brain indicated a brain infarct, perhaps a result of contracting Lyme Disease. Literally, part of the brain was dead. Antibiotic treatments were fruitless in their simplistic and oft-hailed approach to treatment of the disease.

It became obvious to the Does that disease-focused treatments were not winning this battle with Lyme, and what they needed was health-restoration treatments which sought to reinstate the integrity of the body, thereby allowing the body's natural state of homeostasis to return. The Does had an innate sense that the quality of life they sought lay in a more nontoxic and natural approach to healing that worked with the inherent design of the body. After reading Dr. Jernigan's book, *Beating Lyme Disease*, the Does traveled to our clinic, Hansa Center for Optimum Health, in Wichita, Kansas, to pursue restoring their own health and to re-establish a state of balance between body, mind and spirit.

Periodic treatments over six years at Hansa Center enabled the conclusion of the nightmarish wheelchair days, and although there had been many return trips to the clinic in Kansas, which always made her feel better, there was still something fundamental that was not being addressed.

Jennifer felt as if every tissue of her body was on edge, she awakened as many as 20 times every night, and her need for sunlight was becoming peculiar to everyone close to her. Using Bio-Resonance Scanning™, our testing kept revealing that she was in a state of balance while being exposed to different light stimuli. Even though she was no longer in a wheelchair, working full-time, and avidly participating in family life once again, we knew there was no way that Jennifer's body could be processing light 100% correctly. We were not quite asking the correct question (with BRS) to assist her body in processing the light correctly. A vital key was missing to assist her on her full path back to health and wholeness, and perhaps on another return visit, we (both doctors working together) could solve the problem. This knowingness kept prompting us to use BRS in new and more advanced ways to locate the primary underlying dysfunction.

On a return visit, we brought Jennifer and her husband into the treatment room to experience BRS and a new treatment technique, combined in a creative new way, using light. Dr. Jernigan had just developed the technique and called it NeuroPhotonic Therapy (NPT). The Does flew in from out-of-state for the treatment, so we assured them that this was not the same old color therapy they had done before. This had actually been used to restore strength in the muscles of a stroke victim, stop brain seizures, correct chronic ligamentous laxity, improve cognition, and so much more, often in one treatment. The theory is that photons of a specific frequency and wavelength would be registered as a specific color, such as red, by the classic visual mechanisms of the eye and brain, but some of the photons would travel through the body's liquid crystalline matrix, much like light passing through fiber optic cables. Every tissue in the body is indeed a part of an intricate web of interconnecting liquid crystalline pathways. We can send the photons into the body and use our BRS technique to monitor any problems they may cause in the body. If the photons reach all of their correct destinations without interference, then we will not detect any abnormal frequencies. If the photons are not able to flow undisturbed throughout one's body, we will see local and global frequency disturbances on all levels of the organism.

The NeuroPhotonic Therapy apparatus was placed over Jennifer's eyes. We were supremely confident we would find Jennifer's body greatly aggravated by the photon stimulation. No one we had ever tested showed light processing correctly, not even apparently-healthy young children who were born without drugs and had never been exposed to any conventional medicines. We also knew that even with all of the improvements we had facilitated in Jennifer over the years, there was still something missing…something everyone had missed! To our amazement, the application of NPT (high-intensity frequency light stimulation) resulted in no detectable aggravation to Jennifer's body.

Dr. Joseph empathically sensed that there was an energetic blockage at the vertex of Jennifer's cranium. Subsequent testing with Bio-Resonance Scanning at this location showed several energetic blockages. The energetic blockages were apparently impeding the ability to correctly test her for light coherence within her structure. Once the blockages were cleared, her entire body began to short-circuit, revealing the underlying light metabolism disturbances.

Over the next two hours, high-intensity photons of varying frequencies were sent into the body, each of which set off unique aggravations. Bio-Resonance Scanning enabled the rapid identification of corrective therapies (homeopathic sarcodes, essential oils, solfeggio tuning forks, bioenergetics, and low-level Erchonia® laser therapy frequencies) that would realign the liquid crystalline pathways. A fascinating finding is that while many modalities were necessary to align the pathways, each correction was made with a single application, the results of which were immediately obvious physically and virtually instantaneous.

To support the movement of light through the body, we introduced anthocyanidins, plant-based pigments obtained from appropriately harvested and prepared fruits and vegetables. The body uses these pigments to correctly process and conduct light through the crystalline matrix.

With the correction of each neurophotonic aggravation, Jennifer reported feeling an increasing sense of calmness settling into her being. She was fascinated and slightly frightened by the fact that every photonic stimulation (color) would initially throw her body into a mass of quaking and quivering nerves and muscles; however, when corrected, the same color would be like food to a starved body, bringing strength and integrity to her system. Many times it would take half an hour for her body to get "filled" with the color it had been blocked from receiving for so many years. Witnessing the intensity of her initial reactions to the light stimulus may have intimidated others; however, now that the problem was finally revealed, BRS and NPT rapidly restored integrity.

During the treatment, we discussed the importance of light and how it is processed in the body. Jennifer and her husband began to relate stories of how Jennifer would continually search out sunlight. Being one of the top executives at the corporation in which she worked, she had been able to choose the office space she wanted. She was drawn to choose the sunniest office in the building, though unable to say why at the time. She had strategically positioned her desk to get maximum exposure to the sun as it traveled across the sky.

Considering that her fair skin and red hair predisposed her to freckles rather than the classic Hawaiian Tropic tan, Jennifer had an unreasonable need for daily sunlight on her skin. When faced with the option to eat lunch or run home to sunbathe, depending upon how much sun she had been exposed to that day, she would often opt for the later. "I sometimes get frustrated with her unreasonable need to sunbathe," complained her husband. "We can be on vacation with the family, and everybody will be ready to go do something, but she will have to stop and sunbathe before we go anywhere."

Jennifer's home reflected the success that comes from intelligence and hard work. It was one of the largest homes in the city, but its square footage was not its most distinguishing feature. Anyone entering the home was accosted with a sensory overload of brilliant fluorescent colors throughout. It was apparent that this was the home of a "light and color junkie!"

When they built their house, Jennifer and her husband had worked with the architect to design a floor plan for the house that would facilitate the complete saturation of natural light. By design, the home was striking in its openness. No walls would block light from reaching the furthest corner. Many picture windows and roof-mounted sun-tunnels had been strategically positioned to allow sunlight to flood into the home and bounce off the fluorescent greens, pinks, and blues, filling the rooms with an ethereal glow. The rooms were alive with the vibrations of photons of varying light frequencies bombarding the body of anyone in the space. It seemed that Jennifer's entire life revolved, like the planet earth, around the sun.

It appears that the body uses light as a stimulatory nutrient. Light is the glue that holds all of the atomic particles and molecules together. The eyes are the primary photoreceptors and most crystalline structure in the body, providing the most direct pathway for light to flow into the body's organ circuits. It would seem that due to the brain infarct, the only light Jennifer's body could receive was the small amount of light it could get from the secondary and less crystalline photoreceptors of her skin. She was literally starving for light. This is likely why she had been craving sunlight for so long. This is also likely why she picked scintillating colors to paint the inside of her house. Her body needed intense color stimulation on the skin to feed the tissues through light's photoelectrical and photochemical cascades. Future contact with Jennifer proved to be positive – she now sleeps through the night, has decreased in compulsive sun cravings, and is maintaining an overall sense of wellbeing with strength and vitality she has never known before.

---

[59] Atema, J. 1973, 'Microtubule theory of sensory transduction', *Journal of Theoretical Biology*, vol. 38, pp. 181-190.

[60] Pankratov, S. Meridians conduct light, *Raum und Zeit*, vol. 35 (1991), pp. 16-18.

[61] Kim B. 1963 On the kyungrak system. J Acad Medi Sci 10:1-41.

[62] Pankratov, S. pp 16-18.

[63] Johng H, Yoo J, Shin H, et al. Use of magnetic nanoparticles to visualize threadlike structures inside lymphatic vessels in rats. eCAM Original Article, Biomedical Physics Laboratory, Seoul National University (Seoul, Korea 2006).

[64] Oschman J L, *Energy Medicine; The Scientific Basis*, (Churchill Livingstone, New York, NY 128-131 2000).

[65] Ho M. *The Rainbow and the Worm: The Physics of Organisms* (World Scientific Publishing Co., River Edge, NJ 2003).

[66] Bajpai R. 2003 Preface to the International Institute of Biophysics, Symposium on Biophoton, *Indian Journal of Experimental Biology* vol. 41.

[67] Popp FA, Chang JJ, Photon sucking and the basis of biological organization. Intern. Inst. Biophysics (2001).

[68] Frohlich: Long range coherence and energy storage in biological systems. Int. J. Chem. 2:641-649 (1968).

[69] Popp FA, Nagl W. A physical (electromagnetic) model of differentiation. Cytobios 37:71-83 (1983).

[70] Grote J, Heckman E, Hagen J et al. Deoxyribonucleic acid (DNA)-based optical materials. Optical Materials in Defense Systems Technology, SPIE vol. 5621, pp. 16-22 (2004)

[71] McCraty R. The energetic heart: Bioelectromagnetic interaction within and between people. Boulder Creek, CA: HeartMath Research Center, Institute of HeartMath, Publication N. 03-016 (2003).

[72] Cohen D Magnetoencephalography: detection of the brain's electrical activity with a superconducting magnetometer. *Science* 175:664-666 (1972).

[73] McCraty R, Atkinson M, Tomasino D, Modulation of DNA conformation by heart-focused intention. Boulder Creek, CA: HeartMath Research Center, Institute of HeartMath, Publication N. 03-016 (2003).

[74] Popp, A. About the Coherence of Biophotons. Macroscopic Quantum Coherence, Proceedings of an International Conference. Boston Univ. , pp 1-5 World Scientific (1999).

[75] Popp FA, Molecular Aspects of Carcinogenesis. Thieme Verlag, Stuttgart, Germany pp. 47-55 (1976).

[76] Popp FA, Ruth B, Bahr W, et al. Emission of visible and ultraviolet radiation by active biological systems. *Collective Phenomena* vol. 3, pp. 187-214 (1981).

[77] Ho Maewan, The Rainbow and the Worm; The Physics of Organisms 2nd ed. World Scientific, New Jersey (1998) p. 163.

[78] Sheldrake R, *A New Science Life*. Los Angeles: J.P. Tarcher (1981).

[79] Bohm D. Wholeness and in Implicate Order. London: Routledge & Kegan Paul (1980).

[80] W, Popp F A, Warnke U (eds) Bioelectrodynamics and biocommunication. World Scientific, Singapore, ch 3, pp 81-107
[81] Oschman 128-31.
[82] Bischof M. *Biophotons: The Light in Our Cells*, (Neuss, Germany 1995).
[83] Horowitz L G, *DNA; Pirates of the Sacred Spiral*, (Tetrahedron, Sandpoint ID 2004).
[84] Microsoft Encarta Encyclopedia, 2003.
[85] Frohlich H. Long-range coherence and energy storage in biological systems. Int. J. Quantum Chem. 2: 641-649 (1968).
[86] Wijk R, Aken J, Photon emission in tumor biology, Cellular and Molecular Life Sciences, Birkhauser Basel, Utrect, Netherlands (1992).
[87] Chang J, Yu W, Sun T, Popp FA, Spontaneous and light-induced photon emission from intact brains of chick embryos, *Science in China* (Series C) 40(1): 44-51 (1997).
[88] Jernigan, D. *Beating Lyme Disease* (Somerleyton Press, Wichita KS 2004).
[89] Rattemeyer M, Popp FA, Nagl W. Evidence of photon emission from DNA in living systems. *Naturwissenschaften* 68:572 (1981).
[90] Rein G, McCraty R. Modulation of DNA by coherent heart frequencies. *Proc. 3rd Annual Conf. of the Intern. Soc. Study Subtle Energies & Energy Medicine*, Monterey, CA. (1993).
[91] Fröhlich H. Coherent electric vibrations in biological systems and the cancer problem. *IEEE Transactions on Microwave Theory and Techniques* MTT 26: 613-617 (1978).
[92] Oschman 128-131.
[93] Horowitz.
[94] Pankratov 16-18.
[95] Andreev E, Beloy M., Sitko S. The manifestation of natural characteristic frequencies of the organism of man. Reports to the Academy of Sciences of the Ukrainian SSR No. 10, Series b, *Geological Chemical and Biological Sciences*, pp 60-63 (1984).
[96] Smith C. Biological effects of weak electromagnetic fields. (1994).
[97] Callahan P. *Tuning into nature*, (Devin-Adair, Greenwich, CT 1975).
[98] Popp F A, Ruth B, Bahr W et al Emission of visible and ultraviolet radiation by active biological systems. Collective Phenomena 3:187-214 (1981).
[99] Popp F A, Li K H, Gu Q Recent advances in biophoton research. *World Scientific*, Singapore (1992).
[100] Dorland's Illustrated Medical Dictionary, WB Saunders, Copyright 2004.
[101] Slawinski J, Photon Emission from Perturbed and Dying Organisms: Biomedical Perspectives, Res. In Comp. Med. 12:90-95 (2005).

Section 2
Detoxification

9

~

Why Detoxify if I Have Lyme Disease?

Recall that earlier we discussed research indicating that the majority of symptoms in Lyme Disease are caused by the release of toxins by the spirochetes. And the Herxheimer reaction is a worsening of your symptoms due to the die-off of bacteria which break open, spilling their guts into your tissues. If that were not bad enough, your daily accumulation of toxins just from living, eating, and breathing is staggering! These toxins are jamming up the machinery of the cells, interfering with the regulation of the body. Toxins are a universal problem. There is virtually no one on the planet who does not need to detoxify the body on a continual basis. There is no one who should not be working to eliminate the sources of toxins in the home and life.

I hear frequently that doctors are telling their patients that it's great if they feel horrible while on antibiotics for Lyme Disease. Some believe that indicates good treatment. I think it's poor treatment. You suffer terribly because the doctor didn't bother to make sure your body was able to efficiently eliminate the die-off toxins. Detoxification of the body must be a part of any effective Lyme protocol, or one risks permanent damage to nerve and joint tissue from the toxic irritation.

Today more than 77,000 chemicals are in active production in this country. Our exposure to these chemicals is greater than at any time since the beginning of the Industrial Revolution. More than 3,000 chemicals are added to our food supply, and more than 10,000 chemicals in the form of solvents, emulsifiers, and preservatives are used in food processing and storage. Ethyl alcohol, isopropanol, wood rosin, shellac, propylene glycol, silicone, ammonium hydroxide... You're eating it for breakfast if you're eating grapefruit, melon and fresh oranges from the supermarket... Thiabendazole, mineral oil, methylparabin, dimethyl polysiloxane, benzimadazole... You're eating these for lunch if you had supermarket tomatoes, avocado, apples... Fungicides botran, 2-6 dichloro-4-nitroaniline, orthophenylphenol... Sound like a good balanced dinner? You're eating these yummy ingredients in sweet potatoes, onions, and limes from your local supermarket. Fungicides are put into wax to provide a longer shelf life; even peeling won't get rid of them, you eat them. They cause cancers, birth defects, damage to the immune system, and other diseases.

When ingested, these chemicals can remain in the body for years, altering our metabolism, causing enzyme dysfunction and nutritional deficiencies, creating hormonal imbalances and lowering our threshold of resistance to chronic disease.

Besides food borne chemicals, we are continually subjected to poor air quality, chemically contaminated water, household cleaners, paint fumes, pharmaceutical drugs, pesticides, heavy metals (including mercury) and the list goes on and on. Today, studies show that most of us have between 400 and 800 foreign chemical residues stored in the fat cells of our bodies. This occurs gradually over the course of our lives. These chemicals enter into the body either through the skin, lungs, or they are eaten. Most of the time, these chemicals are bio-accumulative, meaning miniscule amounts accumulating over the course of years. These chemicals and heavy metals make up the "total toxic burden." When the amount of toxins exceed the body's ability to excrete them, our body will begin to store these toxins. This bio-accumulation seriously compromises our physiological and psychological health and leads to chronic disease.

Environmental Protection Agency (EPA)

Since 1976 the EPA has been conducting studies to determine the presence of toxins in the fat cells of the body. This study is called the National Adipose Tissue Survey (NHATS). The results of this study are staggering. Across the United States, the EPA took samples of people's fat cells (adipose) and analyzed the samples for the presence of various toxins. In 98% of the samples they found many toxins, including benzene, PCBs, DDE (a metabolite of DDT pesticide), dioxins, toluene, and chlorobenzene, all of which are highly damaging to the immune system and compromise every tissue in the body. The EPA only looks for 100 out of the potential thousands of different toxins that could be present in the fatty tissue samples. Twenty different toxins were identified in over 75% of all the samples.

So, from this and other studies you can see that it is no so much a matter of "if" you have toxins in your body, rather how much! Remember that our goal is not to just get rid of Lyme spirochetes or your symptoms, but to remove anything that may be blocking your body's healing mechanisms. True health is not the absence of pain or symptoms, otherwise aspirin would be the ultimate longevity medicine.

Toxicity Symptoms

The following is a partial list of known symptoms often related to toxicity: allergies, acne, anxiety, burning skin, brain fog, chronic fatigue, chemical sensitivities, depression, eczema, frequent colds or flu, feeling "sick all over," insomnia, loss of dexterity, low body temperature, memory loss, mood swings, muscle and joint pains, and poor concentration. The list of potential toxicity symptoms for Lyme sufferers is the entire list of possible Lyme Disease symptoms since the symptoms are the result of the bacterial toxins.

As a result of this widespread environmental contamination, doctors are faced with increased rates of toxin-related cancers, neurological diseases, reduced immune function, allergies, and the newer diagnoses of multiple chemical sensitivities, chronic fatigue syndrome, and fibromyalgia. Doctors are finding their usual treatments are not as effective as in the past due to the presence of these many toxins in people.

Did you know that few people actually die of cancer? Authorities say that they actually die of toxemia, produced by an excessive buildup of toxins.

Did you know that you can not simply take supplements and laxatives to eliminate all of the toxins? You must be guided through a total body protocol to truly achieve detoxification. Consider the skin for a moment. Did you know that your skin is one of your largest organs of elimination? Your skin should be releasing two pounds of waste acids every day! Most people have spent their entire life blocking this process through lotions and powder and toxic antibacterial, deodorant soaps. So as you can see, two pounds of waste per day that is not being eliminated through the skin is going to add up and tax the body severely.

Toxins, Lymphatic Drainage, Elimination Organs, and the CRT Test

The CRT (Computerized Regulation Thermography) test is one of the most reliable methods of determining the degree of toxic load on the body. If your doctor conducted this test, he probably showed you areas of your body indicating toxins effecting proper organ thermal regulation on your CRT test. He most likely also found that your lymphatic system was blocked or otherwise demonstrating dysregulation of some form on the CRT. Problems in the lymph system are common when the body is toxic.

Everyone has experienced a swollen lymph node at some time in his or her life. A lymph node is part of a chain of nodes all over the body, which is an integral part of your immune system. Lymph channels that conduct lymph fluid, connect lymph nodes. Every lymph node has special immune cells, like little "pac-men" that swallow up, and help the body break down toxins, and microbes. Lymph fluid flows through the channels and gathers toxins from the tissue spaces between cells and in the tiny blood vessels called capillaries. The lymphatic system can be likened to an efficient plumbing system. When plumbing is clogged, then the bathroom gets a backlog of hazardous waste. As long as the lymphatic system is flowing freely through the body, it can filter out toxins. Once the lymphatic system is clogged, the liver, kidneys, skin, and lungs have to work much harder to keep the body clean. Eventually, these organs of elimination become fatigued and can no longer deal the toxins.

As people age or become less physically active, the flow of lymph is impaired. Sometimes the lymph nodes are blocked due to permanent scarring from repeated infections. Proteins begin to concentrate in the lymph vessels and nodes, which become clogged (blocked), stagnant (hyper-regulating), and inflamed. From here the organs of the body begin to show toxin strain and eventual overload which leads to illness from accumulated toxins.

Women: The lymph channels and nodes of the armpit become congested, as do the breasts, when underwire bras are worn. Studies by several researchers found that the majority of women who wore their bras over 12 hours daily were 21 times more likely to develop breast cancer compared to those wearing them less than 12 hours a day. Women who also wear their bras to bed had 125 times greater breast cancer risk. The underwire bras create a dam, causing a blockage of the flow of lymph through the armpit and breasts, which leads to the accumulation of toxins.

10

~

Lyme Toxins and a Toxic World

Considering toxins, we must recognize that these are poisonous substances that are irritating, and sometimes permanently damaging, to the tissues of the body. Neurotoxins damage the most sensitive tissues in the body, the brain and nerves. Toxins of any type must be avoided and eliminated at all costs. In this section, we will exhaustively discuss the primary types of toxins that I guarantee you have: microbial toxins and environmental toxins. Microbial toxins, like the neurotoxins of Lyme Disease, require a different and more targeted treatment approach than the more common environmental toxins.

Fifty percent of the health restoration every Lyme sufferer is looking for will come from effectively eliminating toxins and reducing the sources of the toxins (i.e. bacteria and toxic lifestyle products). The other fifty percent of healing will revolve around restoring structure, function, and optimal coherence within the body, mind, and spirit.

Bacterial Toxins: The Primary Cause of Your Symptoms

Research and clinical studies have determined that there are neurotoxins released by the *Borrelia burgdorferi* (Bb) spirochete[102,103]. Neurotoxins are nerve poisons. Based on the research, these toxins are the cause of most (if not all) of the symptoms of Lyme Disease. It is also believed that tissue damage is not caused by Lyme bacteria directly; the bacteria are not "eating" your tissues. It is the accumulation of Bb toxins in your body that is most likely responsible for the symptoms experienced by Lyme sufferers.

In the scheme of facilitating healing in the body, mind, and spirit, toxins are poison in the body. In that the body, mind, and spirit are all interconnected and interdependent, if the body is poisoned, then the mind and spirit must necessarily be poisoned as well! These toxins are a major interference to your body's ability to heal itself.

An astonishing new finding was released by John Travis in the July 2003 *Science News*[104]. Travis reported that research performed by John F. Prescott found that certain antibiotics, such as fluoroquinolones (the class that includes the name-brands and generic brands of Levaquin™, Cipro™, Tequin™, and Avelox™), actually are known to be able to trigger a type of virus called bacteriophages (viruses that can infect bacteria) to change the genetic sequencing of the bacteria. This causes the infected bacterium to start producing toxins. These viruses can act as genetic delivery vans, invading bacteria (such as spirochetes) often lying dormant, until activated by a change in the host (your body) environment. Once activated, these viruses insert their toxin-generating genes into the bacterial chromosomes. These viruses can turn basically harmless bacterium into killers through this genetic sequencing of toxins.[105]

Not only are toxins released through the die-off of bacteria, and not only can antibiotics actually increase the production of the toxins, but these viruses can cause the bacteria to rupture, spilling their toxins into your body.[106]

When a doctor uses an antibiotic to kill some Lyme spirochetes in a patient, there is often a resultant **Jarish-Herxheimer reaction** (Herx) -- a worsening of the patient's symptoms in response to the increased release of bacterial die-off toxins. The toxins are deposited into the bloodstream and are circulated throughout the body until they can either be eliminated or become lodged in areas of weakened tissues. As neurotoxins, they are preferentially taken up by nerve tissue. These lodged toxins are one of the reasons that symptoms can persist even after the actual Bb infection is gone; the toxins can remain as an irritant in the tissues for years.

In truth, a severe Herxheimer reaction is a sign of poor elimination pathway drainage, poor organ support, <u>and poor treatment by your doctor</u>! The body of most chronic Lyme sufferers is a toxic dump to start with; if the doctor does not get the pathways of elimination open and working, the body gets even more toxic when the bacteria begin to die and their toxins release. Many doctors think good treatment is indicated by the fact that you feel worse than usual, which they believe confirms that they selected an effective antibiotic.

Most of my chronically ill patients cannot afford to feel worse just from the treatment! The person with Lyme Disease has already suffered enough and does not need to go through a Herx just to prove they have Lyme Disease.

Herxheimer reactions are not confined to antibiotics. One of the more popular herbal remedies on the market causes such a severe Herx that the recommended dose is only one drop. I have spoken to hundreds of readers of my previous books from all over the world who have taken natural products and/or pharmaceuticals which apparently have released toxins, and now they not only still have their old symptoms, but they have many new symptoms as well. Remember, no matter what the cause, whether the resulting Herx is a true bacterial die-off or is a direct toxic effect of the remedy/medication, elimination of these toxins must be given just as high a priority as the actual infection.

Chronic Lyme sufferers do not have adequate detoxification mechanisms to detoxify these Bb toxins.

Development of My Herbal Formulas

I worked for many years, sifting and sampling many of the world's finest detoxification products, with mediocre results at best. When I presented research at the 1999 International Tick-borne Diseases Conference in New York City, I took a break one day and wandered through China Town. In my wanderings, I found an herbal pharmacy with a huge assortment of exotic herbs and medicines from China, all held in drawers that covered a long wall from floor to ceiling. Every drawer had three bins, each holding something different. Since I was on a quest to find the elusive solution to address the specific toxin of Lyme spirochetes, I was inspired to use Bio-Resonance Scanning™ (BRS, a real-time, non-computerized testing technique I developed) to test these herbs for efficacy against Lyme. The BRS testing required only a few moments and resulted in four herbs, out of the hundreds available, that tested beneficial. The Chinese pharmacists were quite certain I was doing some sort of magic with my BRS testing and literally huddled together in a corner to watch me. My six foot-seven inch frame and the BRS testing must have been a rare spectacle to them. I think they were glad to hand over the bags of herbs and be rid of me.

Upon arriving home, I prepared my herbs in a hydro-alcoholic extract as I had been taught by the Anthroposophical medical doctors in Eckwalden, Germany. With great elation, I discovered that the final product tested highly beneficial for some of my Lyme patients that had previously hit a plateau in their healing. The new formula took these patients to another 25% improvement! I and they were ecstatic. It wasn't the end-all solution, but it definitely was a step in the right direction.

Unfortunately, in their rush to be rid of me, the Chinese pharmacists, who spoke no English, must have written down the wrong Pinyin (the English derivation of the Chinese name for an herb) for the herbs. When I ordered more from another supplier, the herbs I received were not the same and would not work. Formula lost! Not to worry -- in those days, no one knew what the exact Lyme neurotoxin was; it took me five more years to identify ammonia as the primary toxin, even though I could detect the general frequency of the Lyme toxin with BRS during the days of the Chinese Apothecary. This is how I ultimately found better remedies for real people in my clinic.

I am convinced that today's newest formulations, the Neuro-Antitox II formulas, are the most advanced Lyme-ammonia detoxification products available. I also identified the herbs in these formulas using BRS. The herbs Silphium and Pale Spike Lobelia were both growing in my own pasture, and it was simply my inborn curiosity, or more likely Divine inspiration, that led me to uproot these herbs and test them! Like all of the different formulas I developed, the primary herbs cannot be purchased from any herbal supply house. Jernigan Nutraceuticals must grow, harvest, process, and bottle them each year. Each formula is the result of striving to help real people (over 3,000 patients) in my clinic, after trying, with minimal results, all the big-name, heavily marketed, nutritional supplements.

Testing for Treatment Efficacy -- FACT

Direct Resonance testing, a clinical research technique, along with the Functional Acuity Contrast Test (FACT) seems to verify that the Neuro-Antitox II formulas reach all of the hidden reservoirs of ammonia in the body, even crossing the blood-brain barrier, restoring integrity to the body, mind, and spirit.

A Direct Resonance Test functions based upon the fact that every bend, rotation, or atomic bond of a given molecular structure, such as NH3, has a certain resonant frequency.[107] When two substances similar molecular frequency come in close proximity to each other they will tend to vibrate "sympathetically" through harmonic resonance.[108] The FACT test is a very good test for detecting the presence of neurotoxins in the brain. It is also known as a Visual Contrast Test (VCS) and is acceptable in a court of law, usually to document the exposure to neurotoxic chemicals in a workman's compensation case. The FACT test has been successfully used in medical diagnosis and subclinical neurotoxicity detection. It is produced by the Stereo Optical Company, is simple to use, and can be used indefinitely without ever wearing out. If your doctor does not use this test, let him know about it, because it is well researched, and you can track your progress on a weekly basis if you so desire. As brain neurotoxin levels go down, your test should improve. To perform the test, you simply hold the apparatus in front of you, as the instructional sheet will indicate, and the degree that you can visually see certain images on a card determines the level of neurotoxins.

The basic FACT testing device:

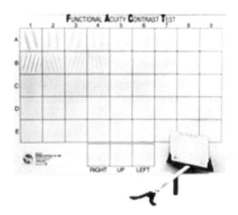

The Jernigan Lyme FACT Scoring System

After years of testing with the FACT device, I have developed a quantifiable scoring system to determine the severity of neurotoxicity in Lyme sufferers.

The FACT test is performed using first the right eye, and then the left. To determine the average score, simply record the last correct (readable) answer for each row A-E for each eye. Each number is multiplied by 11, so if you were able to read each box in row A all the way to number 9, then the score would be 99, if it was 7 then it would be 77 and so on for each eye. Add up the numbers and divide by 10. The resulting number is your average score. Ideally you would be above 75%. Another way to determine neurotoxins is that no row would show a drop of two or more levels. A drop of two or more levels means -- if Row D was scored at 7, then if Row E scored a 5 or less, this indicates a problem area in the brain is still high in neurotoxins.

FACT test scores lower than 70% represent excessive interference of neurotoxins. In a review of Lyme patient FACT tests scores in our clinic, the average initial score was 62%, demonstrating that neurotoxins were quite severe. These people were given Neuro-Antitox Formula to help reduce the levels of toxins, along with Borrelogen, as well as the detoxifying therapies and treatments in the clinic to help the body reduce the source of the neurotoxins (spirochetes), and to increase the tissue integrity so that all the organs of elimination are working at optimum. Improvements were detected within one week! Within 8-12 weeks, the FACT test scores soared to an average of 87%, with some patients scoring 100%! To my knowledge, these results are unparalleled in medicine. Some people report that with other treatments, such as prescription Cholestyramine, every FACT test was worse than the one before, indicating a progressively worsening neurological condition.

Keep in mind that it is often not enough to just take some remedies to detoxify the body. As you will read in the Perfect-7 protocol, it takes a lot of work to do all this at home! Even with much of work at home, you may not be able to overcome the many and various circuit problems that will enable your body to finally detoxify and heal.

If you don't remember anything else I say, hear this. No matter what type of Lyme treatment you ultimately choose, be it antibiotics or natural herbal supplements, you must clear the toxins as quickly and efficiently as possible and support the organs of elimination. To not do so may result in a temporary or ongoing worsening of your condition and predispose you to Post-Lyme Syndrome!

It can get confusing to read about the many general body detoxification nutritional and botanical supplements that are plentiful on the nutraceutical market. These products are designed to be general detoxifiers of the liver and intestines. While these products are a very good idea for almost everyone, they are not designed to handle Lyme neurotoxins, nor do many, if any, of them actually cross the blood-brain barrier to reach the ammonia and other toxins in the brain.

If your primary symptoms are in the brain, then many of these detoxifying supplements, foot pads, and cleanses will not work. Purchase your own FACT testing device or have your doctor do the testing for you, and you will see if the detox protocol you have chosen is working for the Lyme-specific neurotoxins.

We must remember that symptoms will not completely disappear just with the elimination of Lyme toxins; health and healing entails much more than the absence of toxins. The toxin-damaged tissues must be restored, the diseased mindset must be reset to that of positive affirmative health, and the spirit must learn and live the new insights gained during the illness.

Lyme Leaky Brain Syndrome (LLBS)

Although many people have heard of Leaky Bowel Syndrome (LBS), few know of Leaky Brain Syndrome. I coined this term after I made the first discovery of the presence of ammonia in Lyme Disease patients and then studied other illnesses that also resulted in hyperammonemia in the brain. Leaky Brain Syndrome is caused by the damaging effects on the blood-brain barrier (BBB) from the accumulation of Lyme-induced ammonia in the brain. The damage to the BBB from Lyme-induced ammonia has subsequently been confirmed. Using radioactive tracers, researchers have shown that laboratory animals, when infected by Borrelia, lose the protection of the blood–brain barrier after just two weeks.[109]

Ammonia in the brain is a primary cause of neurological and psychological hypersensitivity. Ammonia alters the permeability of the BBB, enabling larger molecules, such as common amino-acids, to cross. When these random molecules touch the brain tissues they set up hypersensitivities, otherwise known as cerebral allergies. The symptoms of these cerebral allergies are unique to which part of the brain is being affected. Ammonia-induced Leaky Brain Syndrome is one of the primary causes of Multiple Chemical Sensitivities, Cognitive dysfunction, Chronic Fatigue Syndrome, and a myriad of other chronic conditions.

There are only a few ways ammonia can become a problem in the brain. Severe liver disease is a well recognized producer of global or systemic ammonia. As far as I know, I was the first to discover, quite unexpectedly, that Lyme spirochetes could cause ammonia to accumulate in localized areas of the brain.

I first became aware of brain-ammonia problems while treating a gentleman from England who came to me after being diagnosed with Lyme Disease (another name is Neuroborreliosis). Quite surprisingly, my testing revealed Trypanosoma gambiense as his primary microbial challenge. T.

gambiense causes African Sleeping Sickness (ASS). Only after subsequent study did I find that the symptoms of ASS are caused by the neurotoxic effects of ammonia produced in the brain by the microbe. Interestingly, the patient said that for years he had told doctors that it felt like someone was pouring ammonia over his brain!

The severe debilitation this man was experiencing reminded me of some of the symptoms of many of my extreme Chronic Fatigue, Fibromyalgia, MS, ALS, and Lyme patients. Subsequent testing revealed that all of these people had localized ammonia accumulations primarily in the brain, heart, liver, and gums, caused by the bacteria *Borrelia burgdorferi* (Bb), the causative agent in Lyme Disease.

It would seem that Bb release ammonia, which is converted to glutamine, by way of the glutamine synthetase pathways, leading to **localized** swelling of astrocytes (brain cells). This ammonia-induced glutamine accumulation may cause dysfunction of astrocytes, leading to impairment of vascular reactivity other than through a decrease in Arginine availability for Nitric Oxide Synthetase (NOS), and resulting in increased production of nitric oxide.[110]

We do know that that many neurological problems are caused by either congenital or acquired hyper-ammonemia.[111] Therefore, finding ammonia as an issue in Lyme Disease, an illness marked by significant neurological problems, is of great clinical significance.

All of the ammonia-related pathological changes predispose Lyme sufferers to cerebral allergies, due to alterations in the blood brain barrier, subsequently allowing larger molecules, such as common dietary amino acids, to pass through to the brain. Neurotransmitter receptors and function are impaired. Possibly the most common symptom is altered brain energy metabolism, leading to cognitive brain dysfunctions, the total fatigue of the mind when forced to read, talk, or think for extended periods.

Research on the effect of ammonia on the immune system revealed that the bactericidal (bacteria killing effect) action of macrophages was significantly diminished in the presence of ammonia.[112] When it comes to ammonia's effect on the immune system's response to viruses, the research is just as bleak. The levels of ammonia produced in our system reduce human lymphocyte viability. Lymphocytes are the body's primary response to viruses.[113]

The weaking of the body's immune response from the effects of ammonia is likely the primary reason that so many people with chronic Lyme Disease suffer from the progressive worsening effects of multiple coinfections which seem to "come out of the woodwork."

Direct Resonance Testing (DRT) has been used to test for the presence of ammonia in the brain, heart, and liver of over 1000 chronic-illness patients; all patients were positive for ammonia over these areas. Several other doctors have confirmed this finding using the Direct Resonance Testing.

Aggravating Factors in Lyme Leaky Brain Syndrome (LLBS) and Lyme Disease Symptoms

- Weather Conditions
- Diet
- Herpes Viruses
- pH Balance
- Smoking
- Severe constipation
- Eating a high-protein or a low-protein diet
- Using medicines that increase blood ammonia levels, such as heparin, some diuretics (such as furosemide), acetazolamide, valproic acid, neomycin, tetracycline, diphenhydramine, isocarboxazid (Marplan), phenelzine (Nardil), and tranylcypromine (Parnate), heparin, and lactulose

Weather-related Worsening of Symptoms

Depending upon the severity of infection and tissue environmental issues -- including pH, temperature, oxygen levels, and emotional state -- the amount of ammonia could cause variable and cyclical worsening of symptoms. Localized astrocyte (brain cells) swelling would be aggravated by changes in barometric pressure, due to the fact that any intracellular swelling is going to swell more when there is less atmospheric pressure on it. In the case of falling barometric pressure before a storm, a worsening of symptoms occurs. This variable worsening of symptoms is described in medical science by the term allodynia. Allodynia results when a pain signal doesn't reach the brain and therefore pain is not felt by the person. Allodynia explains why the "old-timer" knows it is going to rain before the weather man. The old-timer's knees may have mild swelling due to arthritis, but the knees don't hurt until the barometric pressure falls just before a thunderstorm. As the barometric pressure falls, there is less pressure on the swelling in the knees allowing them swollen tissues to swell even more. Increased swelling causes the pain signals to be stronger, reaching the brain, and therefore being experienced as true pain. It may help to compare this to a balloon. If you measure the diameter of a balloon in clear weather, it will be smaller than before a storm because there is more atmospheric pressure pushing in on all sides. Now imagine the brain cells (astrocytes) and other inflamed tissues becoming more swollen and inflamed with changes in barometric pressure. This same phenomenon can be seen many times when one travels to a higher altitude. For this reason, living or traveling in the mountains can aggravate Lyme-related symptoms. A possible logical conclusion may be to move to a lower altitude to relieve some of the symptoms while healing.

Atmospheric-related worsening of symptoms, as seen with moon phases as well as prior to storms, are a common complaint in Lyme Disease. Understanding this can help preserve sanity since it can be very disconcerting to have a sudden worsening of your symptoms and wonder if the treatments have suddenly stopped working. Keep in mind that any time a symptom worsens even due to something temporary like the weather, it is aggravating the tissues, and the symptoms may not clear up simply because the storm passes.

For those who want to be proactive and avoid increased symptoms related to atmospheric/barometric changes, possible preventive measures may include purchasing a barometer that also shows the phases of the moon. With careful charting, you may notice that your symptoms generally get worse at a certain level of the barometric pressure. If you observe the barometer falling to that level, or you hear the weather man saying the barometric pressure is falling, you will want to begin increasing your systemic proteolytic enzymes, such as TPP Protease by Transformation Enzymes, or Wobenzym-med™ from Longevity Plus. Both of these products are the safest anti-inflammatory remedies for people suffering with Lyme Disease. Prescription corticosteroids and NSAIDs (Non-Steroidal Anti-Inflammatory Drugs) are contraindicated for anyone with Lyme and therefore should not be used. Another great product, and the only one I know that has been developed to specifically address weather-related and chemical sensitivities, is the German homeopathic remedy, Solum Uliginosum, which comes also as massage oil. Any good sports cream or ointment rubbed into affected joints and muscles ahead of time may also help to avoid a worsening of your pain. Staying ahead of your symptoms in these situations helps keep you from literally taking two steps forward and one step back, which would prolong your complete recovery. Whatever you do, do not use NSAIDs or steroids such as prednisone to treat Lyme-related pain.

Obviously, the best way to combat any of the Lyme Disease symptoms is to directly address the toxins (using

Neuro-Antitox II Formulas™) and reduce the cause of the toxins, Lyme spirochetes.

Dietary Worsening of Lyme Symptoms

High protein foods such as grains and meat contain an amino-acid (the breakdown unit of protein) called L-arginine. L-arginine in foods and as a nutritional supplement should not be taken in the presence of ammonia. Research reveals that ammonia + arginine + manganese = increased nitric oxide (NO) up to 53% in astrocytes (brain cells), leading to increased brain swelling. "Manganese in excess is neurotoxic and causes a CNS disorder that resembles Parkinson's disease (manganism). Manganese highly accumulates in astrocytes, which renders these cells more vulnerable to its toxicity."[114]

When localized brain swelling increases, the symptoms increase dramatically, and the perception of fatigue can escalate to critical. Armed with this knowledge, health care professionals would be wise to instigate a protein-poor diet for Lyme patients during treatment to minimize aggravations from arginine.

While not absolutely necessary for most people, it is a good recommendation for those people with severe brain toxicity and the symptoms to match to decrease your intake of arginine-rich foods. Foods that are high in arginine, and therefore should be avoided until ammonia tests are negative and symptoms are improved are carob, coconut, chocolate, dairy, gelatin, oats, meat of any kind, peanuts, soybeans, walnuts, white flour, wheat, and wheat germ. Dietary arginine is found in wheat germ and flour, buckwheat, granola, oatmeal, dairy products (cottage cheese, ricotta, nonfat dry milk, skim yogurt), beef (roasts, steaks), pork (Canadian bacon, ham), nuts (coconut, pecans, cashews, walnuts, almonds, Brazil nuts, hazel nuts, peanuts), seeds (pumpkin, sesame, sunflower), poultry (chicken and turkey light meat), wild game (pheasant, quail), seafood (halibut, lobster, salmon, shrimp, snails, tuna in water), chick peas, and cooked soybeans.[115,116])

Many people suffering with Lyme Disease also have various viral issues as well, such as Human Herpes Virus-6, Epstein Barr Virus, and others. Arginine feeds viruses. The amino acid L-Lysine blocks Arginine's ability to feed viruses, so it will benefit everyone to boost the dietary intake of L-Lysine. If you must have meat, fish is the best choice. It is high in L-Lysine, which may be adequate for combating the effects of the arginine in the fish.

Lysine rich foods include legumes, eggs, lima beans, potatoes, and brewers yeast. You may also purchase L-Lysine as a nutritional supplement from a health food store.

The trace mineral **Molybdenum** (pronounced ma-lib-denum), available in capsule form, can dramatically aid in the detoxification of the toxins caused by the dysfunction of multiple tissues in chronic illness. Molybdenum is very useful for detoxifying the toxin aldehyde from the die-off of Candida-type yeast. This is important to Lyme sufferers since aldehydes are considered neurotoxins. Aldehydes are also the toxin responsible for the hangover experienced by drinking excessive amounts of alcohol. I know of many Lyme patients who complain of this hung-over feeling without having drunk any alcohol.

Even though every Lyme sufferer should use Molybdenum to get rid of the aldehyde toxins, each should also drink plenty of purified water to keep the everyday metabolic toxins flushed out of the tissues.

It is our experience that Molybdenum will not detoxify the specific Bb toxin, but taking it will help slow the degeneration of tissues and related symptoms from the toxic overload.

Viral Worsening of LLBS

The Centers for Disease Control (CDC) report that about 92% of Americans would test positive to having the antibodies to at least six strains of Herpes viruses. This means that even without any Herpes symptoms (cold sores, canker sores, ulcers in the mouth and genital tissues), you likely have these viruses in your body.

Lyme Disease researchers have found that a common virus in chronic Lyme is the *Human Herpes Virus-6* (HHV-6). The Herpes viruses, especially the *Herpes simplex*, synthesize or produce arginine-rich protein. Herpes viruses need arginine in order to continue replicating.[117] This is another good argument for minimizing your intake of arginine-rich foods.

With the knowledge that Lyme spirochetes increase ammonia, and mixing arginine with ammonia leads to increased brain swelling and energy deficits, addressing viruses becomes a very important issue in healing from Lyme Disease.

Dietary supplementation with the amino-acid L-Lysine helps to block the Herpes virus from replicating by several different mechanisms. L-Lysine limits the absorption of L-arginine in the gut, it promotes the rapid, enzymatic breakdown of L-arginine, and it generally antagonizes the growth-promoting actions of arginine on the Herpes viruses.[118]

I developed the frequency-matched products Virogen™ and Microbojen™ to provide the body's crystalline matrix (See Chapter 3 for more info on the crystalline matrix) with the specific information necessary to facilitate the control and ultimate destruction of viruses. Clinical experience suggests that a general recommendation would be to start out using L-Lysine (from foods or in capsule form) for 4-6 months, and at the same time, use Virogen for 2-3 months, and then switch to Microbojen for 2-3 months, still maintaining the same dose of L-Lysine. Ideally, you will find a doctor to test you on all of your nutritional supplements before implementing any protocol.

Supplemental vitamin C is a good idea, but not all vitamin C is created equal. In high doses, some will cause diarrhea. Ester C is a good form of C, is readily available in health food stores, and it will not cause diarrhea. My favorite form of oral vitamin C is an advanced, highly bio-absorbable product called Beyond C™, made by Longevity Plus. Your physician can give you high-dose intravenous vitamin C, which has been shown to be beneficial in many viral conditions.

pH Aggravations of Lyme Ammonia

Ammonia is very alkaline. Many doctors have been taught that most sick people have acidic bodies. The reality is not that simple. People may be predominantly acidic but may also be extremely alkaline in the areas of ammonia accumulation. This is why many people worsen when they are given dietary recommendations such as fresh fruits and vegetables, which work to alkalinize the body. It appears that alkalinizing these people is only aggravating the already over-alkaline ammonia regions of their body: the brain, heart, and liver. The ammonia conditions must be cleared before addressing the more acidic regions of the body.

The alkalinity of ammonia is also another reason that one must be careful when using therapeutic magnets to heal. Before anyone knew about Lyme ammonia, it was generally thought that using only the negative polarity of a magnet over the body would be beneficial. It appears that this thinking is all wrong when ammonia is present. The negative polarity will increase the alkalinity even more, creating more problems in those areas, since too much alkalinity is just as bad as too much acidity. Much caution is warranted with the use of magnets.

In the hands of a trained health care professional, 4x6x1" ceramic, positive polarity magnets used for <u>five minutes</u>

only over these areas of ammonia can help counteract over-alkalinity in the tissues. Too much positive polarity over an area will cause the area to become acidic. Caution: positive polarity should never be used near any type of cancerous tissue!

Rapid Testing for Ammonia

Direct Resonance Testing (DRT) for ammonia is a simple test that a lay person or healthcare practitioner can perform in one minute, for less than 20 cents. It is recommended that anyone with any chronic condition be tested in this way.

To perform a DRT, you will need a vial or small bottle of pure ammonia. A muscle strength challenge should be performed to identify a strong muscle, preferably using the deltoid muscle with the patient's thumb pointing towards the feet. The muscle should "lock" and be strong immediately when challenged, without being spongy. Once a good strong muscle has been identified, hold the vial of ammonia over various areas of the brain, heart, liver, and teeth, testing to see if the previously strong muscle goes weak when the ammonia is held over any of these areas.[119] Due to the temporary neuromuscular interference caused by the harmonic resonance of ammonia in the vial with any ammonia present in the tissues, the strong muscle will go weak.[120,121] The most effective treatment can be identified with the same test method, by adding the corrective substance, such as one of the Neuro-Antitox II Formulas™. To determine the best corrective substance, hold the vial of ammonia and the remedy over the same spot where the strong muscle went weak. If you have found the proper corrective substance, the former weak muscle test now will go strong. You will likely find that general liver and intestinal detoxification supplements will do nothing to clear out ammonia.

ALS (Lou Gherig's Disease) and Lyme Ammonia

Every occurence of ALS that I have tested through Direct Resonance Testing has Lyme Disease as its instigator. Uniquely, ALS patients all have *global* accumulations of ammonia. Most people with typical Lyme have ammonia only in the liver, heart, brain, and gums; ALS has ammonia in every part of the body! This fact is being released to the world only now in this book.

In most people with typical Lyme, the ammonia is converted virtually instantly into nitric oxide in the extremities, muscles and joints. In ALS, the conversion of ammonia into nitric oxide appears to be blocked by some unknown biochemical defect.

The first time I tested a person with ALS, I was shocked to find global ammonia accumulations. Upon questioning, every ALS sufferer I have treated has told me that when they perspire, they smell ammonia. One woman said that when her husband with ALS would exit their infrared sauna at home, his towels reeked of ammonia, but no other doctor had ever recognized this factor.

Another fascinating finding is that the muscle fasciculations of ALS (the worming, twitching of the individual muscle that leads to the death of the nerve ending) have been dramatically improved when the patient soaks in a bath with four ounces of Neuro-Antitox II Formula! This finding is remarkable -- if one could completely stop the muscle fasciculations, the nerve-endings would not continue to die, and the ALS would be brought to a halt. However, the reality is still that the cause of the lack of biochemical breakdown of ammonia must be corrected, the source of ammonia (Lyme spirochetes) must be brought to controllable levels, and the tissues must be repaired.

So far, the "cure" for ALS is still elusive, but the Lyme-ammonia connection is a profound revelation.

Good results are also being reported in ALS using intravenous (IV) glutathione, peroxide drips, and IV phosphatidylcholine.[122]

Parkinson's Disease and Ammonia

I am not aware of much research on the effects of ammonia on Parkinson's Disease, but one source for a reference to and ammonia connection to Parkinson's is worth mentioning here. Federico, P. and Zochodne, W. *Reversible parkinsonism and hyperammonemia associated with portal vein thrombosis.* Acta Neurologica Scandinavica 103 (3), 198–200. 2001.

Environmental Toxins: Jamming the Machinery of the Body

Today more than 77,000 chemicals are in active production in this country. Our exposure to these chemicals is greater than at any time since the beginning of the Industrial Revolution. More than 3000 chemicals are added to our food supply, and more than 10,000 chemicals in the form of solvents, emulsifiers, and preservatives are used in food processing and storage. Ethyl alcohol, isopropanol, wood rosin, shellac, propylene glycol, silicone, ammonium hydroxide -- you're eating it for breakfast if you're eating grapefruit, melon, and fresh oranges from the supermarket. You're eating thiabendazole, mineral oil, methylparabin, dimethyl polysiloxane, and benzimadazole for lunch if you had tomatoes, avocados, or apples.

Do fungicides, botran, 2-6 dichloro-4-nitroaniline, orthophenylphenol sound like a good balanced dinner? You're eating these yummy ingredients in sweet potatoes, onions, and limes from your local supermarket. Fungicides are put into wax to coat fruit and vegetables to provide a longer shelf life; even peeling won't get rid of them. You eat them. They cause cancers, birth defects, damaged immune systems, and other diseases.

When ingested, these toxic chemicals can remain in the body for years altering our metabolism. They cause enzyme dysfunction and nutritional deficiencies, creating hormonal imbalances and lowering our threshold of resistance to chronic disease.

Besides food borne chemicals, we are continually subjected to poor air quality (anything you can smell is a chemical floating in the air and you are breathing it into your body), chemically contaminated water, household cleaners, paint fumes, pharmaceutical drugs (66% of drugs tested by researchers could be found still biologically active in most municipal tap water, so you could be taking your neighbor's heart medicines or chemotherapy drugs), pesticides, heavy metals (including mercury), and the list goes on and on. Today's studies show that most of us have between 400 and 800 foreign chemical residues stored in the fat cells of our bodies. This occurs gradually over the course of our lives. These chemicals enter into the body either through the skin, through the lungs, or they are eaten. Most of the time, these chemicals are bio-accumulative, meaning miniscule amounts accumulate over the course of years. These chemicals and heavy metals make up the "total toxic burden." When the amount of toxins in the tissues exceeds the body's ability to excrete them, the body will begin to store these toxins. This bio-accumulation seriously compromises our physiological and psychological health and leads to chronic disease.

I was told by a patient who was a Vietnam war veteran that during the Vietnam war, military personnel realized that if an American soldier was killed, they didn't have to do anything special with the body for over a week since the American diet and lifestyle is so full of preservatives. If a Vietnamese soldier was killed, they knew they must bury the body almost immediately because decomposition would occur rapidly, due to the lack of preservatives in their bodies.

Virtually all mainstream brands of toothpaste are

preserved with formaldehyde. Interestingly, formaldehyde is hidden under about 26 different names to keep you from knowing you are using it. Did you ever wonder why your toothpaste has a "Warning" label on it? That is because of the formaldehyde and the neurotoxin fluoride, which was recognized for many years as one of the most toxic minerals known to man!

In the past, the government required any product with a known toxic chemical like fluoride or formaldehyde to carry a "Skull and Crossbones" picture on the label. However, companies complained that no one would buy toothpaste that has a skull and crossbones on it. After much lobbying, the government changed the label requirements based upon how toxic one or more of the ingredients are, as follows:

>**Caution**: One or more ingredients meets the definition of "eye-irritant."
>**Warning**: As little as one teaspoon can kill an adult.
>**Danger**: Contains an ingredient that will kill an adult with five drops.

Evaluate your personal care products, and stop poisoning your healing process. You cannot continue putting toxins on your skin and eating toxic foods and realistically expect to not suffer the consequences.

Since 1976, the EPA (Environmental Protection Agency) has been conducting studies to determine the presence of toxins in the fat cells of the body. This study is called the National Adipose Tissue Survey (NATS). The results of this study are staggering. Across the United States, the EPA took samples of human fat cells (adipose) and analyzed the samples for the presence of various toxins. The EPA only looks for 100 out of the potential thousands of different toxins that could be present in the fatty tissue samples. Twenty different toxins were identified in over 75% of all the samples. In 98% of the samples, they found many toxins, including benzene, PCBs,

DDE (a metabolite of DDT pesticide), dioxins, toluene, and chlorobenzene, all of which are highly damaging to the immune system and compromise every tissue in the body. From this and other studies, you can see that it is not so much a matter of "if" you have toxins in your body, but rather how much. Remember that the goal is not to just get rid of your symptoms, but to remove anything that may be blocking your body's healing mechanisms. True health is not merely the absence of pain or symptoms.

The following is a partial list of known symptoms often related to toxicity: allergies, acne, anxiety, burning skin, brain fog, chronic fatigue, chemical sensitivities, depression, eczema, frequent colds or flu, feeling "sick all over," insomnia, loss of dexterity, low body temperature, memory loss, mood swings, muscle and joint pains, and poor concentration.

As a result of widespread environmental contamination, doctors are faced with increased rates of toxin-related cancers, neurological diseases, reduced immune function, allergies, and the newer diagnoses of multiple chemical sensitivities, chronic fatigue syndrome, and fibromyalgia. Doctors are finding their usual treatments are not as effective as in the past, due to the presence of these many toxins in people.

Did you know that few people with cancer actually die of the cancer? Authorities say that they actually die of toxemia, produced by an excessive buildup of toxins.[123]

You cannot simply take laxatives to eliminate all of these toxins. You must be guided through a total body protocol to truly achieve detoxification.

All of the Lyme detoxification recommendations will still address most of these environmental toxins. However, just like in Lyme Disease, we must reduce the source of the toxins! You cannot continue putting toxic products in or on your body and expect to not get sick.

Skin Toxins

Consider the skin for a moment. Your skin is the largest organ of elimination. It should be releasing two pounds of waste acids every day! Most people have spent their entire lives blocking this process through lotions and powder and toxic antibacterial, deodorant soaps. As you may guess, two pounds of waste per day that is not being eliminated through the skin is going to add up and tax the body severely.

DEET is a well-documented toxin used in most insect repellants. Unfortunately, there are very few better substances to reliably repel mosquitoes, ticks, and other biting insects. Now consider that the newest way that drug companies are delivering pharmaceutical drugs is using transdermal patches to enable more efficient delivery of the medicine than if you ingested it. If you swallow a pill, a certain amount of the medicine will be broken down by the digestive juices in the stomach and small intestines. The skin, however, has no digestive juices to break down the medicine, so higher concentrations of the medicines actually enter the body.

If putting chemicals on the skin enables greater concentrations of them to enter the body than if we had eaten them, would anyone voluntarily eat DEET? What about your underarm deodorant, soaps, perfume/colognes, hairspray, hair dyes, lotions and creams? How about the laundry detergents and softeners in your clothes that find their way into your body? Remember, anything you can smell is an out-gassed chemical floating around in the air that you breathe into your body. Read the labels on your makeup products. Propylene glycol is another name for antifreeze, just like you put in your car. What are all of those unpronounceable words on your shampoo labels? If your shampoo has the ingredient DEA, then you are getting more nitrites soaking into your scalp and into your body from one shampooing than you would get from eating a pound of bacon!

Take a look at the flea and tick sprays, dips, and collars

for your pets. The label says not to get it on your clothes or skin, yet your pet may contact your carpet or furniture, and you may want to actually pet your animal without ingesting chemicals. All of these poisons are known to be bio-accumulative, meaning miniscule amounts cross the skin and accumulate to pathological amounts that poison various tissues in the body.

You may think you are only getting a chemical just under your skin, but the reality is that every chemical has an affinity for a specific tissue and will accumulate over time and repeated exposure. A chemical you get on your hands may end up in your brain. Other chemicals may end up in your pancreas, such as is known of virtually all herbicides, pesticides, and heavy metals.

NanoDerm™ Lotion: There IS a Solution

Imagine a non-toxic product that you could put on your skin that creates an invisible barrier to virtually any organic or inorganic toxin for more than five hours. I am very pleased to be introducing a new product to the world, a lotion I am calling Nanoderm Lotion™, which literally creates an invisible, hypoallergenic, and nontoxic skin barrier that will still enable the skin to perspire, but it will <u>not</u> allow virtually any type of chemical to penetrate the skin! Once applied, it cannot be felt on the skin, has virtually no odor, and it will not rub or wash off for eight hours. Nanoderm Lotion™ will continue working, to some degree, for as long as 24 hours, but it is maximally efficient for the first eight hours.

For years, I have searched for a nontoxic substitute for DEET-containing insecticides. Some herbal products and oils seem to work, but nothing worked as as well as DEET. Now with Nanoderm Lotion™ protecting you, you can apply it to the skin and let it dry and then spray on the DEET products. You could drench you clothes with DEET and never have any of the chemicals penetrate the body.

Nanoderm Lotion™ is so amazing that you can even handle any acid or chemical with NO penetration or irritation. You can literally pour hydrochloric acid directly on the Nanoderm-treated hand and not be affected. If the hydrochloric acid runs off of your hand, it will burn a hole through even aluminum foil.

Imagine the possibilities! You could apply Nanoderm Lotion™, and no smell will "stick" to you. Onions, garlic, rotten fish, grease, make-up, and personal care products will all just wash off with no residual smell and no chemical penetrating the skin.

Poison Ivy and other rash causing plants will not cause any effect because their oils and irritating chemicals cannot penetrate the Nanoderm-treated skin! The poison simply washes off with normal soap and water. Of course, any untreated skin will still be affected.

The people needing Nanoderm Lotion™ span virtually all occupations. Anyone who shakes people's hands, comes in contact with body fluids, uses any smelly substance, solvent, or chemicals, anyone with contact dermatitis, latex glove allergies, cleaning service people, mechanics, morticians, surgeons, forensic pathologists, butchers, fishermen, food product handlers, soldiers in the military, and the list is endless.

If the toxin-blocking abilities of Nanoderm Lotion™ were not enough, it also contains APS (All-Purpose Solution) and other proprietary ingredients that make it one of the world's most effective, nontoxic, and natural antimicrobials to block the penetration of viruses and bacteria through the skin. In independent laboratory studies, Nanoderm Lotion™ kills even the hospital strain staph bacteria called Multi-Resistant Staphylococcus Aureus (MRSA).[124]

Nanoderm Lotion™ is non-greasy and contains 14 different moisturizers and emollients that make it safe for all skin areas. Nanoderm will also help alleviate the pain of raw and cracked skin due to constant exposure to the elements.

Nanoderm will not penetrate the skin layers either, yet

forms an undetectable barrier on the skin so you are protected from virtually any chemical toxin, an especially important factor now that biological agents are becoming another threat to our health.

In this toxic world in which we live in, this is truly the most remarkable product on the market anywhere in the world! Even if you do not use Nanoderm Lotion™, you must keep in mind that you should never put anything on your skin that you would not eat. Whether simple hand cream or soap, whatever you apply or absorb into the skin will absorb into the body in higher concentrations than if you ate it! Nanoderm is the primary way to reduce the external sources of toxins.

Detoxing During Pregnancy and Breastfeeding

Toxins are a huge problem for virtually every person on the planet! I can tell you with certainty that you, too, have accumulated toxins, as have I. It was reported in a leading cardiology medical journal that we all have about 1000 times more heavy metals (lead, mercury, nickle...) in our body than people did at the beginning of the Industrial Revolution. It was also reported that people with heart disease have over 25,000 times more mercury metal that the rest of the population.

Pregnancy presents a very real dilemma when it comes to the treatment of Lyme Disease and undergoing a detoxification program. Toxins from the mother can be transmitted to the fetus, leading to potential problems in the child, and may increase the risk of miscarriage.

A healthy woman's body will naturally test the developing fetus during the first 7-12 weeks for any problems. If any major problems are detected, it will abort the pregnancy. This is a natural design to ensure that only healthy children are born.

However, pregnancy and breastfeeding is NOT the time to start an *intensive* detoxification program! Many, if not most, toxins are bound up or lodged in the tissues of the mother's body. The last thing we want is to liberate those toxins into actively circulating around the body. Once liberated, the toxins could end up crossing the placenta and will almost definitely enter the breastmilk.

So what do we do when a mother is suffering from the effects of Lyme-specific toxins, which may still end up crossing the placenta or end up in the breast milk? The logical and best solution is to only seek to *break down* the specific toxins of Lyme spirochetes without liberating too many other toxins. The key word here is *break down*, as opposed to *chelating* (the grabbing onto and pulling the toxin out of the tissue and into circulation in the body fluids).

As we have presented, clinical research suggests that the primary toxin of Lyme spirochetes is ammonia. The excess ammonia causes several chemical chain reactions, all resulting in dysfunctions in the tissues which you experience as symptoms.

In a healthy body, ammonia is broken down into urea and easily eliminated through the normal pathways in the body. The Neuro-Antitox II Formulas are unique in that they appear to facilitate the restoration of the body's ability to rapidly break down the ammonia molecules into harmless urea long before it or its metabolites can reach the fetus or get into the breast milk.

The Detox Bath #1 with warm (but not hot) water is also safe to use during pregnancy -- it helps break down and pull toxins directly through the skin, but it will not tend to mobilize toxins into active circulation.

As in all toxin-related problems, the source of the toxins must be reduced, or otherwise the toxins will be an ongoing problem.

Before undertaking any detoxification program, check first with your doctor, ideally one who can do Applied or Clinical Kinesiology (usually these are Doctors of Chiropractic) or some sensitive testing like Electrodermal Screening.

Whether using antibiotics or natural supplements to address the Lyme Disease, you must be on Neuro-Antitox II to help remove the toxins.

The First-Timers Response

One of the biggest revelations I have experienced in my years of being a doctor is that the cleaner the body, mind, and spirit becomes, the more sensitive one becomes to putting the "bad stuff" in the body. Your body tries to tell you when something you are doing is bad for it. Usually the first few times you do something, bad your body responds with an unpleasant reaction.

The first time you smoke a cigarette, you feel nauseous, light-headed, fuzzy, and green. This is your body's true reaction to cigarettes. If you keep smoking, eventually this passes and the body begins to feel that smoking is a normal thing.

If you have been drinking pop or soda every day for years and decide to stop for a few months, when you go back and drink one, your body will feel queasy and sluggish, and the pop will taste syrupy, sometimes soapy. This is your body's true response to pop.

You see, God gave us these sensations of pain and discomfort to alert us to those things that we should not be doing. Pain is a guidepost, not merely a sign of a deficiency of Tylenol® or any other medication.

If you undergo a dietary fast or the Master Longevity Cleanse presented in this book, you are in effect cleaning the tissues of the body. Once truly clean, your body will be able to let you know when foods and other substances are not good for it. If you eat or drink something and it makes you feel anything but normal and vibrant with health, then your body will immediately let you know. Listen carefully, because your body will only tell you a few times before it will adapt to the garbage, and you will gradually become sicker and have less vital energy.

For those of you who desire to know more about how to achieve a truly clean "temple," which is actually a clean body, a clean mind, and a clean spirit, I recommend you read my book, *Everyday Miracles by God's Design*.

From this truly clean state, true health and true joy of living can be experienced. You can now live life purely in the moment you are in. You perceive all the good in life because all that poisoned the perspectives of your body, mind, and spirit are gone.

[102] Klinghardt, D. 2002. *The Klinghardt Neurotoxin Elimination Protocol*, 2nd Annual Conference of Applied Neurobiology; Treating Lyme and Co-infections, Bellevue, WA, Dec.
[103] Cartwright, M.J., A Novel Toxin (Bb Tox 1) of Borrelia burgdorferi.
[104] Travis, J. 2003. *Phages behaving badly; Viruses can control how dangerous some bacteria are.* Science News, July 12, Vol. 164.
[105] Travis, J. 2003. *Phages behaving badly; Viruses can control how dangerous some bacteria are.* Science News, July 12, Vol. 164.
[106] Waldor, M. 2002. *Molecular Microbiology*, May.
[107] Oschman, J.L. 2000. *Energy Medicine; The Scientific Basis*, Butterworth Hieneman.
[108] Allen H.C. and Cross, P.C. 1963. Molecular Vib-rotors. John Wiley, New York.
[109] Schutzer, S.E., ed. Lyme Disease: Molecular and Immunologic Approaches, Series 6. Current Communications in Molecular and Cell Biology. Plainview, NY: Cold Spring Harbor Press, 1992.
[110] Toshiki, O, et al. 2000. Interaction of glutamine and arginine on cerebrovascular reactivity to hypercapnia *Am J Physiol Heart Circ Physiol* 278: H1577-H1584.
[111] Albrecht, J. 1998. Roles of neuroactive amino acids in ammonia neurotoxicity, Neurosci Res.Jan 15;51(2):133-8.
[112] S.P. Targowski et al. *Effect of ammonia on in vivo and in vitro immune responses.* Infect Immun. 1984 January; 43(1): 289–293.
[113] Flescher, E., Fossum, D., Talal, N. *Polyamine-dependent production of lymphocytotoxic levels of ammonia by human peripheral blood monocytes.* Immunol Lett. 1991 Apr;28(1):85-9
[114] Rama Rao K, Reddy P, et al, Manganese induces cell swelling in cultured astrocytes. NeuroToxicology Volume 28, Issue 4, July 2007, 807-812.
[115] Cooper, M.D., M.P.H. and Kenneth, H. *Advanced Nutritional Therapies* Nashville: Thomas Nelson Publishers, 1996.
[116] Murray, N.D., Michael, T., and Pizzorno, N.D. *Encyclopedia of Natural Medicine* Rocklin, California: Prima Publishing, 1991.
[117] (Griffin et al. 1981) – where is this reference??
[118] (Miller 1984) – where?
[119] Andreev, E.A., Beloy, M.V., and Sitko, S.P. 1984. The manifestation of natural characteristic frequencies of the organism of man. Reports to the Academy of Sciences of the Ukrainian SSR Number 10, Series b, Geological, Chemical, and Biological Sciences, pp 60-63.
[120] Adolf, E.F. 1979. Look at physiological integration. *American Journal of Physiology* 237:R255-R259.
[121] Frohlich, H. 1978. Coherent electric vibrations in biological systems and the cancer problem. IEEE Transactions on Microwave Theory and Techniques MTT 26:613-617
[122] Bains, J. and Shaw, C. *Neurodegenerative disorders in humans: the role of glutathione in oxidative stress-mediated neuronal death.* Brain Research Reviews Volume 25, Issue 3, December 1997, 335-358.
[123] Diamond, John MD, and Burton Goldburg. *Alternative Medicine; The Definitive Guide to Cancer.*
[124] Microbiological Report, Micro Quality Labs, N. Hollywood CA, 2006.

Section 3
The Perfect-7 Treatment and Detox Protocol™

11

~

The Perfect-7 Treatment and Detoxification Protocol™

Through the years, many people have called our clinic for advice about what they should do at home to heal. Often they cannot find a doctor in their area that is able to address all of their needs. While no two people are exactly the same and therefore cannot be treated exactly the same, there are many things that I have found to be almost universally needed in every Lyme sufferer.

The following recommendations are just that -- my recommendations, not a prescription, and in an ideal world you would always find a doctor who already practices all the techniques outlined in this book, or you would come to our clinic. You could also give a copy of this book to your local doctor so that he or she can help you implement as many of the items as possible.

I say this as a worst case scenario -- if you cannot find a good doctor in your area and wish to be proactive in taking responsibility for your own health at home, the following general protocol is what I have found works the best.

First of all, please do not get into the trap of taking fistfuls of every nutritional supplement that sounds like it may help. Many people I have helped were taking 60-70 different natural and pharmaceutical products that were given to them by celebrated "natural physicians." I am dismayed at how allopathic (symptom-based) much of natural and alternative medicine is becoming. The reality is that the collection of remedies should be greatly streamlined in a synergistic combination of remedies that restore optimal coherence of the body's primary issues. It is not necessary to take a different remedy for each and every problem a doctor can find. The allopathic mentality of "seek and destroy" for bacteria and every other detectible microbe has found a gradual home in natural medicine. Plant medicines are containing more "isolated and concentrated" active ingredients. This sounds eerily like the isolated and concentrated pharmaceutical drugs of allopathic medicine. History has already taught us time and again that when you remove the natural buffers found in medicinal plants, and when using highly concentrated isolates, you will often see adverse side effects.

The goal of supplementation is not to take remedies for the rest of your life, but instead to provide your body with those specific things that will restore the body's ability to completely heal. Nor should it take a year or more for you to start feeling significantly better. If you are truly correcting the bottom-line problems with any supplement, eventually the problem would be corrected and you would no longer need the extra assistance.

Second, you must know in your heart that God truly did design the human body to heal itself of virtually any illness. I have seen miraculous recoveries from seemingly permanent damage. Several years ago, we treated a lady from Alaska who had not had the use of her entire right leg and foot for over a year (from the effects of Lyme Disease). Within 10 seconds of treatment with a specific technique using the Magnetic Resonance Bio-Oxidative Therapy, she was able to lift her knee up to her chest, walk on her toes and heels, and climb stairs! She and her husband were just amazed and ecstatic, as was I. The correction has remained without further treatment of that specific problem ever since. This was achieved because of the restoration of the body's normal crystalline matrix, which is necessary for nerve conduction and subsequent muscle control.

Recall the discussion of the crystalline matrix nature of the body in Chapter 8. The point is that when the body has the <u>specific</u> information and building blocks it needs, the body will do the rest. Don't just take some of everything in the health food store; find a doctor who can determine what your body primarily needs. In the Alaskan lady's case, it was not a nutritional supplement that her body needed to restore the normal function of her leg; it simply needed the stimulation that the Magnetic Resonance therapy provided.

It is not expected that Lyme microbes and your symptoms will miraculously go away within a short period of a week or month of doing this protocol, although it is often reported. Do not let the absence of immediate apparent benefit disappoint you. It took your body a long time to get into this condition, and it may take months to years of doing the right things to fully restore the quality of life you seek. Feeling good or feeling bad during your journey does not indicate that you should stop doing the right things.

Healing at Home With the Perfect-7 Protocol

We have treated thousands of people of all ages who suffer with mild to profoundly serious Lyme Disease. The great success we have experienced is most likely due to our ability to effectively address the primary source of the toxins, the many microbial co-infections of Lyme Disease, and then our ability to successfully and rapidly target the breakdown and elimination of the specific microbial toxins, as well as restore the many organ circuits of the body.

The following protocol is called the "Perfect-7 Treatment and Detoxification Protocol," and it has been the backbone of our treatment process for years with nearly all of our patients. Notice that it is not called "Perfect-7 LYME Treatment and Detoxification Protocol." This is because we are treating people, not bacteria; we are treating a completely integrated organism called a human, not pieces and parts of a body; we are restoring optimum coherence of the body, mind, and spirit, not the numbers on a blood test!

Following sections of this book will discuss each step in further detail.

The Perfect-7 Treatment and Detox Protocol™ Steps

This page is the Perfect-7 at its most basic. More details and suggestions for each step are in following sections.

1. Restore the body's regulation of microbes.

2. Detoxify Lyme-specific neuro- and environmental toxins.
    - Neuro-Antitox II Formulas™
    - Dr. Jernigan's Detox Coffee, Detox Cocoa, or Detox Tea

   Overall detoxification:
    - Dry Skin Brushing
    - Infrared Sauna
    - Dr. Joseph's Colon Cleanse™
    - Hydrogen Peroxide/Epsom Salt Detox Baths
    - Dr. Jernigan's Mustard Foot Bath™
    - Strengthening/Nutritive Bath
    - Master Longevity Cleanse
    - Liver/Gallbladder Flush
    - Non-Toxic Personal Care & Household Products

3. Break Up Bacterial Biofilms and Inflammation:
    - TPP Protease®
    - Beyond Chelation-Improved™

4. Support the Bio-energetic fields of the body against Electromagnetic Pollution and Geopathic Stressors, using essential oils and BioPro™ products.

5. Address all structural interferences to optimize integrity.

6. Align Lifestyle to optimize health.

7. Identify and address all emotional triggers.

The Perfect-7 Treatment and Detox Protocol™ Summarized

1. **Restore the body's regulation of microbes:**
   - **Borrelogen™, Lymogen™, and/or Microbojen™** to facilitate the body's ability to reduce the *source* of the microbial toxins, the Lyme bacteria, *six* days per week (choose one day off).

2. **Detoxify Lyme-specific neurotoxins and environmental toxins:**
   - **Neuro-Antitox II Formulas™** are the only frequency-matched formulas specifically developed to target the body's ability to break down and remove the Lyme-specific toxins, *six* days per week.
   - **Dr. Jernigan's Detox Coffee, Detox Cocoa, or Detox Tea** to speed colon peristalsis and urine eliminative output. Drink 2-3 cups per day.

   Overall detoxification will be facilitated for all types of chemical toxins by:
   - **Dry Skin Brushing** (Daily)
   - **Infrared Sauna** (30-45 minutes, 3-6 times per week)
   - **Dr. Joseph's Colon Cleanse™** (1-3 times per week)
   - **Hydrogen Peroxide/Epsom Salt Detox Baths** (3-4 times per week)
   - **Dr. Jernigan's Mustard Foot Bath™** (3-4 x per week)
   - **Strengthening/Nutritive Bath** to be used on the one day per week that no supplements of any kind are taken. This will help the body regenerate and replenish its energy since detoxifying is a strain on the body.
   - **Master Longevity Cleanse**
   - **Liver/Gallbladder Flush**
   - **Personal Care & Household Products** that are toxic should be replaced with non-toxic products from Young Living or another reputable company.

3. **Break Up** Bacterial Biofilms **and Inflammation:**
   - **TPP Protease®** (by Transformation Enzymes) is a systemic proteolytic enzyme used to break up fibrin and hypercoagulation, and reduce inflammation. 2-3 capsules, 3 times per day on an empty stomach. An

empty stomach means at least 45 minutes before eating and at least 1 hour after eating to ensure all the proteolytic enzymes can get absorbed into the body while the stomach is not busy digesting the protein in the diet.
- **Beyond Chelation-Improved™** (from Longevity Plus), 1-2 packets per day, *six* days per week. This botanical and nutritional support will grab onto and pull out biological and environmental toxins. It also contains anti-microbial High-Allicin Garlic, as well as Calcium Disodium EDTA, which research indicates may help in removing the biofilm of various bacteria.

4. **Support the Bio-energetic fields of the body against Electromagnetic Pollution from cell phones and electrical appliances, as well as Geopathic Stressors:**
    - Follow the Essential Oil Protocol in Chapter 25.
    - Use BioPro™ Home Harmonizers, BioPro™ Personal Harmonizers, BioPro™ Cell Chips and BioPro™ Universal appliance chips.

5. **Address all structural interferences to optimize integrity:**
    - Your Doctor of Chiropractic and/or local natural health practitioner will be able to facilitate proper alignment in this area.
    - Neurological and low body temperature corrections are also important.

6. **Align Lifestyle to optimize health**:
    - Choose healthy ways to "Redesign you life" to promote greater integrity. Read Chapter 33.
    - Adopt smarter dietary choices. Read Chapter 35.
    - Exercise to stimulate flexibility and increase overall vitality – Aqua Aerobics, Tai Chi, and Pilates are often easiest and most fulfilling to integrate, even for the chronically ill.

7. **Identify and address all emotional triggers:**
    - Emotional conflicts and their triggers may be reactivating the symptoms (Read chapters 37 and 41).
    - Use the Essential oil protocol listed in Chapter 25.

I recommend that you follow this protocol for two months beyond the disappearance of your symptoms. For your convenience, the supplements mentioned are available as a kit, and ordering information is provided in the back of this book.

The following sections contain further explanation for each of the Perfect-7 steps.

Other Notes: After completing the recommended duration of Borrelogen, Lymogen and Microbojen, other botanicals can be implemented in Step 1 of the Perfect-7 Protocol. These may include but are not limited to Immuni-T^3 by Longevity Plus, APS Solution from Ancient Formulas, the herb Teasel, and Ionic Silver. Continue each of the other steps (2-7) the same no matter what you use to address the body dealing with the microbes.

Additional Remedies for unique symptoms

While the Perfect-7 Protocol is designed to address the widest possible range of issues, in order to achieve lasting health, there are many symptoms that you may want to more specifically address. Using even more remedies may be disappointing to some people, but consider this example. If a patient goes to a medical cardiologist, he is primarily concerned about the heart. Even so, he will often place a person on three or more related medicines. Because Lyme disease affects virtually every organ, gland, and tissue in the body, it should not be surprising that more synergistic remedies may be needed, depending upon the case.

If your core temperature is low, read Step 4, and implement as many of the corrections mentioned as possible. If you have unique symptoms, you can often handle them by implementing the suggestions in Chapter 41, Remedy Suggestions and the Associated Emotional Conflicts for Specific Symptoms.

Step 1
Restore the Body's Regulation of Microbes

12

~

Borrelogen™, Lymogen™, Microbojen™

As we discussed in Chapter 3, no matter the treatment, it may be assumed that the microbes will immediately strive to survive. They will either attempt to morph or change their shape to survive, and/or they will attempt to change your internal environment. Borrelogen has been clinically tested for nine years, as well as laboratory tested, and from that we know that even as good as I believe Borrelogen is, some of the microbes will likely become resistant to the changes it makes in your body's energy. Therefore, we must employ a better strategy. The most effective strategy we have discovered is rotation of the remedies in the following manner.

1. Take Borrelogen for two months.
2. Take Lymogen for two months (Trade steps 1 and 2 and start the protocol with Lymogen if Bartonella is also a concern.)
3. Switch to Microbojen for two months.
4. If you are still struggling with Lyme symptoms, take the Borrelogen and Lymogen <u>at the same time</u> for 2 months. If you choose this step, do not reduce doses –

use the same recommended doses for taking either separately or together.

By this time in following the protocol, along with employing the rest of this book, you should be well on your way towards the quality of life you seek. Even if you feel dramatically better soon after beginning this protocol, it is not wise to discontinue this plan, since history has shown us that most people who feel better early on and quit the treatments experience a reoccurrence of their symptoms, and their blood tests remain positive for Lyme.

Borrelogen™

Borrelogen is a frequency-matched botanical formula specifically tailored to provide the body with the bio-information needed to facilitate the body's own energetic antimicrobial control mechanisms. Borrelogen was frequency-matched to address the body's needs to deal with multiple strains of Borrelia burgdorferi, both U.S. and European. It factors in the many pleomorphic phases, such as cystic or L-form. Also factored into this one remedy are the common co-infections, such as Babesia microti, Ehrlichia, and Rocky-Mountain Spotted fever. The independent laboratory testing of Borrelogen conclusively demonstrated its Lyme antigen-releasing ability to be far superior to any commonly seen with antibiotic therapy. (Lyme antigens are the dead pieces of Borrelia bacteria appearing and counted in urine.) This research on Borrelogen is provided in Appendix G. Borrelogen was also tested by an independent pharmaceutical laboratory to be non-toxic up to 150 times the maximum recommended dosage. This "Acute Oral Toxicity" test was performed by Toxicon Laboratories, in Bedford, Massachusetts, on male and female rats, following standardized FDA protocols.

Recommended Borrelogen Dosage:
- Teens-Adults: Squeeze 1-2 droppers (one dropper = one squeeze) of Borrelogen under the tongue, swish it around the teeth, and swallow, 3 times per day with or without food.
- 7-12 years of age use 1 dropper, 2-3 times per day.
- Use 10 drops, 2-3 times per day for children under 6 years of age. Always consult your natural health professional before starting any child on any herbal formula.

Borrelogen contains the following botanical ingredients, each of which is added to the formula based upon Bio-Resonance testing, instead of based upon a plant's known actions or historical uses. "Flat-earth" herbalists will likely be confounded by this formula since very few of the herbs in this formula have any direct antibiotic effect. Remember, it is the cumulative frequency spectrum that works to restore the body, not to "bomb" the bacteria, which never works.

Borrelogen ingredients: Phragmites communis rhizome, Morus alba leaf, Baptisia bractiata, Fiddle-leaf fig folium, Chrysanthemum moritolium flower, Platycodon grandiflorum root, Prunum armeniaca kernel, Glycerrhiza uralensis root, Baptisia australis, Mentha hapocalyx, Ophiopogon tuber, Una-de-gato, Morus rubra fruit, Cuscuta, Scindapsis aureus, Ipomoea quamoclit, Dracaena dermensis, Crystal Clear™ distilled water and 20% pharmaceutical grade alcohol.

If taken as directed within the Perfect-7 protocol, virtually no Herxheimer reaction should be expected, even by extremely sensitive people. However, sensitive individuals may want to work up the recommended dosage, starting with only a few drops to see how your body reacts before increasing the amount. If you feel worse, your organs of elimination likely are not working well and need to be supported. This is why it is important to follow the detoxification recommendations outlined in Step 2.

If you are feeling worse upon starting any appropriate and effective Lyme treatment, it is likely due to the increased movement of Lyme toxins from bacterial die-off. This problem is often remedied by significantly increasing your dosage of Neuro-Antitox II Formula™, which should <u>always</u> be taken with Borrelogen, in order to break down and bind up more of these toxins. Incorporating all of the steps in the detoxification part of the Perfect-7 protocol will greatly minimize aggravating symptoms from increased toxins and weakness in the tissues of the body. The less Lyme toxins you have, the fewer symptoms you should experience. Of course, there remains the possibility with all drugs and all natural remedies that a true allergic reaction may be occurring if you feel very poorly during a treatment. Only a trained health care professional can determine if what you are experiencing is an allergic reaction, drug toxicity reaction, or if the aggravation is from weaknesses in the organs of elimination.

Lymogen™

I developed Lymogen™ due to the increased demand for a frequency-matched remedy that would provide the body with the bio-information necessary to facilitate the body's integrity when dealing with all of the various U.S. and European strains of Lyme Borrelia, all the normal Lyme co-infections, as well as varioubsed upon the presence of any antibiotic-like herbs, but upon the complex and synergistic frequencies of the combination of herbs. Keep in mind that when I am speaking of complex frequency spectrum, it should be understood that all medicines, pharmaceutical and natural, broadcast their unique frequencies based upon their specific molecular structure. Even Rife machines are based upon broadcasting frequencies.

Step 1: Restore the Body's Regulation of Microbes

Of course it should be understood that there is so much more to restoring health than killing bacteria. Simply broadcasting a cookbook set of frequencies, one frequency at a time or even five or six frequencies at a time, is like saying you can speak French when all you know is, "Bon Jour." To restore the optimum bio-communications of the body, one must broadcast all of the bio-information necessary on all levels.

The incredible range of frequencies found in each of the different herbal combinations in the Lymogen™, Borrelogen™, and Microbojen™ combine to answer every question and issue the body might have, in order to create perfect integrity throughout the entire body when challenged by these microbes. Using frequency-matched remedies is like speaking French fluently, using precise grammar and perfect word choice as well. No other formulations in the world are developed from this philosophy.

Borrelogen™ has a longer history of clinical experience, but Lymogen™ is exciting because it is incorporating all the advanced understanding I have gained over the last nine years since the first development of Borrelogen. Lymogen is a completely unique remedy which, when rotated with Borrelogen, provides an amazing "one-two punch" that is unsurpassed in its promoting of long-term health.

Lymogen™ Ingredients: Extracts of Fructus Bruceae, Lycium chinense root bark, Portulaca oleracea herb, Aloe vera juice powder, Salvia miltiorrhiza root, White Peony Root, Scuttellaria root, Coptis chinensis rhizome, Oldenlandia herb, Dioscoria opposite rhizome, Fresh Ginger rhizome, 5% Apple Cider Vinegar.

Recommended Dosage: Always put in water or juice.
- Teens-Adults: Squeeze 1-2 droppers (one dropper = one squeeze) in 3-4 ounces of water or diluted juice, swish it around the mouth, and swallow, 3 times per day with or without food.

- 7-12 years of age use 1 dropper in 3-4 ounces of water or diluted juice, 2-3 times per day.
- Use 10 drops in 1-2 ounces of water or diluted juice, 2-3 times per day for children under 6 years of age. Always consult your natural health professional before starting any child on any herbal formula.

Adverse Reactions

If taken as directed within the Perfect-7 protocol, virtually no Herxheimer (toxin die-off) reaction should be expected, even by extremely sensitive people. However, sensitive individuals may want to work up the recommended dosage, starting with only a few drops to see how your body reacts before increasing the amount. If you feel worse, your organs of elimination likely are not working well and need to be supported. This is why it is important to follow the detoxification recommendations outlined in Step 2.

If you are feeling worse upon starting any appropriate and effective Lyme treatment, it is likely due to the increased movement of Lyme toxins from bacterial die-off. This problem is often remedied by significantly increasing your dosage of Neuro-Antitox II Formula™, which should <u>always</u> be taken with Borrelogen, in order to break down and bind up more of these toxins. Incorporating all of the steps in the detoxification part of the Perfect-7 protocol will greatly minimize aggravating symptoms from increased toxins and weakness in the tissues of the body. The less Lyme toxins you have, the fewer symptoms you should experience. Of course, there remains the possibility with all drugs and all natural remedies that a true allergic reaction may be occurring if you feels very poorly during a treatment. Only a trained health care professional can determine if what you are experiencing is an allergic reaction, drug toxicity reaction, or if the aggravation is from weaknesses with the organs of elimination.

Microbojen™

Microbojen is the broadest-acting formula I have developed. The spectrum and complexity of the microbes factored into this frequency-matched formula far surpasses any real-life scenario of possible infection, short of biological warfare. It is a well-balanced and gentle formula for all of its power in facilitating the body's own integrity in the presence of an amazing array of the world's worst microbes.

Recommended Dosages:
- Teens-adults: Take 1-2 droppers, 2-3 times per day in water, with or without food.
- 7-13 years of age: 1 dropper, 2 times per day in water.
- Use 10 drops, 2-3 times per day for children under 6 years of age. Always consult your natural health professional before starting any child on any herbal formula.

Like all of the Jernigan Nutraceuticals formulas, Microbojen™ is frequency-matched to provide the body with the information and building blocks it needs to overcome and control specific problems. None of the formulations of Lymogen™, Borrelogen™, or Microbojen™ treat disease in the classic sense of the term. They are not "antibiotics," although they provide the body with the specific informational frequencies needed to overcome and control microbes. They are instead designed to work with God's design of the human body, instead of "doing for the body what the body should do for itself," as most prescription drugs do.

Microbojen was initially developed in an effort to prepare for the worst-case scenario of biological warfare. Bio-Resonance Scanning™ was used to simulate the worst condition we could think of. We simulated that "if" a person had, all at the same time, the following microbes, what corrective frequencies would the body need to overcome them?

We tested for a hypothetical person infected with Lyme Borrelia, smallpox, anthrax, HIV, hepatitis B and C, West Nile Virus, Epstein-Barr Virus (EBV), Cytomegalovirus (CMV), Mycoplasma fermentans incognitus, and Bubonic plaque, *all at the same time.*

Obviously, this is an unlikely event; however, by formatting the test for such a condition, it is likely that the resulting botanical formula, Microbojen, will be highly effective against a wide range of the world's worst "designer microbes." The end result of this research, Microbojen, just so happens to test amazingly well against an equally evil microbe -- Lyme spirochetes and their partners, Babesia microti, Ehrlichia, and the many viruses found in chronic sufferers.

Microbojen ingredients: Tragopogon (tota), Isatis root, Lasiosphaera fungus, Scrophularia root, Oldenlandia herb, Moutan peony bark, Phellodendron bark, Poria cocos sclerotium, Glycerrhiza uralensis, Crystal Clear™ Distilled Water, and 20% pharmaceutical-grade alcohol.

Step 2
Detoxify Lyme Toxins

13

~

Neuro-Antitox II Formulas™

These Neuro-Antitox products were developed to detoxify the body of the Lyme-related toxins. This is a must-have for any type of treatment to limit feeling worse from the bacterial die-off (Herxheimer reactions). You may select the specific formula you need based upon where your worst symptoms are -- nerves and brain (Neuro-Antitox II CNS/PNS), muscle and joint pain (Neuro-Antitox II Musculo-Skeletal), heart symptoms (Neuro-Antitox II) or the Basic Formula. As a general recommendation, take 1-3 droppers, 2-3 times per day, with or without food. It may be that you have to use more than one formula if there are problems in multiple areas, in which case 1-2 droppers are recommended from each corresponding Formula.

Recommended Dosages:
- Teens-adults: Take 1-2 droppers under the tongue, 2-3 times per day, 10 minutes away from food or drink.
- 7-13 years of age: 1 dropper, 2 times per day.
- Use 10 drops, 2-3 times per day for children under 6 years of age. Always consult your natural health

professional before starting any child on any herbal formula.

Neuro-Antitox II CNS/PNS™

CNS/PNS is for those suffering primarily from problems in the brain, meninges, and peripheral nerves from Lyme toxins and heavy metals. Indications include, but are not limited to, cognitive disturbances, dizziness, vertigo, disturbances in vision, neuritis (nerve inflammation), neuralgia (nerve pain), numbness, palsies, and headaches.

Ingredients: Silphium laciniatum extract, Pale Spike Lobelia extract, sarco-bioenergetic potencies in P6, 12, and 30 of cerebrospinal fluid, dura mater, cerebellum, optic nerve, substantia nigra, cerebral cortex, cranial nerve VIII (vestibulocochlear n.), myelencephalon, temporal lobe, occipital lobe, quadrigeminal plate, lumbar plexus, brachial plexus, periodontium, Crystal Clear™ Distilled Water, and pharmaceutical-grade alcohol.

Neuro-Antitox II Musculo-Skeletal™

Musculo-Skeletal is for those suffering primarily from muscle and joint problems as the result of Lyme toxins and heavy metals. Indications: Muscle and joint pain and weakness, sensations in the extremities of burning, tingling, radiating pain, swelling, arthritic, and rheumatic conditions.

Ingredients: Silphium laciniatum extract, Pale Spike Lobelia extract, sarcobioenergetic potencies in P-6, 12, and 30 of connective issue/fascia, cartilage, intervertibral joints (cervical, thoracic, and lumbar), humoral joint, elbow joint, intercarpal joints, knee joint, interphalangeal joint, bamboo, rhus toxicodendron, Crystal Clear™ Distilled Water, and 20% pharmaceutical grade alcohol.

Neuro-Antitox II Cardio™

Use Cardio for those suffering primarily from heart problems from Lyme toxins and heavy metals. Indications: angina, palpitations, hypertension, arrhythmia, valve problems, shoulder and arm pain, shortness of breath, chronic fatigue.

Ingredients: Silphium laciniatum extract, Pale Spike Lobelia extract, sarcobioenergetic potencies in P6, 12, and 30 of cardiac plexus, cardia, myocardium, endocardium, mitral valve, tricuspid valve, and aorta. Other ingredients: Crystal Clear™ Distilled Water, and 20% pharmaceutical grade alcohol.

Neuro-Antitox II Basic™

The Basic formula is good for global detoxification of the Lyme toxins, heavy metals, and for those who are unsure which specific Neuro-Antitox II Formula to take. This formula does not contain any sarcobioenergetic potencies.

Ingredients: Silphium laciniatum extract and Pale Spike Lobelia extract, Crystal Clear™ Distilled Water, and 20% pharmaceutical-grade alcohol.

The chief ingredient in all of these formulas is a novel-use botanical, Silphium laciniatum. Out of 5000 different natural botanicals, minerals, nutraceuticals, and pharmaceuticals tested using Bio-Resonance Scanning™, Silphium tested superior to them all for detoxifying the Lyme-specific neurotoxins. The Neuro-Antitox II formulas also contain the next best substance identified as a synergistic (supportive) botanical along with the Silphium, Pale -- Spike Lobelia. The only difference between the Musculo-Skeletal, and CNS/PNS formulas is the use of Sarco-bioenergetic Potencies™, which may act as driving agents (to direct the Silphium and Pale Spike to the specific tissues where they are needed, instead of just circulating around the body randomly).

The Basic formula does not have any of these Sarcobioenergetic Potencies™ and is therefore good when you are not sure which formula you need, or for more global symptoms.

The combined effect of these key ingredients makes the Neuro-Antitox II Formulas an absolute necessity in any well-rounded treatment plan.

To minimize any Herxheimer reaction, I recommend that Neuro-Antitox II dietary supplement be taken for at least one week before beginning any antibiotic or other medical/alternative treatment. Remember, Herxheimer reactions are caused by toxins, and the Neuro-Antitox II Formulas are designed to mop up, bind up, and break down these Lyme-related toxins to eliminate any adverse reactions to the Lyme bacteria die-offs.

Besides Silphium laciniatum's function as an amazing anti-neurotoxin, it was successfully used in times long passed to treat various cancers, all forms of asthma, and bronchitis, and it was effective in breaking down mucus in the tissues. Resonance testing reveals that Silphium may also bind heavy metals and break down isopropyl alcohol and benzene accumulations, adding to its phenomenal arsenal of beneficial effects.[125]

Overall detoxification can be supported by simply drinking eight ounces of purified water every hour to keep the everyday metabolic toxins flushed out of the tissues. Some patients have difficulty drinking water, so putting fresh lemon juice or Ningxia Red™ wolfberry juice in the cool (but not cold) water makes it easier to drink more water per day.

14

~

Dr. Jernigan's Detox Coffee™, Detox Tea™, and Detox Cocoa™

Dr. Jernigan's Detox Coffee™

Since coffee is one of the world's favorite beverages, it was my desire to develop a proprietary detoxification formula that actually tastes like coffee, while gently detoxifying all of the major organ systems of the body. It is designed to be gentle enough to use two servings per day and detoxify the body gradually.

It is caffeinated to help stimulate the rapid transit of waste out of the colon. Caffeinated coffee achieves this through stimulating peristalsis, the wave-like movement in the muscular walls of the large intestines that pushes fecal material out. Those people wishing to avoid caffeine should opt for the Detox Herbal tea or Detox Cocoa.

While the Neuro-Antitox II™ Formulas are the primary detoxification remedies for Lyme-specific toxins, they are not designed to support all the organs of elimination like the Detox Coffee, Tea, or Cocoa.

Ingredients: Coffee, Natural coffee flavor, Milk ext., Red clover extract, Dandelion ext., Black Walnut Hulls, Artichoke ext., L- Glutathione, N-Acetyl Cysteine, Grape seed ext., L-Carnitine Fumarate, Schisandra ext., Shavegrass ext., Vitamin C, Bladderwack, Whole Aloe Powder, Cascara Sagrada ext., Papaya leaf, Inositol, Citrus Bioflavonoid, L-Methionine, Rutin, Choline, Slippery Elm Bark, Marshmallow Root Pwd, Artemesia Powder, Pau D' Arco powder, Gentian Root, Senna leaf ext., Buckthorn Bark, Alpha Liporic Acid.

Dr. Jernigan's Detox Herb Tea™

This tasty, naturally decaffeinated, herbal tea is designed to gently, but efficiently, detoxify the body and promote a healthy immune system. Two servings a day is all a person should need to receive the healing benefits of this beverage.

Ingredients: Hibiscus flower, Dandelion root, slippery elm bark, Burdock root, Red clover flower, Alfalfa, Rose hip, Milk thistle, Yellow dock root, Siberian ginseng, Chamomile flower, Echinacea augustifolia root, Corn silk, Sarsaparilla, Chicory root, Licorice root, Ginger, Cascara Sagrada, and Shavegrass.

Dr. Jernigan's Detox Cocoa™

Not everyone is a coffee or tea lover, so I developed the Detox Cocoa for the chocolate lover. All of the same ingredients found in the Detox Coffee are in this formula as well, except cocoa was substituted for the coffee, and I added Stevia extract as a sweetener.

I didn't use just cocoa in the formula, but I also added concentrated Cocoa Polyphenols to boost the healing quality. Cocoa Polyphenols are the primary ingredient that has been shown by research to create all the healing properties in dark chocolate. Cocoa polyphenols improve health by:

(1) Improving blood flow, via vasodilation,
(2) Reducing Platelet aggregation,

(3) Improving insulin sensitivity,
(4) Improving cognitive performance, by increasing blood flow to gray matter,
(5) Possibly reducing overall mortality from all causes, and
(6) Acting as antioxidants.[126]

Ingredients: Cocoa powder, Cocoa Polyphenols, Milk ext., Red clover extract, Dandelion ext., Black Walnut Hulls, Artichoke ext., L- Glutathione, N-Acetyl Cysteine, Grape seed ext., L-Carnitine Fumarate, Schisandra ext., Shavegrass ext., Vitamin C, Bladderwack, Whole Aloe Powder, Cascara Sagrada ext., Papaya leaf, Inositol, Citrus Bioflavonoid, L-Methionine, Rutin, Choline, Slippery Elm Bark, Marshmallow Root Pwd, Artemisia Powder, Pau D' Arco powder, Gentian Root, Senna leaf ext., Buckthorn Bark, Alpha Liporic Acid, Stevia extract.

15

~

Dry Skin Brushing for Enhancing Skin Elimination

Your skin is the largest eliminative organ. Healthy skin should eliminate two pounds of waste acids every day. Skin brushing before dressing, and before every bath, will remove the top layer of dead skin that would otherwise block the effective elimination of toxins through the skin.

You can look closely at the iris (colored part of the eyes) in the mirror and tell how well your skin is eliminating. If you can see a darker ring around the very most outer edge of the iris, you have what is called a scurf ring. Seeing a scurf ring always indicates that your skin is not eliminating toxins well, and it is being reflected on the iris of the eye. It is not a disease of the eye but simply a reflex sign of an overload of toxins at the level of the skin. You can observe your eye and watch it improve as you progress with your detox protocol.

You will need:
- Natural Fiber Skin Brush with a long handle. (NEVER USE A SYNTHETIC BRISTLE BRUSH -- these can cause an adverse electrical charge on the body.)

Instructions:

- Use this brush dry, without any soaps or water, prior to bathing or dressing. It should take you about 5 minutes or so, brushing your entire body, except the face.
- Brush in all directions, but generally moving towards the heart. Imagine you are brushing the lymph fluid up from your feet, up the legs toward your heart.
- Do the same with the upper body, starting at the hands and moving lymph fluid up the arm towards the shoulder and on to the heart.
- Reach to the lower back area and brush the lymph up the spine and sides, moving it up and over the shoulders to the heart.
- Your skin may at first be very sensitive, and you may think that you are scratching and hurting the skin. Make sure you are not damaging the skin, but after a week or so of doing this you will usually find that it feels good.
- You may be able to find a special face brush to use on your face.

16

~

Infrared Sauna Therapy

There are not many therapies that can equal the vast range of healing benefits than is documented with infrared sauna therapy. Studies from all over the world report such a wide range of illnesses that are benefited by this therapy that to include a complete list would requires several pages. Some of the conditions benefited are listed below.

In the realm of assisting chronic or frequently occuring infectious illness, infrared sauna therapy is a vital part of any good treatment program. This is because of its ability to detoxify the body of heavy metals and toxins that are locked up in the fat cells.

Heavy metals and toxins are known to promote an environment in the body that is a microbe heaven. They cause overcooling of the body, hypersensitivities and allergic tendencies, and direct toxic effects on the body as a whole.

When many people hear the word "sauna," they immediately conjure up images of steamy sweat rooms that are intensely and uncomfortably hot. Infrared saunas are nothing like the old steam or dry convection heat saunas. Infrared saunas operate from between 100°F and 130°F, which is still very comfortable for most people, compared to the intense heat of traditional saunas (180° F to 235° F).

While studying Biological Medicine, I was impressed to find that some of the world's most successful Biological Medicine Hospitals and Clinics in Germany, Switzerland, and the U.S. use the infrared saunas for almost all of their patients. In today's highly toxic world, there is almost no person who would not benefit tremendously from the health promoting effects of this therapy.

Infrared saunas work by emitting far infrared energy, which penetrates the body just over four and a half inches! The deep penetration of heat is much more efficient than traditional saunas.

Infrared is a fascinating technology. Scientific research has now resulted in saunas that emit a finely tuned infrared energy output that closely matches the body's own radiant energy. What this means is that almost 93% of the infrared waves are absorbed into the body. With this much absorption of the infrared waves, the body heats up, but the air in the sauna remains cooler. The cooler environment of the sauna is much more pleasant to sit in, and the air is not so hot to breathe.

So many of the chronically ill patients I see know that they should work out and do aerobic exercise as part of living a balanced life; however, the illness they suffer usually prevents them from performing truly meaningful workouts. Many are too sick, too tired, too depressed, too overweight, in too much pain to work out, or working out would cause them to feel even worse. If you are one of these people, I've got exciting news for you! In 30 minutes of sitting, infrared sauna therapy has been shown to burn up to 250% more calories than spending 30 intense minutes on the best aerobic exercises, rowing machines, and long-distance marathons. It not only burns more calories, but it has also been shown to have many of the same cardiovascular benefits as well!

Rowing and running marathons, the best aerobic exercises in the world, will burn 600 calories in 30 minutes at their peak. Sitting in an infrared sauna for 30 minutes can burn 900-2400 calories! Just one infrared session of 30 minutes could burn the equivalent amount of calories as running six to nine miles!

So who do you know that would benefit from detoxification, weight management, cardiovascular conditioning, and increased rate of healing? Almost everyone!

Some of you may be wondering how infrared saunas can burn so many calories. According the Guyton's Medicinal Physiology textbook, the body requires 0.586 kilocalories (kcal) to produce 1 gram of sweat. An infrared sauna can cause a person to lose two to three times more sweat than a traditional sauna. The Journal of the American Medical Association reported that, "A moderately conditioned person can easily sweat off 500 grams in an infrared sauna, consuming nearly 300 kcal – the equivalent of running two to three miles. A heat conditioned person can easily sweat off 600-800 kcal with no adverse effect. While the weight of water loss can be regained by rehydration, the calories consumed will not be."[127] For those needing more convincing, note that NASA, after extensive research, determined in the 1980's that infrared stimulation would be the ideal way to maintain cardiovascular conditioning of astronauts in the weightless environment of space during the long space flights.

I use the infrared saunas on almost all my patients. Most people are fine with 30-minutes sessions three or more times per week for several months, or year-round. Some people who feel they are coming down with a cold may benefit from staying up to one hour.

People with heart disease are concerned that they cannot get in the sauna. Researchers in Finland report that there is abundant evidence to suggest that blood vessels of regular sauna-goers remain elastic and pliable longer due to the regular dilation and contraction of blood vessels induced by sauna use. As a matter of fact, German researchers found in type I and II essential hypertension (high blood pressure) that after a session in the infrared sauna, each person had a significant decrease in arterial, venous, and mean blood pressure that lasted for at least 24 hours. This finding is thought to be from the persistent dilation of peripheral blood vessels, and also due to the improvement of the viscosity (liquidity) of the blood.[128]

Research performed in the U.S., Germany, Japan, and China has shown infrared sauna therapy to benefit people suffering from the conditions listed below. (This benefits people, not diseases. Biological Medicine only treats people, since it is understood now that to treat the disease does not work as effectively.) Always seek the advice of a healthcare professional before starting any therapy.

If you choose to purchase your own, our favorite saunas are made by High Tech Health. Their company uses poplar wood that will not outgas during the prolonged heat of the sauna. The Paracelsus Klinik of Switzerland, famous for high-quality cancer treatment, also uses this same brand of sauna, and we highly respect their health opinions.

The following pages list conditions that have been benefited by use of the infrared sauna.

Infrared Sauna has helped people with:

- Acne/Blackheads
- Arthritis
- Asthma
- Backache
- Bell's Palsy
- Benign Prostatic Hypertrophy
- Brain damage (accelerated healing of)
- Bronchitis
- Bursitis
- Cancer
- Cancer pain
- Children's overtired muscles
- Chron's Disease
- Chronic Fatigue Syndrome
- Cirrhosis
- Colds/flu
- Cold hands and feet
- Cholecysitis (inflammation of the gallbladder)
- Cystitis
- Dandruff
- Diabetes
- Diarrhea
- Duodenal ulcers
- Ear diseases
- Ear infections (acute and chronic otitis media)
- Eczema with infection
- Edema
- Electromagnetic pollution (effects improved)
- Exudates
- Fibromyalgia
- Gastritis
- Gastroenteric problems
- Gout arthritis
- Headaches

- Heavy metal toxicity (i.e., mercury, cadmium, lead, aluminum)
- Hemorrhoids
- Hepatitis
- Hypertension (high blood pressure)
- Hypotension (low blood pressure)
- Inflammatory conditions and infiltrates
- Keloids
- Leg and decubital ulcers
- Low core body temperature
- Lyme Borreliosis
- Nervous tension
- Neurasthenia
- Neuritis
- Nosebleeds (reduced)
- Obesity
- Pediatric pneumonia
- Pelvic infections
- Peripheral Occulsive Disease
- Post-surgical infections
- PMS and menopausal symptoms
- Pneumonia
- Rheumatoid Arthritis
- Sciatica
- Short-term memory loss (improved)
- Skin tone (improved)
- Sore throats
- Strained muscles
- Stretch marks
- Tinea (fungal infections)
- Tinitus (ringing of the ears)
- TMJ
- Trigger points (relieved)
- Varicose veins

17

~

Dr. Joseph's Colon Cleanse™

Dr. Joseph developed this product after years of clinic patients using a very basic coffee enema recipe. This recipe is also now bottled for your convenience. Some of the ingredients are difficult to find unless you have a large health food store nearby, and when purchased individually they can be expensive and of questionable "therapeutic" potency. For all of these reasons and for consistency of action, Dr. Joseph decided to have her own recipe packaged for your and my convenience

However, we will give you the exact recipe for those of you who would rather get started using your own ingredients.

If you are using **Dr. Joseph's Colon Cleanse**™ kit, simply follow the instructions on the label.

To make your own recipe at home:
- Combine and stir gently all the ingredients listed below in a stainless steel pot or glass container.
- Cover for 4 hours at room temperature.
- Over very low heat, bring the liquid to 98 degrees (use a thermometer).
- Remove from heat, strain and pour into enema bucket for immediate use.

Combine the following:
- 4 cups of room temperature, distilled water
- 2 tsp. organic, raw (green and unroasted), ground coffee
- 3 Milk Thistle teabags (available from most health food stores)
- 11 drops Liquid Iodine (made by Biotics Research) -- except for people with Iodine allergies
- 2 Tablespoons Liquid Chlorophyll or fresh wheat grass juice
- 2000 Mcg of liquid B12 (ideally in the form of Methylcobalamin)
- 1 tablet broad-spectrum probiotic (ideally pick a product that has six or more different types of temperature- and pH-stable, friendly flora)
- Do not exceed more than three of these colon cleanses per week. Maximum benefit is likely achieved after using this cleanse for three weeks.
- Repeat every two to three months.
- <u>Do not use if you have a known allergy to any of the ingredients.</u>

Supplies you will need:
- 1 Enema bucket or bag with hose
- K-Y Jelly (A lubricant available in any pharmacy)

Dr. Joseph's Protocol:
- **Read the complete protocol listed here before you begin.**
- Start the Colon Cleanse on a weekend or day off from work.
- Add 2 teaspoons of ground, unroasted, organic coffee (not instant or decaffeinated) to 4 cups of distilled water. Boil for 5 minutes uncovered to drive off oils,

then add the 3 teabags of Milk Thistle, cover, lower heat, and simmer for an additional 15 minutes.
- Strain and allow liquid to cool to body temperature. (Test temperature on forearm to be sure.) Add the remaining ingredients and mix thoroughly.
- Pour mixture into enema bag. Lubricate rectal enema tube with K-Y Jelly.
- Hang enema bag above you but not more than 2 feet from your body. The best level is approximately 6 inches above the intestines.
- Lying on your right side, draw both legs close to the abdomen. It may be best to lay on a towel to catch any spillage or leakage.
- Gently insert tube no more than 3 inches into rectum (for an adult).
- Open the stopcock and allow fluid to flow into the colon very slowly to avoid cramping. Relax and breathe deeply to let liquid flow in. If you feel that you cannot take in very much fluid, it may indicate that the liquid is too cold. You also may want to release into a toilet what you cannot hold in any longer.
- Take in the rest of the fluid when possible. Often fear causes us to clamp down at the rectum. Relax and purposely ease the stress by concentrating on your steady breathing.
- Retain the solution for 12-15 minutes. It can help to have a book or magazine to distract yourself so time doesn't do that trick of standing still! If you have trouble retaining or taking the full amount, lower the enema bucket/bag to the floor to relieve the pressure.
- Watch the tube for backwashing. If this occurs, close the stopcock and raise the enema bucket a little. Relax further, open the stopcock, and feel yourself allow in the fluid. After about 20 seconds, slowly start raising the bag toward the original level. You can also pinch the tube to control the flow.

- Release into the toilet.
- Upon waking the next morning, if you experience headache and/or drowsiness, you may drink a cup of Dr. Jernigan's Detox Coffee™, Detox Tea™, or Detox Cocoa™, and/or do Dr. Jernigan's Mustard Foot Bath™ to detoxify the body even further.
- Keep all equipment perfectly clean between sessions.

Facts concerning Dr. Joseph's Colon Cleanse

The unroasted, organic coffee in this colon cleanse helps to purge the colon and liver of accumulated toxins, dead cells, and waste products. Roasted coffee has been subjected to a lot of heat, and therefore much of the medicinal ingredients have been destroyed by the heat.

The rectal use of coffee may seem strange at first, but research by Max Gerson, M.D., reveals that the coffee enema is effective in stimulating a complex enzyme system involved with liver detoxification (called the glutathione-S-transferase enzyme system). During the coffee enema, there is a 600% increase in the activity of this enzyme system, which ensures that free-radical activity is greatly reduced and that the activity of any carcinogens is blocked.[129] Dr. Gerson used coffee enemas as a routine therapy for many hundreds of cancer patients. He later started the Gerson Institute, which is still in operation today, serving the chronically ill. While not a cancer treatment, the coffee enemas serve a very important purpose in gently enabling the body to detoxify itself, and therefore increase the survivabililty and quality of life of everyone using it.

Coffee is known to contain choleretics, which are substances that increase the flow of toxin-rich bile from the gallbladder. The coffee enema is thought to be among the only pharmaceutically-effective choleretics noted in the medical literature that can be safely used many times daily without toxic effects.

The **Milk Thistle tea** is a botanical that has been shown to protect the liver from toxins. The active constituents of milk thistle are known collectively as silymarin. Silymarin is believed to function to protect liver cells from toxins by binding to liver cells, acting as an antioxidant and scavenger of free radicals, and stabilizing liver cell membranes. It is said to be able to reverse some of the fatty deposits of lipotrophic toxins that lead to greatly diminished liver function. Milk Thistle may help the liver tolerate toxic medications when these medications cannot be avoided.

Vitamin B12 (Methylcobalamine) is a form of B12 that is more protective and specific to restoring optimal neurological functions. There are other forms of B12 that are more common in supplements, such as cyanocobalamine and adenosylcobalamine; however, only the methylcobalamine seems to direct its action so willingly on the brain and nervous system. It may directly or indirectly facilitate the detoxification of neurotoxins.

Probiotics are a generalized name for friendly bacteria, also known as the intestinal flora. Many people are familiar with the common probiotic called Acidophilus. While it is great to supplement with acidophilus bacteria, such as is in natural, cultured yoghurt, it is definitely not enough to replace this one type of friendly bacteria. It must be understood that when a patient is on antibiotics, as many as 400 different strains of friendly bacteria are killed by the drug. By "friendly," I mean that the bacteria help digest your food and actually produce chemical substances which you absolutely should never be without. Recent research has shown that the friendly bacteria actually modulate your immune responses, produce enzymes that can eliminate lactose intolerance, stop diarrhea, fight rotaviruses and other viruses, and stop food allergies, eczema, and asthma by stimulating interleukin and TH1 cells. Most pertinent to this book is that friendly bacteria can actually block and break down potent toxins in the sinuses and gut![130]

18

~

Hydrogen Peroxide/ Epsom Salt Detox Bath

This is one of my absolute favorite bath therapies. It is the first thing we do for our own family whenever we feel we are developing a cold or illness. Not only does it detoxify the body and relieve pain, but it seems to also stop many infections quickly and help the body regain balance. Through medical studies, this therapy has been shown to relieve pain that did not even respond to narcotic medicines.

You will need:
- 4-6 cups Epsom Salt (Magnesium Sulfate)
- 32 to 64 fluid Ounces of Hydrogen Peroxide (3%, as found in grocery stores)
- 2-4 Tablespoons of Ginger (fresh grated preferably, wrapped in a thin piece of cloth or in a tea ball. An old piece of nylon hose also works well.)

Instructions:
- This and all bath therapies work best by first dry skin brushing the entire body (see Chapter 15, Dry Skin Brushing). This removes the layer of dead skin that may otherwise block the absorption of energy and nutrients from this bath and stimulates the blood and lymph fluids to rise to the skin to accept the healing effects of the bath.
- Fill tub with warm water. Add the above ingredients.
- Soak for at least 20 minutes. The beneficial effects of this bath are cumulative and increase in effectiveness the more you use them.
- Recommended taken for at least seven consecutive days, or as recommended by your doctor. Continued use daily, or as needed, is fine.
- **Do not use if you are pregnant.**

Actions of Bath Ingredients

- **Hydrogen Peroxide** – a simple, nontoxic molecule of H_2O_2 that is beneficial in oxidizing (breaking down) toxins as well as killing anaerobic microbes. It will also detoxify pesticides and petroleum-based toxins and oxidize metals. Hydrogen peroxide is also naturally produced by macrophages in the body to kill harmful bacteria. Most harmful bacteria are anaerobic and cannot survive in the presence of oxygen or hydrogen peroxide. Cancer cells are often very sensitive to increases in oxygen and cannot survive in oxygen-rich environments. When hydrogen peroxide is applied topically to a cut, the resulting bubbling is from the rapid release of free oxygen and, more importantly, from the killing of the bacteria in the cut. Friendly bacteria are aerobic and need and thrive on oxygen.
- **Epsom Salts (Magnesium Sulfate)** – Recent research has shown that when one soaks in a bath of magnesium

sulfate, both magnesium and the sulfate independently increase measurably in the blood and urine. Magnesium sulfate helps stabilize Hydrogen Peroxide so that its ultimate breakdown into H_2O and free oxygen is more gradual and functional to the process of benefiting the body. This research documents the very real beneficial aspects of this bath therapy. The Epsom Salt Council reports the following about the benefits of Magnesium in Epsom Salt baths.

- **Magnesium**, a major component of Epsom Salt (magnesium sulfate), is the second-most abundant element in human cells and the fourth-most important positively charged ion in the body. Magnesium also helps to regulate the activity of more than 325 enzymes and performs a vital role in orchestrating many bodily functions, from muscle control and electrical impulses to energy production and the elimination of harmful toxins. The National Academy of Sciences, however, reports that most Americans are magnesium deficient, which may account for our society's high rate of heart disease, stroke, osteoporosis, arthritis and joint pain, digestive maladies and stress-related illnesses, chronic fatigue and a host of other ailments. The Academy estimates the average American male gets just 80% of the magnesium required for good health, while females get only 70% of their recommended levels. Nutritionists say Americans' magnesium levels have dropped more than 50% in the past century.

Raising magnesium levels may:

> Improve heart and circulatory health, reducing irregular heartbeats, preventing

hardening of the arteries, reducing blood clots, and lowering blood pressure.
- Improve the body's ability to use insulin, reducing the incidence or severity of diabetes.
- Flush toxins and heavy metals from the cells, easing muscle pain and helping the body to eliminate harmful substances.
- Improve nerve function by regulating electrolytes. Also, calcium is the main conductor for electrical current in the body, and magnesium is necessary to maintain proper calcium levels in the blood.
- Relieve stress. Excess adrenaline and stress are believed to drain magnesium, a natural stress reliever, from the body. Magnesium is necessary for the body to bind adequate amounts of serotonin, a mood-elevating chemical within the brain that creates a feeling of wellbeing and relaxation.

o **Sulfate:** The "sulfate" part of Epsom Salt (magnesium *sulfate*). This form of sulfate must not be confused with "Sulfa" drugs, to which some people are allergic. People who are allergic to sulfa drugs will not react to the sulfate in Epsom Salt. The benefits of sulfate in the body are summarized by Dr. Rosemary Waring of the School of Biosciences, in Birmingham, England:[131]

- Oral supplementation of Sulfate cannot be easily absorbed across the gut walls; therefore, by soaking in this bath, sulfate can be more efficiently supplemented. Sulfate is essential for many biological processes.

- ➤ Sulfate is needed for formation of proteins in joints; decreased sulfate levels are common in the plasma and joint synovial fluids in cases of arthritis. Sulfate is also low in people with irritable bowel syndrome.[132,133]
- ➤ Sulfate in necessary for sulfation, a major pathway in detoxifying drugs and endogenous (toxins from within the body) or exogenous (environmental) toxins.
- ➤ Sulfate is necessary for the repair and formation of brain tissue. Reduced levels of sulfate can lead to faulty neurological connections and subsequent dysfunction.
- ➤ Sulfate is needed for proper digestion and for proper utilization of digestive enzymes.
- ➤ Sulfate is essential for the production of mucin, a protein which lines the intestines. Mucin stops food and drugs from sticking to the lining of the intestines. It also blocks the transport of toxins from the gut into the bloodstream.

- **Ginger** - functions to open up the pores of the skin and increase the blood flow at the surface of the skin, so that the oxygen from the hydrogen peroxide can do its work in detoxifying poisons and kill bacteria and fungi. The pores open wider so that the magnesium sulfate can be more readily absorbed. Ginger is invigorating and can stimulate perspiration for the elimination of toxins.

19

~

Dr. Jernigan's Mustard Foot Bath™
May also be used as a Hand Soak

I developed this product after years of raiding the spice cabinet in my own kitchen for the ingredients for footbaths. Not only are kitchen spice bottles expensive, but they are generally small bottles and of questionable "therapeutic" potency. For all of these reasons and for consistency of action, I decided to have my own recipe bottled for our mutual convenience. I will also give you the recipe for those of you who would rather get started using your own spices. This is NOT recommended for use in a full body bath, due to the cayenne pepper in places you definitely don't want it!

Whisk or stir into warm (not hot) water to cover just above the ankles:
- 1 Tbsp. Dry Mustard Seed powder
- 1 tsp. Cayenne Pepper powder (Ideally use 90,000 heat units)
- ½ tsp. dry Ginger powder
- ½ tsp. dry Rosemary powder

This foot soak is used as relief from general aches and pains, toxic headaches, and overall toxic conditions. It also seems to increase blood and lymph circulation, as well as the overall sense of wellbeing. To get further results out of your mustard bath, you may either soak your hands only, or soak the hands immediately after completing the footbath using the same water.

Sit in a comfortable chair and soak your feet for 20-30 minutes in this mixture.

If following up with a mustard hand soak, rinse off and dry your feet then place the hands in the footbath water for another 20-30 minutes. You may do this 2-3 times per day if desired, for weeks to months, and definitely in periods of intense toxicity and pain.

Hot/Cold Contrast Mustard Foot Bath
Variation on Dr. Jernigan's Mustard Foot Bath™

The Contrast Mustard Foot Bath can be used to help stimulate the warmth organization of the body, resulting in the improvement of the body's core temperature. To use this therapy:
- Soak the feet in the warm ("just below hot") water of the Mustard Foot bath for one minute.
- Soak feet in cold water for 30 seconds.
- Repeat 3-5 times in a session, 2-3 times per day, for several weeks.

Note: It is important to your healing process to keep your feet warm at all times. To continue the warming effects of the contrast foot bath or the regular mustard foot bath, wear wool/silk blend socks.

20

~

Strengthening/Nutritive Bath

As its name implies, this bath can be very healing, especially in people with low vitality, low body temperature, and low reactivity. It is indicated for individuals with poor, slow, or no response to appropriately applied healing efforts. Often so much effort is given to detoxification that the body becomes strained and tired from being constantly challenged. This bath should be used at least once a week to assist the body in recouperating from this strain. Once again, this formulation is available as a product that I developed for the sake of convenience, but if you want to assemble it yourself, the recipe is below.

You will need:
- Goat milk – 1 quart to a half gallon (If raw milk is not available, pasteurized goat milk from the healthfood store is acceptable.)
- Sea Salt – 1 cup (preferably sun-evaporated)
- Succanat or turbinado sugar (raw cane sugar available from health food stores)
  1 cup (Optional: Replace with 1 cup of Ningxia Red™ Wolfberry juice)
- 1-2 egg yolks, beaten

- Lemon – 1
- Equisetum (Horsetail) herb powder – 3 tablespoons

* Optional -- Sip an 8 oz. glass of water mixed with 1-2 ounces of Ningxia Red™ Wolfberry juice while soaking in the bath. Wolfberry stimulates the anabolic metabolism (the building up of the tissues) and helps strengthen the body in times of exhaustion, convalescence and weakness. It is very beneficial, either diluted or undiluted, for infants who fail to thrive. Ningxia Red™ Wolfberry juice is the most concentrated form of wolfberry on the market. It has more different types of live enzymes than can be named, as well as many regenerative and strengthening properties. It is likely one of the top three of the most powerful antioxidants in the world, slowing the effects of aging in the cells and tissues in the body. It is consumed daily by the longest-living people in the world in the Ningxia Province of China.

* Bathing by candlelight can add to the soothing, balancing and strengthening effects of this bath.

Instructions:
- This and all bath therapies work best by first dry skin brushing the entire body (see Chapter 15, Dry Skin Brushing). This removes the layer of dead skin that may otherwise block the absorption of energy and nutrients from this bath and stimulates the blood and lymph fluids to rise to the skin to accept the bath.
- In a warm bath, add and whisk in the above ingredients; use extra if the tub is larger than standard.
- Score the skin of the lemon while holding it under the bath water to better release the oils, and then cut into quarters and squeeze out the juice, leaving the lemon quarters in the water.
- Soak for at least 20 minutes.

- Do not rinse off; simply towel dry (use no soap or shampoo).
- This bath can be used any time, but is most beneficial before bedtime since sleep is the time when the body focuses on healing, regenerating, and recouperating.

A good way to preserve the benefits of this bath after drying off is to apply Solum Uliginosum Oil (from the Wala company of Germany) all over the body. The peat and other ingredients in this phenomenal oil create a shield of sorts to protect the body from adverse electromagnetic and geopathic stress, thus preserving and retaining the healing energy of the bath.

It is a good idea for people of low vitality to do this bath just before going to bed, but may be equally beneficial to in the morning as well.

- Equisetum herb (Horsetail) contains about 29% nanoparticle silica -- silica in its purest form is quartz. The entire body is permeated by silica, but it is found in higher quantities in the sensory organs, skin, and connective tissue. Silica helps guide healing effects of the Nutritive bath across the skin and into to the body. Silica then directs these healing forces to where they are needed in the body. Silica brings light and warmth to the tissues, and indeed into the entire being. The nanoparticle silica of Equisetum has a healing effect primarily on the vitality-regulating mechanisms of the kidneys.

Eliminative Organ Support

The liver, kidneys, intestines, lungs, and skin are usually very overloaded in Lyme Disease. I recommend you use all of the various Detox Baths in this book. My favorite is the Epsom Salt/Hydrogen Peroxide Detox Bath for overall daily use, but listen to your own body to determine which one seems to work the best for you. Ideally, use the Strengthening/Nutritive Bath after every 4-5 Detox Baths. You may want to skip the Detox Baths for a few nights and add the Solum Uliginosum Oil or Rosemary oil to the water to revitalize your body since detoxifying can be tiring to the body.

Constipation and poor elimination is usually at the heart of the many symptoms related to toxins associated with Lyme Disease. Laxative tea combined with coffee enemas and skin brushing (see Chapters 14, 15, and 17) will greatly relieve this toxic condition. Remember, you were not completely well prior to being bit by whatever gave you Borrelia burgdorferi. Prior total body problems had to be present in order to manifest infectious disease. Also do the ilio-cecal Valve / Valve of Houston Reactivation 2-3 times per day (See therapies section).

Practice all of the principles in this book for balanced living in regard to the body, mind, and spirit. I recommend that you read this book several times, and keep reading it, until you know it inside and out and can apply all of the balanced living suggestions on a daily basis.

21

~

The Master Longevity Body Cleanse

There are few, if any, other total body cleanses that will do more good for you than this cleanse. I developed this cleanse protocol after years of using a modified version of a classic lemon juice, cayenne pepper, and grade-B Maple syrup recipe. This new cleanse still ultilizes lemon juice, cayenne pepper and grade-B Maple syrup, but it also incorporates Chinese wolfberry juice concentrate.

This longevity body cleanse program is light years better than the old "Master Cleanse." If you are going to spend the time and effort to do a cleanse of this type, you might as well benefit from more than simply cleansing the tissues. The potential for detoxifying *and* healing is so much greater, and now that I get excited just knowing my patients are starting this cleanse.

The new cleanse still provides the beneficial limonine from the lemons of the old Master Cleanse, but it also provides the therapeutic-grade lemon oil added in the Wolfberry Ningxia Red Juice®, made by Young Living Essential Oils. Every nutrient, mineral, vitamin, carbohydrate, and amino-acid needed by the body is provided by Ningxia Red®. Those people with blood sugar concerns can adjust the cleanse by adding more or less of the juice.

It is a good idea to do this cleanse for 7-21 days (with a maximum of 40 days), during which no other food should be consumed. I prefer 14-21 days of the cleanse, followed by foods from the "highly beneficial foods" group for your specific blood type, listed in the book by Dr. D'Adamo, *Eat Right for Your Type*. None of these foods should be consumed more than one time in a four-day period. The basic concept is to rotate your foods in order to avoid maladaptive syndromes and food allergies in the future.

Don't be afraid to use this cleanse. The first three to five days are the hardest for most people, due to lifelong habits and emotional ties to eating. This cleanse will help you in innumerable ways, and it will be well worth the effort. This cleanse could be considered a fast, as mentioned in the Bible, and is a prime time for you to practice meditation and prayer. You will be rewarded with a cleansing of the body, mind, and spirit.

You will need (per day):
- 1 gallon distilled water
- 6 ounces Ningxia Red Juice® (from Young Living)
- 1/8 to 1/4 tsp. cayenne pepper (red pepper), depending on preference
- 12 Tbsp. fresh-squeezed Lemon or Lime juice (about 6 whole fruits)
- 2- 4 Tbsp. of genuine, Grade B Maple Syrup (not maple flavored syrup). You may increase the amount if you are experiencing low blood sugar.
- 1 bottle of Digestive Enzymes (Detoxzyme or Allerzyme, both from Young Living, work well)
- 1 bottle Probiotics (Nutri-West, 120 capsules – should last about 1 month)

- 1 bottle Herbal Laxative

Instructions:
- Combine all of the ingredients listed. Always use fresh-squeezed lemons or limes. It is preferable to use organic lemons when possible.
- Drink a minimum of a ½ gallon to a maximum of 1 gallon of the Master Longevity Combination, spread throughout the waking period of your day. If you get hungry, drink another glass. <u>Absolutely no other food should be eaten throughout the duration of your program</u>.
- Take one capsule of the Herbal Laxative at night to loosen accumulated mucus and fecal matter in the intestines.
- Take one capsule of the Probiotics in the morning and one at night.
- Take 1-2 capsules of digestive enzyme morning, noon, and night.

Other considerations:
- It is best if the Master Longevity Body Cleanse is used at the same time as Dr. Joseph's Colon Cleanse, since it is very important to have 3-5 bowel movements per day to expel all of the now-liberated toxins from the body. Without good bowel movements, toxins can be stirred up and lodge in new areas of the body. You are constipated if you only have one bowel movement per day. When you get the urge to have a bowel movement, go immediately to the stool instead of waiting, as many people are prone to do when they are busy. Do not strain excessively on the stool. Most people are surprised at how much is eliminated in the bowel movements even though they are not eating any food. Much of the movements are the 20-40 pounds of fecal

matter that has been lodged throughout the intestines. In research performed by the world-renowned Sir Bernard Jenson, D.C., who was knighted for his work in natural healing, a study of 600 elderly people, who reported they were having at least one bowel movement every day, found that upon autopsy, all study participants had at least 20 pounds of accumulated matter lodged in the intestines.[134]

- Observe your bowel movements so that you can report what they look like to your doctor – note color, diameter, firmness, size, quantity, parasites, recognizable food that went undigested.

- Upon successful completion of the Master Longevity Body Cleanse, you will have a clean body. It will respond differently than before the cleanse. You should absorb more nutrients from your food and gain more vitality from the food you eat. However, your clean body will also let you know immediately, with various symptoms, when you have eaten something full of food additives, toxins, or otherwise of low-vitality quality.

Expectations of the Master Longevity Body Cleanse:
- Eliminate and break up toxins lodged in any tissue of the body.
- Relieve strain and stress on the organs and glands of the body.
- Re-establish proper fluid balance.
- Cleanse all body/ tissues and purge poisons out of the body.
- Break up mucus.
- Strengthen and build the blood.
- Stimulate and build the immune system.
- Reverse the aging process, increase longevity.

- Eliminate food and/or other allergies.
- Normalize the metabolism, including blood sugar and cholesterol.
- Relieve the body of the burden of having to work to digest food while you heal.Inhibit tumor growth.

Facts about the Master Longevity Cleanse

This cleanse has all of the nutrition needed during this time. There is no need to take vitamins during this cleanse; in fact, vitamin supplements can frequently hinder getting the best results from the cleanse.

Rest and take life at a slower pace if you have to – most people can go on about their regular business without difficulty.

It can be used 3-4 times per year and will do wonders for keeping the body functioning at maximum health. <u>You may drink distilled water</u> throughout the cleanse. No other drinks or foods are allowed.

Wolfberry Ningxia Red Juice® is the closest to the "fountain of youth" found to date. Not only does it contain high amounts of Chinese wolfberries, but it also contains five of the richest sources of the free-radical fighting antioxidants from wolfberry, blueberry, pomegranate, apricot, and raspberry. Even more, the juice is enhanced with therapeutic-grade essential oils of lemon and orange, both of which contain the phytochemical d-limonene and its derivative perillyl. The lemon and orange oil in the the juice are antiviral, antiseptic, invigorating, a body tonic, antiparasitic, increase white blood cell formation, antidepressant, antispasmotic, digestive aid, and sedatives.

This source of wolfberries comes from the Yellow River in the Ningxia Provence of central China, where it has been used for 5000 years and is listed in the world's oldest medical books. Science has documented that wolfberries are the only known substance proven to increase human longevity.

Wolfberries are consumed daily by one of the longest-lived societies on the planet, with people living in excess of 120 years. It is the most nutrient-dense food ever found, containing 13% protein (no other fruit contains more than 5-6% protein) and 21 amino acids (six times higher in proportion than bee pollen). It also contains over 80 minerals and trace minerals, carbohydrates, and more different enzymes than can be counted.

This juice contains substances which stimulate the two primary phases of liver detoxification. It stimulates a 48% increase in the powerful antioxidant superoxide dismutase (SOD) in the blood, as well as a 12% increase in hemoglobin, not to mention that lipid perodixe levels drop 65%.

The blueberry concentrate in Ningxia Red Juice ® is high in the powerful flavonoid antioxidant proanthocyanadin, which recent research has shown improves brain function.

Pomegranate juice is high in potassium and vitamin C, and research shows pomegranate reduces the LDL (bad cholesterol).

Apricots contain a powerhouse of nutrients, housing three times more potassium than bananas, twice as much magnesium as broccoli, and four times as much niacin as spinach, as well as a having high concentrations of carotenoids.

The raspberry juice contain ellagic acid, a plant chemical that protects cells from genetic mutation that can lead to abnormal cell growth, like cancer. Of interest, raspberries contain over four times more antioxidant capacity than vitamin C and beta-carotene.

Ningxia Red Juice ® is crucial to the success of this cleanse. To substitute anything else is incomprehensible because of its lifegiving benefits. Even after the cleanse, I recommend you drink 1-2 fluid ounces a day, which is the equivalent of eating ½ - 1 cup of fresh wolfberries, the ultimate longevity food.

Lemons and limes are acidic fruits, but they are actually alkalinizing in the body once eaten. More acidic tissues and fluids of the body lead to more dysfunction and illness. Alkalinity is conducive to health and the rebuidling of tissues. These citrus fruits contain substances which stimulate the 2 primary phases of liver detoxification. An essential oil contained in these fruits called limonene, and its derivative perillyl alchohol, is thought to block both tumor promotion and progression. Lemon juice is said to be one of nature's most powerful antiseptics, used internally and externally. (If you find you are extremely acidic, take the following Vinegar Bath to reduce the acid levels in your body: put 1 cup to 2 quarts of 100% apple cider vinegar into a bathtub of warm water, and soak for at least 20 minutes.)

Grade B Maple syrup is the second run of maple sap with more vitamins and minerals plus more maple flavor. Grade B is preferable to Grade A for this cleanse, and it is less expensive as well. It contains Vitamins A, B1, B2, B6, C, Nicotinic Acid, and Pantothenic Acid. The minerals include Sodium, Potassium, Calcium, Magnesium, Manganese, Iron, Copper, Phosphorus, Sulphur, Chlorine, and Silicon. This type of maple syrup is a balanced form of positive and negative sugar and should always be used instead of any substitute.

Cayenne Pepper is necessary for stimulating proper circulation. Interestingly, cayenne is also a hemostatic substance, meaning it arrests bleeding. It is vital in this cleanse in its ability to break up mucus and increase the warmth of the body tissues, which has a softening effect on hardened toxic tissues. It helps to build blood and also adds many B-vitamins and vitamin C.

Digestive Enzymes (Detoxyme by Young Living) are necessary to neutralize any gas and toxins. There are special enzymes for digesting proteins (protease), carbohydrates (amylase), fats (lipase), and fiber (cellulase). Lactase is used to break down lactose, the component in dairy products that are indigestible for many people. Detoxyme contains other enzymes but also includes synergistic therapeutic-grade essential oils of cumin, fennel, and anise. These essential oils relax the lining of the stomach and small intestines, making the detoxification process smoother. They are also beneficial in their anti-parasitic actions. When used during this cleanse, these enzymes and oils will assist in removing much of the undigested matter that can get caked on the walls of the intestines. **Probiotics** (Total Probiotics by NutriWest) – as the sludge of years of fermented, putrid matter and mucus begin to be dislodged from the intestines, the underlying intestinal walls, which normally harbor our friendly bowel bacteria, will need to be re-innoculated with a variety of acidophilus-type bacteria. Among their many health promoting functions, they help:

- Reduce the level of cholesterol
- Curb or destroy potentially pathogenic or harmful bacteria and yeasts such as Candida albicans
- Through their production of lactic acid, they preserve and enhance the digestibility of foods.
- Help produce important B-vitamins
- Prevent cancer and other chronic illnesses by detoxifying or preventing the formation of carcinogenic chemicals.

22

~

Liver and Gallbladder Flush

This Liver/Gallbladder Flush is a time-tested favorite of doctors around the world and is one of the best methods of cleansing the tissues of the liver and gallbladder.

Detoxification is essential to any chronic illness program. If you do not relieve the body of toxins, the chances of recovery from many illnesses are greatly reduced. This protocol can be a mildly difficult and uncomfortable process; however, a well-rounded plan of treatment such as this should minimize any discomfort.

The Liver/Gallbladder Flush can be repeated monthly, but at the minimum one should do it every six months. The liver refers more pain to more different parts of the body than just about any other organ. It will be well worth the effort; many people feel greatly improved after doing one of these flushes. The Liver and Gallbladder Flush can be done before, during, or after the Perfect-7 Treatment and Detox Protocol™.

You will need:
- One gallon of Apple Juice – Organic, unfiltered, and unsweetened
- One box of Baking Soda
- One pint of Epsom Salts (Magnesium Sulfate)
- One bottle of Calc-Acid (by Nutri-West) or Calcium Phosphate
- One bottle of Phos-Drops (by Nutri-West)
- One bottle of Total Liver Detox (120 Tablets, by Nutri-West)
- One bottle of Molybdenum (by Jernigan Nutraceuticals)
- Cold-pressed, Extra Virgin Olive Oil
- Bentonite Clay (purified for human consumption)
- Whipping Cream (1 pint)
- Fresh Fruit (Preferably miscellaneous berries)

Follow these instructions completely:
- Add 1 ounce of Phos-Drops to 1 gallon of Apple juice and mix well.

Over the next 4 days:
- Drink all the juice between meals at the rate of 3-4 glasses per day.
- Keep the apple juice chilled to avoid fermentation, but let it come to room temperature first before drinking it.
- Always rinse your mouth out using 1 teaspoon of Baking Soda in 1 glass of water, or brush your teeth with Baking Soda, after drinking the juice to prevent the acid from damaging your teeth.
- Otherwise, eat normally and add coffee enemas as usual.
- Take 2 Total Liver Detox tablets 3 times every day until the two bottles are empty.
- Take 1 Molybdenum capsule 3 times every day until empty.

Step 2: Detoxify Lyme Toxins

On the fourth day:
- Continue drinking the Apple juice/Phos-Drops combination.
- Take 2 Calc-Acid immediately before breakfast, and 2 immediately before lunch.
- Drink about 2 pints of pure water that morning.
- 2 hours after lunch, take 1 tablespoon of Epsom Salts dissolved in warm water; add juice if desired.
- 5 hours after lunch, take 1 tablespoon of Epsom Salts dissolved in warm water; add juice if desired.
- 6 hours after lunch, eat a dinner of Whipping Cream and fruit. The whipping cream contracts the gallbladder. Any fruit is acceptable, but berries are best, either fresh or frozen.
- Take 1 Calc-Acid with your dinner of cream and fruit.
- Half an hour before bedtime, put 1 tablespoon of the Bentonite in 1 glass of water, mix well (start by adding water slowly), and drink.
- At bedtime, drink ½ cup of Olive Oil; a small amount of orange, grapefruit, or lemon juice may be added, if desired.
- Immediately go to bed and lie on your right side with your knees drawn up; hold this position for 30 minutes.
- For maximum detox with the minimum discomfort, you may opt for the Magnetic Resonance Bio-Oxidative Therapy (MRBT) ceramic magnets.
    - Place one of the 4x6x½" ceramic magnets over the liver (over right lower ribcage and overhanging the abdomen a bit).
    - Place the other ceramic magnet over the navel, running lengthwise across the abdomen.
    - Strap these magnets in place with the negative polarity side facing the body, and sleep with these on for at least 3-7 nights.

- You may feel nauseated during the night due to the release of stored toxins from the gallbladder and liver; this is normal and will pass.
- Observe your first few bowel movements, which should be rather loose, so that you can describe them to your doctor. You may see floating pellets, which many doctors believe to be gallstones which were softened and passed painlessly during the night.

On the following day:
- Eat normally.
- Take 2 Calc-Acid with breakfast, 2 with lunch, and 1 with your evening meal.
- Continue taking all of the Total Liver Detox and Molybdenum until gone.

---

[126] Faloon W. A Novel Method to Protect Your Aging Arteries, Life Extension Journal, Winter 2007/2008.
[127] Journal of the American Medical Association, Aug 7, 1981.
[128] Meffert B, Hochmuth O, et al, 2006, *Effects of a multiple mild infra-red-A induced hyperthermia on central and peripheral pulse waves in hypertensive patients*. Springer Berlin / Heidelberg.
[129] Gerson M, *A Cancer Therapy: Results of Fifty Cases*, 1990, Gerson Institute.
[130] Brudnak, Mark A.; The Probiotic Solution: Nature's Best-Kept Secret for Radiant Health, Dragon Door Publications, 2003.
[131] Waring, R. Sulfate and Sulfation, School of Biosciences, University of Birmingham, United Kingdom.
[132] Emery, P., Bradley, H., Gough, A., et al. Increased prevalence of poor sulphoxidation in patients with rheumatoid arthritis. Ann. Rheum. Dis. 51:318-320 (1992).
[133] Bradley, H., Gough, A., Sokhi, R. Sulfate metabolism is abnormal in patients with rheumatoid arthritis. J Rheumatol 21(7)1192-1196.
[134] Jenson, B, *Dr. Jenson's Guide to Better Bowel Care: A Complete Program for Tissue Cleansing Through Bowel Management*. Avery; Rev Ed edition (September 1, 1998.

Step 3
Break Up Bacterial Biofilms and Inflammation

23

~

TPP Protease®
Made by Transformation Enzymes

Take 1-3 of these smooth, coated pills, 2 times per day on an empty stomach. Take them at least 1 hour after eating and at least 45 minutes before you will eat again. They are about the size of an aspirin and are usually easy to swallow. These are systemic enzymes, so we don't want them to be used up simply coming in contact with food in your small intestines. TPP Protease should be continued for the duration of treatment until full restoration of quality of life is restored. It is a very effective anti-inflammatory product as well as a potent immune system booster. In that most pain involves inflammation, improvement in even stubborn pain can often be expected within 24-48 hours. Improvement is often cumulative and improves gradually over time with use of TPP Protease.

Research performed in Europe showed that proteolytic enzymes, such as TPP Protease, helped various antibiotics penetrate the tissues up to 40% better.[135,136] Bio-Resonance-type testing very often demonstrates a complementary/synergistic effect when TPP Protease is used with Borrelogen and Microbojen. It has become a foregone conclusion in many doctors' clinics that it is needed in virtually everyone suffering from any chronic illness, such as Lyme Disease. In Germany, systemic, proteolytic enzymes, such as TPP Protease, are second only to aspirin in over-the-counter sales, with one hundred million people taking it every day, including many European Olympic athletes.

TPP Protease seems to help remove interference to the movement of healing energy and medicines in the tissues. Volumes of research over many years and millions of people bring strong confidence in this well-known systemic enzyme. Its many benefits include immune system support, anti-inflammatory activity, and acceleration of the rate of healing. In my experience, TPP Protease also helps restore the body's warmth organization through breaking up the accumulation of antigen/antibody complexes and by freeing the metabolic processes from their cold, sclerotic, low output. It seems that in Lyme Disease, as in many cold/sclerotic illnesses, the body's chemical reactions (metabolism) are being held captive, and the energy-producing mechanisms of the cellular factories have wrenches in all of their gears. TPP Protease seems to remove these wrenches over time by directly and indirectly breaking up excessive protein accumulations in the intracellular spaces. Excessive protein, as we have said, promotes darkness and cold, and therefore TPP Protease should break up the darkness, allowing the light and warmth metabolism to be restored by the other treatments specifically designed to do so. Dosage is large due to the fact that these enzymes are used up as they work their way through to the farthest reaches of the body. This is not a digestive enzyme -- it is a *systemic* enzyme. Digestive enzymes are used to aid in breaking down the foods you eat. Systemic, proteolytic enzymes go throughout the body and break down fibrin, reducing inflammation, and increasing the rate of healing.

Side effects: With overwhelming research and millions of people using systemic proteolytic enzymes every day, there is virtually no safer product on the market. An expected effect of TPP Protease is the healthy thinning of the blood. This is one of its healthy effects; however, caution is warranted in those using proteolytic enzymes when taking prescription blood thinners, anti-coagulants, or dealing with bleeding disorders

24

~

Beyond Chelation Improved™
Made by Longevity Plus

Use 1 packet 1-2 times per day, with or without food, taken for 6 months to a year or indefinitely.

As you will read below, this Beyond Chelation Improved (BC-I) plays a huge role in de-cloaking these *stealth microbes* so that the body's immune system and the remedies can effectively reach the bacteria.

This product will also support the nutritional needs of the body while it is being stressed by the detoxification process. Beyond Chelation Improved provides the highest quality essential fatty acids, botanicals, minerals, and nutrition needed for optimal function of the brain and nervous system, heart and circulatory system, and virtually every other tissue in the body.

BC-I also contains Calcium EDTA, which will help remove many of the toxins and heavy metals jamming up the machinery of your body. It contains high-allicin garlic, which is a favorite antimicrobial of some of the world's leading medical doctors who treat Lyme Disease naturally.

Beyond Chelation's Effect Against Bacterial Biofilms

Recent research has suggested that various forms of EDTA, such as the Calcium EDTA in BC-I, may help to remove bacterial biofilms. Bacterial biofilms are a mucus-like film excreted by bacteria that shield them from the immune system and from the effects of antimicrobial treatments.

Biofilms form a matrix around the bacteria. As reported in the British Medical Journal *The Lancet*, "This matrix protects the cells within it and facilitates communication among them through biochemical signals. Some biofilms have been found to contain water channels that help distribute nutrients and signaling molecules. This matrix is strong enough that under certain conditions, biofilms can become fossilized. Bacteria living in a biofilm usually have significantly different properties from free-floating bacteria of the same species, as the dense and protected environment of the film allows them to cooperate and interact in various ways. One benefit of this environment is increased resistance to detergents and antibiotics, as the dense extracellular matrix and the outer layer of cells protect the interior of the community. In some cases antibiotic resistance can be increased 1000 fold."[137]

---

[135] Klaschka, Franz. *Oral Enzymes – New Approach to Cancer Treatment: Immunological concepts for general and clinical practice; Complementary cancer treatment.* Grafelfing, Germany: Forum-Med.-Verl.-Ges., 1996. p. 123.

[136] Lopez, D.A., M.D. et al. *Enzymes: The Fountain of Life.* Germany: The Neville Press, Inc., 1994. p. 135.

[137] Stewart P, Costerton J (2001). "Antibiotic resistance of bacteria in biofilms". *Lancet* **358** (9276): 135-8

Step 4
Support the Bio-Energetic Fields of the Body

25

~

Essential Oils Protocol
Oils made by Young Living unless noted otherwise

Essential oils have the highest naturally occurring vibrational energy on earth. If we view the body for what it truly is, it is more like an energetic pond, comparable to a pond of water. Each oil has its own unique complex frequency, based upon its molecular structure. When the oils are applied in specific locations on the body, it is like throwing different-sized rocks into various locations in the pond. Each rock will cause a unique ripple effect that will spread its vibrations throughout the entire pond. In the same way, each oil will cause a different ripple effect that will shift the energetic aspects of the entire body.

These oils will work to shift the crystalline-matrix of your body, making your body's electromagnetic fields more resistant to the harmful electro pollution that is being emitted by computers, cell phones, appliances, microwave cell phone towers, and electrical wiring in the walls of your house. For more information on this topic read *Cross Currents: The Perils of Electropollution, The Promise of Electromedicine*, by Robert Becker, M.D.

University research on the antibacterial, antiviral, and antifungal aspects of some of these oils reveals unparalleled activity in the body. Research has shown that some oils allow no virus to mutate around them. To view this research, as well as how each type of essential oil works and for what illnesses, I recommend the book, *Essential Oils Desk Reference, 3rd Edition*, by Essential Science Publishing.

Many people will think these oils are expensive, but it must be understood that each remedy in the Perfect-7 protocol is like a different tool. You must use the correct tool for the job. Nothing else can do what the oils will do for you.

It takes 60 roses to make one drop of pure rose oil and 30,000 roses to make one fluid ounce! However, rose oil has the highest vibration out of about 100 different plant essential oils. Therapeutic grade essential oils, as made by Young Living Essential Oils, are infinitely better than perfume-grade, chemically extracted oils of cheaper brands. The oils and oil blends in this protocol are the same oils we would use on you at virtually every office visit at our clinic. They *are* that important.

Historically, people leave out this step of the protocol because of the expense. I have seen thousands of people who never dreamed that 10-20 years after they first got sick, they would still be fighting to regain the quality of life they used to have! Determine now to do as much of the Perfect7 protocol as possible. These are the oils I recommend:

- Transformation oil blend
- Frankincense oil
- Valor oil blend
- Palo Santo oil
- Thieves oil blend
- Aconite Nerve oil (Wala)
- Solum Uliginosum Oil (Wala)

Rub 1-4 drops of each of these oils in the corresponding areas listed below, 2-3 times per day. These oils are very aromatic but are usually well-tolerated by even the most chemically sensitive individuals, most likely due to the fact that they are pure plant oils with no solvents and no synthetic or petroleum-based additives. You may want to delay putting on these oils until the end of the day at times that you will be in enclosed spaces with other people. Even though they smell good, everyone around you will smell them as well. Daily use is best, but it is not "written in stone" or an absolute must-do before going out. Definitely use them before bedtime. If you feel itching or experience redness of the skin after applying an oil, simply rub olive oil on the area to soothe the skin. From then on, dilute a drop of the oil you were sensitive to with a drop or two of extra-virgin olive oil or extra-virgin grapeseed oil before applying. If skin sensitivity persists, discontinue the oil that is causing it, but continue with the other oils.

- Frankincense oil -- base of the ears, and ear lobes.
- Transformation oil blend – on the breast bone .
- Valor oil blend -- back of the neck and low back.
- Thieves oil blend – on the big toe and at the base of the toes.
- Palo Santo oil -- on the forehead and any inflamed joints.
- Aconite Nerve Oil -- any area experiencing neuropathy, such as numbness, tingling, or nerve pain.
- Solum Uliginosum oil blend -- all over the body at least once per week, but as much as daily. This oil blend can be applied on top of the other oils or by itself. It can also be added and whisked into bath water in order to coat the entire body, a very helpful way to get it all over the body when there is no one around to help rub the oil in. Soaking for 20 minutes in this bath is best. Aconite Nerve Oil and Solum Uliginosum, from Wala, are imported from Germany and therefore only available through a few companies in the United States. Hansa Center carries both these oils.

26

~

Electromagnetic Pollution and BioPro® Products

Often our patients are surprised to hear me speak so much about the electrical aspects of their body. Conventional medicine focuses strongly on the blood, so many times patients have not been told that the body is electrical. The entire body is controlled through electro-chemical interactions. These electro-chemical interactions of the body are sensitive to the influence of the much stronger electrical fields found in every home, and virtually everywhere in our power line-wrapped earth.

The body operates on 50 cycle direct current electricity, while the electricity in the wiring of your house works on 60 cycle alternating current electricity. This difference can disrupt the normal function of the body.

At no other time do these house appliance electrical fields seem to affect the normal functioning of the body more than while we are asleep. The primary purpose of sleep is to rebuild, regenerate, and repair the body. If we stops to consider that most bedrooms have electricity running in all the walls, the ceiling, and the floor (whether or not the lights are on), we begin to see how many electromagnetic fields are pulsating through the body during this all-important healing time of the day. Electric alarm clocks, electric blankets, and electric heating pads all create even more disruptive fields and should be thrown away.

Computers have become a standard of life in many homes. Research shows that the emitted electromagnetic fields are definitely harmful, as demonstrated by the increased miscarriages associated with prolonged computer usage by pregnant women.[138] I had a patient come for care with symptoms of chronic debilitating fatigue and profound weakness of the muscles. I found that she is a professional editor and author. When I treated her, she rapidly became much stronger in her muscles. When I found out she wrote her books on a laptop computer laid on her body while in bed (due to excessive fatigue and weakness), I decided to test her newfound muscle strength with the laptop laying on her. She immediately could not lift her arms at all! Is electromagnetic pollution a potential problem for all of us? Definitely.

There are several high-tech devices designed to protect against this form of pollution. My favorite devices provide protection against electromagnetic pollution, as verified by independent researchers and doctors all over the world – the BIOPRO Home Harmonizer™ for your house, and the BIOPRO Cell Chip™ should be used on all cell phones and Bluetooth headsets. The cell phone's microwave technology is not safe for lengthy use.

Life is a constant balance between forces weakening the body and the forces of the body trying to restore the lost energy. The electromagnetic forces of our homes, autos, and electrical gadgets are definitely weakening the body.[139] These BIOPRO devices minimize these harmful effects so that your body can restore itself without all of these outside interferences.

Many of the Lyme patients I see have been fighting the illness so long, and antibiotics have so weakened their body, that if their body was a light bulb, it would be very dim indeed.

Step 4: Support the Bio-Energetic Fields of the Body

The BIOPRO devices also provide a way to energize the body 24 hours a day in a way that does not require nutritional supplements or prescription drugs.

27

~

Lyme and Low body Temperature

One of the very common findings I have noticed in chronic Lyme sufferers is a low body temperature, or at least a very unregulated distribution of temperature in the body. I am not promoting the hyperthermia treatments that are being used to kill Lyme spirochetes in some health facilities. I am not necessarily opposed to their use, but this chapter deals primarily with the importance of restoring and maintaining a normal core body temperature. This is true not just in Lyme Disease but also in every degenerative disease of our day.

Your core body temperature is the temperature taken under the tongue and in your armpit. When human physiology books refer to the "normal" core body temperature, it is presented as a range sometimes listed between 97.0-99.0°F . Understand that the "Normal Range" for temperature, or even the normal ranges in blood tests, are based upon the average person of today. That is why "normal" changes periodically, because as our average population continues to get sicker, the Normal Ranges must be adjusted. In this discussion I am speaking about what is an <u>optimal</u> core body temperature: 98.6-99.6°F.

To measure your temperature, use the best quality thermometer that you can afford. It will likely be a digital thermometer. Optimally use a thermometer that can be placed under the tongue with a disposable plastic sleeve over it. Take the temperature under your armpit as well, since many people are so thermally dysregulated that there can be a wide difference between the mouth and armpit. When measuring in the armpit, <u>you must add one degree to the result to get the accurate reading</u>. For those few adventurous souls, if taking a rectal reading, one degree must be taken away from the thermometer reading for the accurate reading.

Much emphasis is usually placed upon fevers; however, a low body temperature is a much more sinister condition. Where a fever can be viewed as an active developmental and corrective process of the healthy body, a low body temperature can never be viewed as a normal or healthy condition, nor is it a mechanism for a learning or developmental process in the body. A low body temperature creates a happy home for viruses and chronic infections, and is a sign of degeneration and gradual cellular death.

Low body temperature is the plague of the 21st century. People with low body temperature have a weak reaction to even the most ideal medicines and therapies. As the body's core temperature becomes cold, the energetic crystalline matrix experiences a systemic collapse as tissues condense and cellular tensegrity, the infrastructure of the intra and extracellular matrix, loses its structural conductivity and integrity. The cooperative and collective intelligence of the human organism is short-circuited as the body temperature cools. As a result, all cellular functions decrease. There is a decrease in the production of all hormones, neurotransmitters, and other body chemicals necessary for normal healthy balance. This follows with an increased susceptibility to infectious disease. As the temperature drops, the acidity of the body increases and the normally predominantly negative polarity of the cells become more positively charged. I will discuss the polarity issues in more detail later.

The colder the body becomes, the more prone the person becomes to depression and other psychological abnormalities and all degenerative illnesses of the body, mind, and spirit. Until the causes of the lowered temperature are addressed and corrected, the best that can be hoped for is only temporary or mild improvement of symptoms and a gradual but steady overall decline in health.

Viruses prefer and promote a cold environment and replicate at a much more rapid rate when the body is cold. Viruses are killed and further replication is impeded by maintaining a warm body. Some bacteria. such as Lyme spirochetes, also prefer and promote a cold environment and can remain in a chronic state as long as their cold environment is maintained. Therefore, in the interest of the prevention and treatment of any viral, bacterial, or chronic illness, this topic must be understood.

The ultimate body coldness is seen in death. When observing a corpse, many clinical gems can be gleaned and correlated to degenerative states of human suffering. In death, the blood and lymph fluid of the body solidify, and the body becomes stiff and cold. In the same way, in many chronic cold illnesses such as Lyme Disease, fibromyalgia, chronic fatigue, diabetes, and cancer, we see that the body becomes progressively colder. As the body cools, the electrical oscillations of the fluids in the body slow down, and there is a shift in the body's polarity, which promotes the overgrowth of potentially infectious microbes and cancer.

We can see the same principle of what happens in the body by observing the dynamics in a water molecule. When the electrical oscillations of a water molecule slow down, it becomes a solid, ice. As we speed up a water molecule's electrical oscillations, it liquefies and ultimately becomes a vapor.

The colder a body becomes, the slower the electrical oscillatory rate, and therefore the thicker, more viscous (syrupy) the body fluids become. The more viscous the fluids become, the more difficult it is for the body to push the fluids through the body. The lymph fluids that are normally supposed to bathe the outsides of all of your cells become progressively stagnant and too thick to move efficiently. Consider the fact that just like your skin is constantly dying and flaking off and being replaced, so it is that every cell in your body is in a constant state of dying and being replaced. Only now the cold, syrupy lymph fluid cannot wash the dead cellular debris away. As a result, the body becomes a toxic waste dump!

Muscles normally have a high demand for energy. Due to the constant contraction and relaxation mechanism of muscle tissue, muscles assist in eliminating their own cellular waste products. In a cold body, however, the liquidity of the fluids inside of the muscles is gone, and the muscles cannot move the toxins and cellular debris. The deeper you go into the belly or center of the muscle, the more difficult it is to move the toxins. All muscular contraction grinds to a halt, like an engine with no lubricating oil, when the tissues are cold. The belly of the muscle develops a knot that can be felt when massaging the muscle. This is the knotted, painful, muscle condition commonly known as "trigger points" of Fibromyalgia Syndrome, which is being diagnosed in millions of people every year. If the low body temperature is allowed to persist and no therapies are applied, even in a palliative manner as in massages to move toxins manually out of the belly of the muscle, the condition follows that of the water molecule. The belly of the muscle, due to the increasing coldness and decreased muscular activity, progresses over time and reaches the point of zero electrical oscillations, at which time the tissue solidifies in a calcified stone in the belly of the muscle.

Interesting research that supports this concept has been performed by Dr. Carolyn McMakin, D.C., using the electrotherapy called Microcurrent. The Microcurrent is applied through direct contact on these trigger points via vinyl/graphite gloves connected to the Microcurrent machine. The trigger points virtually vanish under the gentle touch of the glove when applying the correct electrical frequency.[140] What may be happening here is that the stimulation of the muscle through Microcurrent is externally increasing the electrical oscillatory rate of the thickened fluids in the muscle, resulting in temporarily restoring the normal liquidity of the fluids, allowing the muscles to once again contract and pump out the toxic accumulation. The results are somewhat temporary since the underlying condition that created it in our scenario, the overall low body temperature, remains unchanged. However, used in combination with various other corrective measures, this Microcurrent therapy can speed healing in many cases.[141]

Continuing with other degenerative aspects of the body, we have seen that the body is set up on electrical circuits, all of which are interdependent and interconnected. One circuit in the body cannot fail without ultimately affecting the whole. Therefore, if the muscle is seizing up and becoming progressively rigid and solidified, what do you suppose the organ that is also on that same electrical circuit is doing? It is likely that, to some degree, it is also progressively seizing up and solidifying.

In the many miles of blood vessels, the cold, thick blood is more difficult to push through veins and arteries. Arteriosclerosis, the progressive hardening of the arteries, and the clogging of the blood vessels, is manifesting the exact same problem that is being experienced by every tissue in the too-cold body. Edema in the extremities is seen as the muscular walls of the blood vessels seize up and can no longer maintain tone, so the fluid leaks out of the pores of the vessels.

I look at many older patients (and some not so old) who are experiencing all the signs and symptoms of death in the extremities. They are dying in their extremities first, from the feet and hands up to the torso. To touch their feet is just like touching an icy, stiff, dead corpse. The foot is deathly whitish blue and etched in blue/black blood vessels from devitalized, stagnant blood.

The overcooling of peripheral blood returning from cold legs and feet causes depression of the temperature in the vital organs with slowing of metabolic processes, particularly in the brain and medullary centers.[142] Death occurs when a vital organ reaches the point of being too cold. Your physician can name your disease, and he can draw your blood and show you everything that is wrong with it, but he is simply describing the process I have just outlined. When the core temperature of the body is cold, every organ, gland, and tissue is affected and becomes hypo-functional. Hypo-functional means that there are fewer hormones and less of every chemical involved with normal body and brain function. Even the psyche is affected, leading to potentially any type of psychological problem, especially depression. How many people are told that they have psychological depression from a deficiency of a certain brain chemical? Many! Of course they are deficient in "happy" brain chemicals, possibly due to the overcooling of the body.

It could be said that you are dying in direct proportion to the coldness of your body. Follow this logic: Cells die in direct proportion to the depletion of oxygen. Blood that is overcooled from a cold core temperature is too thick to efficiently carry oxygen, and the lung vital capacity is reduced, leading to shallow breathing. This means that the oxygen to carbon dioxide exchange rate in the lungs is minimal. Now combine the degenerative effects of the oxygen deprivation and the cold temperature, and the fact that all of this and the overgrowth of microbes promote an acidic environment, and you have greatly accelerated cellular degeneration and the onset of life-threatening disease.

There is an optimum body temperature which all chemical reactions in the human body need in order to maintain health: 98.6° F. I can honestly say that I have never seen a new patient come into my clinic with a normal body temperature. Just recently, a 66-year-old woman came in as a new patient with a temperature of 94.6! Her body is not in good balance. She could not feel her feet, and to touch her legs was like touching the legs of a corpse. The legs even looked dead and grey, streaked with blue/black veins of stagnant, devitalized blood. Even in classic hypothermia, as seen in people stranded in blizzards, it is well-known that the circulation of blood in the arms and legs is reduced dramatically, almost to zero, in order to provide protection and warmth to the vital organs. These people will also cease to feel cold and will experience numbness, loss of coordination, mental confusion, and heart rhythm problems. It sounds like I am describing many elderly people and some Lyme sufferers doesn't it?

One way to treat weather-related hypothermia is to give the person warm sugar drinks. Sugar is a cheap, fast-burning fuel for your body and therefore generates a lot of heat in the process. This may be why so many people suffering from lifestyle-induced cold core temperature are plagued with sugar cravings. Many of them consume copious amounts of sugar in the form of soda pops, chocolate, pastries, and various candies. It may be a craving that is driven by the body's desire to generate fast heat to keep the body functioning. Sugar cravings should diminish as the core body temperature problems are resolved.

Keep in mind that the body has been too cold possibly since birth, due to suppressive medicines, vaccines, fever reducers, heavy metal and chemical toxins, and energetically dead foods. The retraining and resetting of the body's thermostat is just the beginning of healing the body of chronic illnesses. The normal body temperature must be held steady, possibly for a year or more in some cases, before the body can undo the damage of a lifetime of coldness.

Track your temperature when you first awaken in the morning, before even getting out of bed. This reflects your core body temperature when it is not being influenced by what you just ate, drank, or your activity level. Many of you will likely be surprised to see just how cold you already are. This is the result of generations of suppressive therapies and an imbalanced life. You must make some choices to save your health.

Many doctors will undoubtedly say that you need to take a thyroid medication to bring up the body temperature; however, this is the same mentality as taking a Tylenol for a headache. If you don't believe me, ask anyone on the prescription thyroid medicines what happens when they go off of the medication. The body returns immediately to the previous cold condition.

Definitely do support the normal functioning of the thyroid, by detoxification, organic iodine, and nutritional support, but see the coldness for what it really is -- a sign of multi-organ system breakdown, and longstanding or even generational imbalance. Besides, it is really the hypothalamus that regulates your core body temperature, along with your degree of motivation and sex drive. The hypothalamus is actually "upstream" from your thyroid and helps the pituitary regulate the thyroid.

The healthy body has daily temperature fluctuations, with the coolest temperature in the early morning hours, and the warmest in the evening between 8-10pm, after having rested for half an hour. Tracking of the difference between morning and evening temperature should reveal, in a healthy person, a difference of at least 0.9° F (0.5° C). People with a low body temperature and an overall degenerative condition will find that this temperature variation is minimal. Another unusual finding of dysregulated body temperature is that the evening is often colder than the morning reading.

The body's best chance at long-term healing increases in direct proportion to the restoration of normal body temperature and its normal diurnal fluctuation.

You and your healthcare team must address your body from every direction and with every balancing tool available. You can never truly overcome this condition with pills. Additional therapies must engage and reactivate and stimulate the rhythmical, metabolic, and nerve/sense aspects of your body, addressing the body, mind, and spirit.

In a cold body, there is always a disruption of the rhythmical aspects of the organism, that part of you that establishes balance between the metabolic and nerve/sense aspects of your body. No other medicine has performed as well as the product I formulated called **Core Warmth**™ by Jernigan Nutraceuticals. The benefits of Core Warmth™ formula are from its ability to restore the thermostatic regulation of the body. It works gently and yet effectively at warming the core temperature so that the blood and lymph fluid of the body can "thaw out" and flow freely through the core of the body, reaching the extremities. It will help relieve obstructions in the energy pathways of the body and promote the circulation. Core Warmth™ will balance the immune system, enabling it to work more efficiently without danger of over-stimulation as is seen in some allergic tendencies and autoimmune dysfunctions. Core Warmth is also beneficial in helping people suffering from Post-Lyme Syndrome (PLS). Core Warmth™ will greatly benefit any of the following "cold body" symptoms: Chronic Fatigue syndrome, chronic pain, achiness, numbness, cramping or heaviness in the muscles, tendons, and joints of the neck, shoulders, back or lower extremities, difficulty moving, rotating or bending, fibromyalgia, severe neck tension, tendonitis, repetitive strain injury, arthritis, rheumatism, sprained ligaments, strained muscles, traumatic injury pain including post-surgical pain, connective tissue disorders, and post-viral syndromes.

Other supporting therapies designed for restoring the rhythms of the body must also be applied. These therapies might include color and sound therapy, hot and cold contrast therapy, life-activity planning, breathing and voice therapy, rhythmical massage therapy, curative movement therapies, and indeed, every other treatment from your doctor will address in some way the rhythmical aspects of your body.

Low body temperature must be addressed to bring the body back to balance. The temperature must be elevated to end the dying process of the body and to help the body eliminate the cellular debris or the "sludge" in the body.

General Treatment Recommendations

- Temperature monitoring and graphing (upon awakening, and between 8-10 pm after a 30 minute resting period)
- **Core Warmth™** by Jernigan Nutraceuticals.
- **Perfect-7 Treatment and Detox Protocol for Lyme Disease**
- **BIOPRO Home Harmonizer™** and the **BIOPRO Cell Chip™** to eliminate electromagnetic interference of the thermostatic regulation and overall function of the body.
- **Solum Uliginosum Oil** (by Wala) This oil and bath essence is great for restoring the warmth organization of the body. They also are beneficial for chemical sensitivities, and those suffering from weather-change related sensitivities. The oil and essence are low-odor products made in Germany. Both can be added to a bath for all-over body application. May be applied as needed.
- **Iodine Skin Test** and Treatment (see Appendix D).
- Chiropractic spinal, pelvic, and cranial alignments combined with specific homeopathic, nutritional, glandular, and myofascial support using Bio-Resonance

Step 4: Support the Bio-Energetic Fields of the Body

Scanning™, or other body circuit balancing technique, as dictated by your healthcare professional.
- **Mini-trampoline workout --** work up to 20 minutes per day (or substitute other movement therapies).
- **Dietary Changes** -- see Chapter 35.
- **Lifestyle modification** – see Chapter 33.

---

[138] Becker R, 1990, *Cross Currents: The Perils of Electro-Pollution; The Promise of Electromedicine.* Tarcher Publishing.

[139] Becker R, 1990.

[140] Addington, John W. *Relief of Fibromyalgia Through Microcurrent Therapy.* ImmuneSupport.com 7-11-2001.

[141] Addington 2001.

[142] Cotran R.S., Kumar V., Robbins S.L., Robbin's Pathological Basis of Disease 4th ed. 1989 pp501.

28

~

Causes of Low Body Temperature

There are many potential causes for a lowered body temperature, each of which must be analyzed and brought into balance by you and your healthcare team. By eliminating the various causes, one can promote health and healing. Potential causes may include:

- Lifestyle
- Diet
- Heavy metal accumulation
- Vaccinations/Immunizations
- Antibiotics/Anti-fever medications
- Symptomatic treatments of all kinds, over-the-counter medicines, herbs, vitamins, prescription medicines
- Electromagnetic pollution
- Synthetic clothing and materials
- Toxic homes and environment
- Over-controlled interior climates of homes and workplaces

Lifestyle Influences on Body Temperature

A sedentary lifestyle and the over-stimulation of the nerve/sense aspects of life lead to imbalance. Too much time and energy is being committed to what can be basically called "living in your head." Balanced living requires one to live to the same degree in your body.

The techno/information age has done us no true favors in regard to maintaining a normal body temperature or in regard to longevity. It seems that everyone assumes that just because there are more centurions alive today, our younger generations will also live longer. I doubt this will be true. While it is true that the human body should be able to live approximately 125 years, today's younger generations are aging faster and manifesting previously considered geriatric or old-age diseases while many are still in childhood. Even with all of the advances in medicine and increased nutritional and dietary awareness, Americans now experience some of the worst health in the world.

Obesity is a problem now in every age group in every developed country. Though obesity is a multi-faceted problem, it can be seen as the body's efforts to insulate the body from the overcooling of its core temperature. Many people have tried different diets to lose weight only to be disappointed. The body may be simply saying, "No way, I need that body fat to help preserve the little bit of heat in the vital organs!"

Scores of people commit the vast majority of their lives in front of the television, computer, reading, dreaming, sleeping, fantasizing, talking, learning, or daydreaming. People are proud of the fact that they exercise three times per week -- what is that? Three hours compared to about one hundred and nine hours per week that are spent on the nerve/senses aspects of the body!

Dietary Effect on Low Temperature

Eating energetically dead food is a drain on the body's energy reserves. Food serves to do more than just satisfy your appetite. Food should also do more than simply provide you with nutrients. Food should bring with it energy! Energy-rich, live food imparts to the body its energy at roughly half the speed of light, long before its nutrient content can be digested, absorbed, and distributed to the body. What most people eat is the dead skeleton of something that was relatively good for you before it was processed and poisoned to death.

Food either contributes energy to your body or steals energy just to process the low-quality nutrients. Even food cooked with love and the intent for good of the receiver has a higher vibrational and health quality.

I want you to understand this one point – our Maker did not design the body to require a Ph.D. in nutrition and diet to feed it and run it perfectly. I truly believe that we are designed to function quite well on a wide range of diets. Our Maker had to know that people in various parts of the world would not have access to the same biodiversity of food. One thing I am sure of is that we are not intended to render our food useless before eating it.

The majority of your diet should be from organically and/or biodynamically grown fruits, vegetables, and meats. Fruits and vegetables should be harvested at peak ripeness on the plant for maximizing its developmental process. These foods are here for your benefit; let them do their job by allowing them to ripen naturally.

You will need to make the conscious decision to either buy your produce from a good health food store/grocery, or to grow it yourself. I recommend that you get out and grow your own produce and learn the different healthy ways to store and preserve it. The very process of preparing the ground, composting, planting, tending, and harvesting is forcing the body to engage the metabolic heat-producing aspects of your being. Gardening in its learning curve, direct contact with the earth, and its rewards through producing life, is very healing to the body, mind, and spirit.

Most of the produce in the grocery store is harvested while still green, and then gassed or chemically treated to achieve the correct color and texture and to extend its shelf-life. The process, however, never allows the food to reach its full energetic or nutritional potential. What little energy this produce has is destroyed by cooking.

Toxic and synthetic foods are one of the most prevalent causes of lowered body temperature. This includes a wide range of food additives in the form of preservatives, dyes, pesticides, fungicides, flavorings and flavor enhancers, and sweeteners. We are being poisoned from conception onward. Our society is dying prematurely all around us. Chronic fatigue plagues almost everyone. It is said that cancer, the ultimate cold disease, will be diagnosed in one out of two people with an estimated one in three dying from it.

Food companies think the current system is a great way to do business. I'm suddenly reminded of the slogan of one leading company, "No one can eat just one." Of course no one can eat just one! In fact, it is difficult not to eat the entire bag in one sitting, with all the chemical additives that are overstimulating your taste buds and appetite centers of your brain. Synthetic foods are good business all the way to the bank, and it also just so happens to support your health insurance company, pharmaceutical companies, and the entire medical community in that it ensures them that there will be a steady stream of chronically dependent people to feed money into their pockets.

Wittingly or unwittingly, each of these entities are part of the problem.

For those who are serious about raising their core temperature and reaping the health-restoring benefits, the following charts outline foods that either promote the cooling or warming of the body. Selecting foods based on this warming or cooling concept has been practiced in Chinese medicine for thousands of years. It was understood that when one had a fever, certain foods would help cool the body; if cold and low vitality is the problem, warming foods would heal this condition.

Cooling Foods to Avoid

These foods should be **avoided** or eaten **in moderation** when working to raise the core body temperature.

Fruit	Vegetable	Legumes/Grains	Herbs/Spices
Apple	Lettuce	Soy milk	Peppermint
Banana	Radish	Soy sprouts	Dandelion greens + root
Pear	Cucumber	Tofu	Honeysuckle flowers
Persimmon	Celery	Tempeh	Nettles
Cantaloupe	Button mushroom	Mung beans	Red clover blossom
Watermelon	Asparagus	Alfalfa sprouts	Lemon balm
Tomato	Swiss chard	Millet	White peppercorn
Bitter melon	Kelp	Buckwheat	Cilantro
All citrus	Eggplant	Barley	Marjoram
Blackberry	Spinach	All wheat	Soy sauce
Green tea	Summer squash	Amaranth	Table salt
Raspberry	Chinese cabbage	Quinoa	
Green grapes	Bok choy		
	Broccoli		
	Cauliflower		
	Sweet corn		
	Zucchini		
	Green bean		
	Bamboo shoots		

Other cooling foods: all seaweeds, blue-green spirulina, oystershell calcium, wheat/barley grass, yogurt, crab/clam, and duck.

Also avoid iced and cold foods and beverages, such as ice cream, cold beer, ice water, and pop. Raw foods also are cooling to the body. Sweets, cow's milk, and dairy products overcool the body. Avoid excessive salt.

Dietary Measures for Raising Core Body Temperature

Each of the following guidelines will assist in resetting and maintaining the body's normal temperature.
- Avoid eating cooling foods as listed above.
- Avoid eating late at night.
- Avoid overly spicy hot foods, since the body will react by attempting to cool the overheated body down.

Foods to Raise Body temperature

Fruits	Vegetables	Legumes/Grains	Herbs/Spices
Strawberry	Fennel	Black beans	Ginger
Peach	Cabbage	Oats	Anise
Apricots	Beets		Dill
Cherry	Chicory		Cumin
Pineapple	Chamomile	**Other Foods**	Parsley
Pomegranate	Horseradish	Chicken	Caraway
Plum	Turnip roots + greens	Trout	Coriander
Pumpkin	Brussel sprouts	Salmon	Cinnamon
	Onions	Lamb	Clove
	Garlic	Chestnuts	All peppers in small amounts
	Scallions	Walnuts	(except white)
	Chives	Raw goat's milk	
	Leeks	Black tea	
	Taro root	coffee	

Neutral Foods

These foods can be eaten without much effect on core temperature issues.

Fruit	Vegetables	Legumes/Grains	Other Foods
Lemon	Cabbage	Polished rice	Honey
Red grapes	Carrot	Corn	Goose
	Mushroom	Pea	Quail meat + eggs
	Cauliflower	Peanut	Olives
	Yams		Beef
	Potato		Chicken
			Jasmine tea
			Oolong tea

Heavy Metal Toxicity and Low Body Temperature

Heavy metals are one of the primary causes of low body temperature and immune system depression. Many microbes cannot be brought back under control until the heavy metals have been removed from the body. High and low-level infections can be ongoing for decades in spite of high dose antibiotics and intravenous antimicrobials when heavy metals are present. Heavy metals promote the over-acidic, low oxygen, low temperature environment which microbes thrive in.

The term heavy metals refers to the over-accumulation of many different types of metals in the fat cells, central nervous system (brain, brainstem, spinal cord), bones, glands, or hair. Heavy metals may include mercury, lead, cadmium, palladium, platinum, arsenic, and nickel, just to name a few.

Of interest concerning low body temperature are the metals palladium and platinum. Researchers from Notre Dame University and Wichita State University, in the most detailed study of its kind, found that the catalytic converters in automobiles are spewing out palladium and platinum in the exhaust fumes.[143] It is now understood that we are driving through an invisible cloud of these metals and are breathing them into our lungs; we are also potentially consuming them in our foods as these clouds of metal are known to deposit up to 150 feet on either side of the roadways. Crops, farm animals, and even your kitchen and home are constantly being poisoned by the fallout of these metals.

Interestingly, palladium is known as "The Depressive Metal," since it is known to cause depression in people. It is also known to cause overcooling of the body. Now consider what maladies are plaguing most of America -- depression and low body temperature. Coincidence, or good science?

A story was published in a recent edition of *Environmental Science and Technology*, reporting that roadside platinum is an allergen that aggravates asthma sufferers and causes other respiratory difficulties.[144] Platinum toxicity has also been associated with cancer and birth defects.[145]

This entire book has been talking about how we must change the body's internal environment so that it is not a happy home for microbes. Heavy metals play a large role in setting you up for chronic and repeated infections. The effects of all the various heavy metals cannot be addressed completely in this book, but you can see that the detoxification of the body is a an ongoing chore. We live in an incredibly toxic environment. Even when you seemingly live a healthy lifestyle, toxins will remain an issue.

The problem with most efforts to detoxify the body, especially in someone with a low body temperature, is the fact that many of these heavy metal toxins are deposited deep within the body tissues. These deep tissues are cold, rigid, and many times too solidified for even the most clever detoxification medicines and therapies to reach. This is difficult for many people to comprehend, but consider how a body with poor lymphatic fluid movement and poor circulation cannot effectively deliver the detoxifying medicines to the various areas of the body.

In order to effectively detoxify the body, it stands to reason that the doctor and healthcare team must address the low body temperature. Restoring the normal body temperature will then restore the normal liquid-fluid flow dynamics that would allow the detoxification medicines to reach and remove the metals and toxins.

Another primary source of heavy metal toxicity is the dental material, primarily mercury, used for the last 100+ years, which is used in many "silver amalgams." These amalgam fillings were so controversial when first introduced in the late 1800's that it split the only dental association of the time, the National Association of Dental Surgeons, into two groups. One group said no one should ever use mercury in the mouth because it is so very toxic and is known to leach out over time, poisoning the body. The other group of dentists

Step 4: Support the Bio-Energetic Fields of the Body

liked how easy it was to work with and how inexpensive mercury amalgams were. In the 1800's, gold was the otherwise preferred dental filling material. The two factions debated the issue until a new dental association was born, the American Dental Association (ADA), our present-day leading dental association, which you see approving most grocery store brand toothpastes. It was the ADA who approved of the mercury fillings, which became the norm of our society.

Of historical interest, the first use of the name "Quack" when referring to a questionable doctor was used to label these dentists using mercury, since mercury was then known as "Quacksilver." Today it is estimated that millions of mercury amalgams are placed in teeth every year in the U.S. alone. One can only marvel at the power and influence various associations in our country have over our standard of living, especially when considering that doctors and dentists have been persecuted and prosecuted, sometimes losing their license to practice in the U.S., for attempting to spread the word about these issues and relieve suffering through the removal of amalgams. Recent legislation has been proposed to outlaw the use of mercury in amalgams.

Some countries, such as Sweden, have banned the use of mercury and will even pay up to 50% of the cost to have it removed from its citizens, stating that the cost of removal is cheaper than paying for the long-term chronic illnesses as the result of these amalgams.[146] (On a related dental note, many European countries do not allow the use of fluoride in water and toothpaste due to limited benefit and excessive health complications.)

Mercury is 1000 times more toxic than lead, while the methyl-mercury vapor coming off of fillings during chewing is 100 times more toxic than elemental mercury.

These "silver amalgams" actually contain up to 50% mercury by weight, 35% silver, 13% tin, 2% copper, and a trace amount of zinc.[147]

German research has shown that mercury from a pregnant mother's amalgams are directly related to high levels of mercury in their fetuses.[148] I have seen many toothless patients who use only dentures and are incredulous that they have heavy metal toxicity still from old amalgams long removed. The teeth were likely removed due to long-term degenerative changes in teeth that were full of amalgams, crowns, root canals, and bridges, all of which were releasing various metals into the bones and tissues of the jaws, and indeed the entire body. Dr. Stephan Edelson, M.D., medical director of the Environmental and Preventative Health Center of Atlanta, Georgia, explains that, "mercury vapor (methyl-mercury) is readily absorbed into the blood because of its solubility in blood lipids (fatty molecules). This process contributes to between 80 and 100% absorption through the lungs from which the mercury is then carried to virtually every tissue of the body, including the brain."[149] Therefore, the burden all of those years of metals leaching from the teeth and from other sources are not relieved by simply removing the teeth. You must understand that it is no simple matter to detoxify the body of heavy metals.

Biological Dentistry is as different from conventional dentistry as doctors practicing Biological Medicine are from conventional doctors. These dentists strive to restore the integrity of the teeth as part of the completely integrated organ circuits. They understand that metals in the teeth create galvanic electricity that blasts through the organ circuits, causing many of today's worst illnesses. Biological Dentists seek to replace potentially harmful dental materials with safe materials that are as close to the normal enamel as possible, or as biocompatible as can be found.

Let's briefly discuss some of the other sources of heavy metals so that you may understand how to avoid further accumulation. Exposure to cigarettes and other tobacco products are a source of the heavy metal toxins lead and cadmium. Lead can also come from old paint in your home,

Step 4: Support the Bio-Energetic Fields of the Body

cooking utensils, ceramic glazes, and solder on water pipes. Aluminum comes from many cooking pots and utensils, as well as antiperspirants and deodorants, aluminum foil, and is found commonly in tap water. Cadmium can be found in some soft drinks, fungicides, various types of plastics, instant coffee, and teas. The continual breakdown of metals in every machine releases an endless variety of metals into the air we breathe; consider atomic particles of titanium coming off of the turbines of approximately 70,000 jet airliners flying over the U.S. at any given time.

The list of metals and their potential for interfering with the proper function of the human body is endless. When considering these issues, you become even more aware of the need to reduce the exposure to potential sources of heavy metal toxins as well as the need to detoxify the body on a long-term, ongoing basis. Stay away from the mindset that you can detoxify for a period of time and be done with it.

With all this in mind, the question ceases to be, "Where did I get all of this heavy metal?" and moves to "How do I now get rid of it?"

General Guidelines for Heavy Metal Detoxification

- First identify the primary heavy metal toxins in your body, either through Electro-dermal screening, Bio-Resonance Scanning, Applied or Clinical Kinesiology, CRT (Computerized Regulation Thermography), or through various laboratory tests, such as Heavy Metal Hair Analysis or Heavy Metal urine tests with a chelation challenge.
- Following all of the guidelines for raising low body temperature is a prerequisite to any successful heavy metal detoxification plan.
- Various nutritional supplements, herbal formulas, and metal chelation products have been tested and reported in peer-reviewed journals and found to greatly reduce

the body's load of heavy metals. Always consult with your healthcare professional, since simply "stirring up" the toxins may just relocate the metals in a more sensitive area of the body and cause a more severe malady. This detoxification should therefore not be attempted as a home treatment.
- Before any type of detoxification treatment is started or any silver (mercury) amalgams are removed, you must make certain that the lymphatic system is open and able to efficiently clear out the toxins that these treatments will be stirring up inside your body. The best way to address the lymphatic system is the ST-8 Lymphatic Drainage therapy. This will be described in more detail later in the book. It is important to continue ST-8 treatments throughout any detoxification program so that the organs of elimination can function without becoming overloaded. The ST-8 will help avoid problems resulting from a congested lymphatic system as well as stimulate the release of metals from every tissue in the body.
- Far Infrared Sauna therapy is one of the best ways to release not only heavy metals from deep within the tissues, but also to release all lipotrophic toxins (toxins stored in the fat cells). Far infrared saunas are not to be confused with regular steam saunas, which many people cannot tolerate and may aggravate some illnesses. Far infrared saunas do not involve excessive temperatures, and the infrared penetrates up to one and a half inches into the body to release deeply embedded toxins and bring them through the skin to be wiped off with a towel.
- Research supports the use of homeopathic metals to induce the release of metals from the body.[150] Usually a low potency homeopathic (6x-12x) is best to cause a release of metals from the body. With this form of detoxification, if the goal is to remove mercury from the

Step 4: Support the Bio-Energetic Fields of the Body

body, your healthcare professional would use homeopathic mercury in a 6-12x potency. If the desire was to remove aluminum, then a 6-12x potency of homeopathic aluminum would be used, and so on.

- Ion-Cleanse Detoxification footbath -- see Chapter 45 for details.
- Drinking distilled water during a metal detoxification program can help remove metals. Distilled water is de-mineralized water. This makes it a good chelator of metals as the distilled water can chelate (pull or attract) metals from the tissues so then the body can excrete them via the urine. (General recommendation is up to 3 quarts per day during detox program only.) Distilled water should only be used during the heavy metal detox program since it may ultimately pull beneficial minerals out of the body when used long-term.

Influence of Sympathetic Treatments on Core Temperature

Any kind of medicine designed to suppress the natural processes of the body can be said to be sympathetic and potentially harmful in the long run. Sympathetic treatments usually counteract whatever the body is attempting to accomplish. This is the proverbial mainstream allopathic (symptom-based) medicine for the most part, although natural medicine as a whole is guilty of much of the same. Such medicines might include antipyretics, antibiotics, decongestants, and pain killers.

Antipyretics are fever-reducing medicines, like most of the acetaminophen type over-the-counter (OTC) drugs. By now, you understand better the role that fever plays in the healthy body. To suppress or artificially bring down a fever, especially in children, really disrupts the body's thermostat, causing it to be too low.

Prescription antibiotics are definitely sympathetic and suppressive treatments that are contrary to maintaining a normal body temperature. Antibiotics, like the name suggests, are "anti" against, and "biotics" means life, so "against life." Many people seem to think a swollen and hot lymph node is a sign that they need an antibiotic. The swollen lymph node is a sign that the body is working and fighting microbial overgrowth. To take an antibiotic is to send the message to the body that it is not needed anymore, and to stop attempting to control microbes. Antibiotics in effect say "step aside body, we will do the work for you." As a result of taking antibiotics, the body is disrupted in mid-stride. The balance is lost. The rhythmical aspects of the body are no longer synchronous. Fluid regulation and transformation and transportation is disrupted, leading to dehydration of the blood and lymph, and ultimately the tissues. Antibiotics kill friendly intestinal bacteria, further creating an internal environment that is cold and dysfunctional.

Natural medicine practitioners are just as guilty many times when they use "natural" antibiotics. Due to their more complex molecular structures, these botanical substances will kill microbes sometimes better than antibiotics. But after everything presented here, is the point of optimal treatment to kill the microbes for the body? No, the body simply requires balance and support so that it can bring microbes under control. I always wonder about the makers and claims of some botanical medicines and colloidal silver-type medicines to "kill every microbe known to man." Did they stop to consider the over 400 species of friendly bacteria (probiotics) known to inhabit the healthy digestive system, that help us digest our food correctly and produce B-vitamins for us? No doubt there will be times when a person has waited too long, and the life or limb must be saved through antibiotics, natural or otherwise. Chronic Lyme is usually not one of these times.

Decongestants are used to dry up mucus, even though the mucus is the body's way of removing toxins and microbes and generally getting rid of substances clogging up the inside of the body, moving it to the outside for expulsion via the nose

Step 4: Support the Bio-Energetic Fields of the Body

and mouth. Decongestants create a condition of dehydration in the tissues. I consulted with one person who had taken a leading prescription decongestant that had caused the entire body to become dehydrated, and the skin was now leathery from an out-of-control fluid disturbance globally. Degeneration of the organs is the end result. In my opinion, there is no time where these types of medicines are a good choice. Natural expectorants and bath therapies to encourage liquefying and moving mucus, combined with addressing the causes of the mucus, is infinitely better and works with the efforts of the body instead of against the body.

Even vitamins and supplements, when used inappropriately, can be a sympathetic treatment that can work against the body's natural tendencies in the long run. This will shock many of you; however, no one takes more vitamins and supplements than the chronically ill. I have seen hundreds of cases where people are taking fistfuls of vitamins in high doses just to feel halfway normal. Most of them have been taking them for years -- if they ever tried quitting, they were soon sick again. If you have to keep taking something, even something supposedly good for you, in order to feel good, then it is a sympathetic treatment only. If it were truly "fixing" the problem, eventually you would no longer need it. If whatever is at the core of the body's problem is not being addressed, it will likely continue to worsen. Granted, most will benefit from supplementation with vitamins at some point, due to the overall poor nutrient content of most of the food we consume.

Many times I have heard of miraculous "cures" from promoters of leading supplement companies; however, in the final analysis, if the "cured" person ever quits taking the supplement, the illness many times returns. The only time I would say this is acceptable is when the person has scarring of organs and surgically removed organs, or otherwise permanent damage; sympathetic treatment is all that is left for these people. True cures from vitamins will be seen only when they are addressing the core of the problem, and when they are thoughtfully applied to support the overall healing process.

---

[143] Cohen E, 2001, *Grit could be a roadside attraction*. Notre Dame Online Magazine.
[144] Hodge V, Stallard M, 1986, *Platinum and palladium in roadside dust*. Environmental Science & Technology. Vol. 20, no. 10, pp. 1058-1060.
[145] The Wichita Eagle, Monday, November 26, 2001, front page story, Denise Neil.
[146] Definitive Guide to Cancer, Goldberg, B., Diamond J. Future Medicine Publishing Inc., 1997
[147] Let the Tooth be Known..., Are Your Teeth Making You Sick, Dawn Ewing RDH, PhD, ND, 1998, Published by Holistic Health Alternatives
[148] Definitive Guide to Cancer,
[149] Definitive Guide to Cancer and Kudsk, F. "Uptake of Hg Vapors in Blood *In Vivo* and *In Vitro* from Hg-containing Air" Acta Pharmacologica et Toxicologica 27 (1969), 49.
[150] Mallick P, Mallick C, et al, *Ameliorating effect of microdoses of a potentized homeopathic drug, Arsenicum Album, on arsenic-induced toxicity in mice. BMC Complementary and Alternative Medicine* 2003, 3:7.

29

~

The Warmth Organization of the Body

Today's society suffers almost uniformly from a chronic condition of dysregulated warmth organization throughout the body. We no longer see the inflammatory diseases so common up until the mid-twentieth century. Plaguing society today are the cold, sclerotic illness, such as chronic fatigue, fibromyalgia, chronic viral and bacterial infections, multiple sclerosis, and the ultimate "cold body" disease: cancer.

Conventional medicine focuses on the microscopic analysis of the body, counting the number of this or that type of cell or microbe. Biological Medicine and Circuit Healing, on the other hand, recognize healing of the body as a completely integrated organism. However, attention can and should be focused upon supporting specific aspects of the human being, such as supporting the restoration of the normal warmth organization throughout the body.

Doctors must become experts at recognizing and addressing the various conditions of dysregulated warmth in the body and extremities. Several possibilities exist. There could be cold hands and feet, warm hands and cold feet, warm oral temperature and cold thorax, local cold spots, or global coldness, just to name a few. Each of these cold conditions should be a clue to the doctor of the unique imbalance in the body, to the same degree as abnormal findings on blood tests.

At times a doctor may get caught up in the microscopic view of the patient and miss the truly vital information gained from simple observation. We must all become masters of reading the signs readily available by observation on the macroscopic scale. One hundred years of microscopic analysis has gained the U.S.A. some of the worst health in the world. The common, but flawed, theme taught in most medical schools is that if one can determine what substance that the body is low or high in, then supplementing with that nutrient or lowering the high substance will correct the illness. This "pieces and parts" mentality is one of the primary reasons our society is failing, and chronic illness of all types is the norm.

Observing and tracking the regulation of warmth throughout the body is one component of the lost "art" in the healing arts. Once one recalls that in the end the body must do the healing, not the medicines, the importance of warmth becomes obvious. Specifically, the electrical oscillatory rate of every healthy cell in the body is sustained by the correct amount of warmth. Too much warmth, either inflammation or fever, increases the electrical oscillatory rate and subsequently increases the breakdown of protein. Too much coldness causes a decrease in the cell's electrical oscillatory rate, the fluids begin to thicken, and the cell degenerates and becomes increasingly dysfunctional and toxic.

It becomes clear that the best medicine in the world for a given condition may not be able to work when the body is too cold. When the body is chronically cold, it becomes non-reactive, ceasing to respond appropriately to medicines and its environment.

The next question must be, "What regulates the warmth organization of the body?" To answer this question, we must understand that there is more to the human body than the eye can see. From an electro-energetic perspective, the body is almost not here. Electrons spinning at billions of cycles per second around a nucleus provide us with the solid feel of the body, but the fact is that the body is, energetically speaking, not very dense. Many types of energy pass freely through the human body, such as quarks, neutrinos, and other energetic particles. Armed with the new realization that we are more electro-energetic than pieces and parts, we can begin to accept that there are varying fields of electro-energy, inseparable within and surrounding the body. These fields of energy have been named for scientific agreement. The etheric field, otherwise known as "ether body," is that electro-energetic level that regulates the warmth organization of the "physical" body.

The challenge of the doctor is to determine how best to recognize and treat the imbalance in the ether body. One may think that simply recognizing the coldness of the body is enough; however, the coldness of the body is a symptom of the disturbed ether body. Treatments must address the imbalances in the ether body. This is the reason that taking thyroid medicines such as Armor Thyroid or Synthroid to combat a cold core temperature is most often purely treating the symptom; they do nothing to correct the ether body.

Generally, we break down the body during the day and rebuild it again at night while we sleep. The only reason we sleep is to repair and regenerate the tissues of the body. Nighttime and sleep is the time of highest etheric field energy. The etheric field governs both the warmth organization and the regeneration of tissue.

Illness and healing are aggravated especially at night due to interference of the etheric field by the chaotic and disruptive nature of the electrical fields emitted by the wiring running in every wall, floor, and ceiling of your bedroom. The wiring in your bedroom can definitely be disruptive to the body, even though we can potentially live over 100 years of age. The idea that living to be 100 years old indicates health is a mistaken impression. Many of these people never wanted or planned to live this long. It is simply living in misery for a very long time. While we obviously can live many years while sleeping bathed in these disruptive electrical fields, in the search for health and healing, one must eliminate every known issue that might interfere with the body's natural ability to regulate its warmth and its ability to regenerate healthy, vibrant tissue.

The electrical fields of your bedroom are one of the primary disruptors of the body's etheric field and therefore must be shielded.

As mentioned earlier, the **BIOPRO Home Harmonizer** is a must in every home. The research shows that the **BIOPRO Home Harmonizer** and BIOPRO **Cell Chip** will protect against cell phone microwaves.

At times the body responds to cold spots or regions within the body by producing an inflammatory reaction to warm it up. This may be seen in pain syndromes that come and go suddenly from no obvious traumatic cause. This body mechanism is inefficient in resolving coldness in the body, not to mention that most people have been conditioned by doctors to fight pain with pain killers. Pain killers promote a chronic cold condition in the body.

Contrast foot baths can be used to great benefit in that alternating cold and hot foot baths seeks to stimulate the body's restorative warmth organization and circulation. To use this therapy, soak the feet in hot water for one minute, and then soak in cold water for 30 seconds. This should be repeated 3-5 times in a session, 2-3 times per day, for several weeks. The effect can be enhanced by adding one teaspoon of **2% copper sulfate** solution to the hot water. Copper is known to be warming to the body; as the old saying goes, "Rubbing a copper penny warms the hand."

Another possible cause of disturbed warmth in the body is the congested and dysregulated fluid organization. The excessive accumulation of fluid overwhelms and basically puts out the fire warming the body. This condition is usually the result of a sedentary lifestyle and poor elimination of wastes through the skin. The best corrective therapy for this common ailment is the regular use of a **Far Infrared Sauna**, which allows for 3-6 times greater sweat production than the much hotter conventional steam and dry saunas. Greater results can be realized by taking 3-6 pillules of the homeopathic remedy **Ferrum phosphoricum 6x** potency, 30-60 minutes before entering the sauna. This improves the warmth reaction of the body and increases sweat production.

Low potency (3-6x) homeopathic **Apis** can be applied locally to fight cold spots and will help restore balanced warmth, negating the need for the body to produce inflammation.

No medicine is better at treating disturbances in the global warmth organization of the body than subcutaneous injections of the German prescription homeopathic medicine **Iscar**, when combined with corrective associated therapies, such as color and music therapy, rhythmical massage therapy, and curative movement therapies.

A primary cause of disturbed warmth organization in the body is the global phenomenon of electro-magnetic, chemical, and heavy metal toxicity within everyone alive. The air we breathe is full of heavy metals, such as titanium, palladium, platinum, and every other conceivable metal and metal alloy from the millions of automobiles, jets, and factories. It is absorbed into even the best biodynamically and/or organically grown foods, as these toxins are carried on the wind to the farthest reaches of the most remote locations on the planet. Until radical improvement and change in industry and society as a whole occurs, we will suffer from toxicity. Environmental toxins are very disruptive to the warmth organization of the body. Until the toxic load in your body is reduced, no success can be expected in regard to correcting the warmth organization, and subsequently the restoration, of your health. There seems to be no relief in sight, and generally ongoing detoxification will always be necessary.

Circuit healing addresses and supports the restoration of all the electro-energetic fields as well as the physical needs of the body. The need for addressing all levels of the body should be obvious, since one can support the etheric body forever, but without decreasing the toxic load, restoration of the body's warmth will not be made manifest.

Step 5
Address all Structural Interferences

30

~

Doctors of Chiropractic

Structural Issues to Address with Your Doctor

- Chiropractic adjustments of the spine, pelvis, cranium, upper/lower extremities.
- Myofascial release of the cellular memory of physical, chemical, and emotional traumas.
- Neurological/hemispheric synchronization and optimizations.
- Neuro-Photonic Therapy™ to address the crytstalline-matrix and bio-information problems.
- Address physical interferences due to low body temperature. Read Chapters 27-29.

Doctors of Chiropractic and Natural Health

I have become aware that many people are surprised that we at Hansa Center, Doctors of Chiropractic, can address people suffering from such a wide range of illnesses. Some people seem to think Doctors of Chiropractic can only deal with stiff necks and low back pain. This is partly due to the political stance that the chiropractic profession has had to maintain in order to exist. However, this is no truer than thinking a Medical Doctor can only prescribe drugs.

Any medical doctor, osteopath, naturopath, or doctor of chiropractic can receive post-graduate training in Euro-America Biological Medicine. I have been asked innumerable times, "Why don't M.D.'s do this?" To answer this, one must realize that most M.D.'s work in hospitals or group practices. These doctors cannot just decide one day to do Biological or natural medicine in these settings. The hospitals and insurance companies dictate what they can and can't do, and rightly so, since the hospitals are ultimately liable for their doctors' actions. Even in small group practices, the safety of the whole keeps one doctor from doing things differently. If all this were not detriment enough, most medical doctors have a "non-compete" clause in their contract with the hospitals that forbids them to practice within a 50 mile radius from any hospital owned by that corporation. In our area, most of the small outlying hospitals have been bought out by large hospital corporations, making it nearly impossible for any of their doctors to set up a Biological Medicine practice in any but the most remote areas.

Doctors of Chiropractic are uniquely qualified to specialize in Biological Medicine due to their intensive education in working with the structure and function of body. They are trained to facilitate healing through natural means instead of relying on drugs to force the body to perform illusions of health.

Doctors of Chiropractic believe that the body has an innate intelligence. Innate intelligence is that part of each of us that knows how the heart should beat. It's the regulatory and control mechanisms behind how the body heals a cut, or how the body knows how to breathe without your conscious participation. Once again, treating **disease** is the realm of the conventional medical doctors – Chiropractic and Biological Medicine have no desire to treat any **disease**, but to focus upon restoring the integrity of the body, mind, and spirit, thereby leading to the disappearance of disease. Of course, there is a place for heroic medicine in the form of drugs, surgery, and other similar needs. In crisis, definitely save the life first and foremost, but once the crisis has been averted, restoring the body, mind, and spirit to maximum integrity through Biological and natural means, working to restore the perfection of God's design, is optimal.

From day one of training, Doctors of Chiropractic are taught the research that proves that the body has an innate intelligence and the body is designed to heal itself. From day one, the Doctor of Chiropractic learns only to facilitate healing, to diagnose different pathologies, and to optimize the neurology, physiology, histology, and chemistry of the body to facilitate healing. Doctors of Chiropractic do not have to unlearn invasive and toxic methods and relearn that God designed the body to heal itself.

As you will see later in this section, Doctors of Chiropractic are fully trained in every area of health and healing. Doctors of Chiropractic must have a Bachelor's degree before being admitted, they must complete their "Pre-Med" elbow to elbow with the other prospective M.D., D.O., D.D.S., and D.V.M students. Once accepted into Chiropractic College, students are taught an almost identical curriculum as every medical professional for four years, up to the point where every doctor must specialize.

It is up to each graduating doctor to determine how they are going to apply the knowledge they have gained. It must be understood that all schooling is an agreed upon minimum amount of information. For a bachelor's degree, you will know at least this much; for a master's degree, this much; for a doctorate, you will know at least the agreed upon minimum also. So, even at the doctorate level, the knowledge is not the ultimate knowledge in the field. That is why doctors must have 35 hours per year of accredited continuing education coursework approved by the State Healing Arts Board. This enables the doctor to learn specialized knowledge in their field of interest. This continuing education in a specialized field may represent over a thousand more classroom hours. Our field of interest and "specialization" is in learning to address the degenerative and chronic diseases, using natural methods. This is called American Biological Medicine.

Keep in mind, no doctor can go any further than they have been taught! Biological Medicine is a specialized training that not every doctor receives; your conventional physician may not know how to advise you regarding its use. You must seek out a doctor specializing in Biological Medicine in your area. One resource for finding these doctors is the Marion Foundation, which can be accessed on the internet or key in a word search for "Biological Medicine."

If you are looking for a Doctor of Chiropractic in your area, you need to call around and say to the receptionist, "I realize that your doctor sees many different problems, but I am curious about which type of patients he or she sees the most?" At the Hansa Center for Optimum Health, we say we attract what we affectionately refer to as our "Humpty Dumpty Bunch," where all the king's horses and all the king's men could not put them back together again.

The profession has different specializations within it just as Medical Doctors do. To name a few, there are Doctors of Chiropractic who specialize as internists, pediatricians, sports medicine, neurology, and obviously my favorite and what I consider the crème de la crème, those specializing in Biological Medicine. You must maintain the integrity of the nervous system and the musculoskeletal system in order for the body to heal itself.

Doctors of Chiropractic are in the top half of 1% of the most educated people in the world and are absolutely qualified to treat the body, mind, and spirit. A Doctor of Chiropractic can be your greatest ally in any illness.

Step 5: Address all Structural Interferences

The following chart compares the number of hours Doctors of Chiropractic and Medical Doctors take in their basic training before they specialize.

Chiropractic Hours	Subject	Medical Hours
456	Anatomy/Embryology	215
243	Physiology	174
296	Pathology	507
161	Chemistry	100
145	Microbiology	145
408	Diagnosis	113
149	Neurology	171
271	X-ray	13
56	Psychology/Psychiatrics	323
66	Obstetrics/Gynecology	284
168	Orthopedics	2
2419	-- Total Hours --	**2047**

31

~

What to Expect with Biological Medicine

If you are suffering from any chronic illness, it is almost guaranteed that you have had "suppressive" therapies used on you. For example: if you went to your doctor for headaches, your doctor would most likely give you a painkiller. After all, you are having a headache due to the fact that your body is deficient in aspirin, right? Wrong answer! The headaches continue to worsen until the aspirin no longer works, so your doctor puts you on something stronger. The cause of the headache remains untouched. You just can't feel it. All you are doing is buying yourself time. You will have to "pay the piper" eventually when all of the different painkillers don't even affect the headaches anymore. Always remember that true healing cannot occur by simply masking the symptoms.

Doctors practicing the principles of Biological Medicine attempt to address the <u>cause</u> of the headache (or whatever problem) by restoring the integrity of the body as a whole: structurally, chemically, energetically, bio-electrically, and by addressing lifestyle, stress issues, and spiritual problems. The resulting relief is sometimes as quick as or quicker than prescription drug painkillers. Sometimes, as the body begins to truly heal from a chronic illness, you may feel worse before you feel better as you body is dealing with the many issues that it had to "put on the back burner" for so long. This is good in most cases, because it means that the causes of your symptoms, instead of the symptoms only, are finally being addressed. Some people call this a healing crisis, but a thoughtful planning of treatment by your physician can limit the severity of these problems. Over-aggressive treatment will undoubtedly cause more severe healing crises.

As mentioned in earlier discussions, in the treatment of chronic Lyme Disease, one may experience something called a Herxheimer reaction, a medical term for an anticipated worsening of your symptoms in reaction to the die-off toxins from bacteria breaking apart. A **Herxheimer reaction is a sign of poor elimination pathway drainage, poor organ support, and poor treatment!** The body of most chronic Lyme sufferers is a toxic dump to start with, and if the doctor does not get the pathways of elimination open and working, the body gets even more toxic when the bacteria begin to die and their toxins dump. Many doctors think good treatment is indicated by the fact that you feel awful, which seems to confirm they selected an effective antibiotic. The "herx" most often indicates a poorly designed treatment program.

Feeling worse during the natural treatments of Alternative and Biological Medicine happens, sometimes because so much of what is wrong in your body are things that your body has adapted to over a long period. If you do not get the appropriate treatment at the initial stages when something goes wrong, the body is forced to adapt to things being out of place and out of balance. When your doctor begins to correct these issues, the body will bring all of these problems "off the back burner" to be finally dealt with. Often you will find that you retrace your symptoms chronologically; the most recent problem will be the first to go, while the first or initial problem will be the last to go. Once you realize that this is what is happening, you can rejoice because you know where you are in your healing. If you stop treatment halfway through this chronological retracing, you can already know much of what you have to look forward to in the upcoming months and years since you have already been there. This said, none of the worsening here is a true Herxheimer reaction, and most patients do not experience a worsening of their condition. Some of the more severely affected Lyme patients I have seen could not tolerate feeling any worse!

Much thought was given in developing the treatment protocol outlined in this book in order to limit or eliminate any "healing crisis" by effectively addressing the needs of the body in states of chronic illness.

Do not be afraid of healing. It took a long time to get to this point, and it is going to take time to heal as well. Remember, as a general rule, you should allow three months of doing things right with balanced lifestyle and proper treatment for every year you have had your condition. Every single atom of your body is replaced at least one time per year. It takes about six weeks for the bottom layer of skin to become the top layer. Old skin cells are constantly dying and being replaced by new ones. You get a new liver, however, every four months. The goal is to remove the problems that are causing the perpetuation of dysfunctional cells so that when the body replaces cells, it is able to replace them with good, healthy cells. Nerve tissue takes the longest to regenerate. When considering that the body's structure and function is driven primarily by its energetic and vibrational properties, any interference with the body's normal crystalline laser-like coherent matrix will result in altered structure and function. So do not look at your illness as a possible quick-fix situation. It is going to take good therapies that do not harm the body plus a whole lot of time.

Keep in mind that many symptoms are blamed on Lyme Disease when the reality is that it may be a mix of Lyme and something entirely different causing some of your symptoms. Parasites, non-related bacterial and viral infections, systemic yeast infections, toxic overload, and poor lifestyle choices can be the cause of some of your symptoms. This is one of the strengths of our treatment protocol outlined here; it addresses many of these common problems.

The true skill of the doctor of Biological Medicine can be seen in his understanding of the interconnectedness of every tissue of the body. The majority of doctors are trained to treat based upon the numbers on a lab test and have only basic training in reacting to symptoms with symptomatic treatments. For example, a conventional doctor will address frequent and burning urination with an antibiotic, an inflamed joint with an anti-inflammatory, or treat a skin rash with cortisone cream or antihistamines. This is not determining cause and effect; it is effect and anti-effect medicine.

The doctor trained in Biological Medicine has learned to read the signs and decipher the clues the body is revealing to form a working set of functional diagnostic conclusions. If the point is to facilitate the body's ability to heal itself instead of simply providing medicines that will counteract the symptoms, then the doctor must learn how to determine where the primary problem is to be found. The doctor's job then becomes one where he works to remove whatever is interfering with the body's ability to heal itself, and to provide the information and building blocks the body needs for optimal function. The beauty of Biological Medicine can be seen in the following patient stories.

Before we get too far along, I want you to realize that many times abnormal findings on blood tests still do not tell the doctor why that aspect of the blood is outside of normal limits, and the tests are therefore simply more clues that should be integrated into the global view of the patient. Although they do not diagnose, blood tests are still a good way to track progress.

Step 5: Address all Structural Interferences

Selected Cases from the Hansa Center

These true cases are selected to highlight the uniqueness of Biological Medicine and to demonstrate various considerations in true healing. The reality is that even in these cases, it usually takes minutes to notice improvements in symptoms but months to years of work to heal completely.)

Case #1: Classic case of a chronic Lyme Disease patient

Miss F. was a vibrant young woman of 17 years of age. She had been diagnosed with Lyme Disease in England, and her conventional medical doctor prescribed numerous antibiotics and a strict regimen of food allergy shots. Miss F. was progressively worsening and had not been able to walk for six months, being confined to the bed due to severe pain in the feet, bilateral knee grinding and pain, debilitating vertigo, headaches, and profound muscle weakness throughout the body. Miss F. could tolerate only a small number of foods and had become dependent upon the food (antigen) allergy shots; if the shots were not taken, all of her symptoms worsened for days, a condition that had only surfaced after beginning the shots.

Miss F. was in a position in which many Lyme patients are placed--their condition is progressively worsening, yet their doctors tell them that they *must* continue with the treatment protocol "for a year or more." The hope of all is that after all the suffering, things will begin to turn around in the end. Miss F. was desperate and beginning to lose hope.

On Miss F.'s first visit, it was determined via Bio-Resonance Scanning™ (BRS) that every organ circuit was working at less than 40% of maximum integrity. As you have read in this book (see Chapter 7, Circuit Healing), most of the muscles of the body share the same dedicated electromagnetic circuitry with an organ. Since every organ circuit was severely compromised, that meant that virtually every muscle in the body would be suffering the same fate. Upon testing the individual muscles, it was found that most of the muscles could barely hold a contraction strong enough to be lifted against gravity!

A complete assessment with BRS enabled the identification of the top ten worst organs or glands, the top ten worst chemical problems, and many other structural and electromagnetic imbalances.

Treatment began the same day. BRS was used to identify the most appropriate treatments to first balance the electromagnetic fields of the body, then to address the many structural problems (such as the eleven different pelvic sprains which were found), and the organ circuits were brought back online energetically by using BRS to select the most appropriate remedies. Many other bio-energetic issues were addressed before the visit was over.

The entire process took about one hour, in this particular case with two of our doctors working on the patient at the same time, both using the BRS to address issues dynamically (at the time of discovery). After both doctors were satisfied that the best initial corrections were done, I instructed Miss F., "Go ahead now and stand up and walk!" To her credit, she was brave -- tentatively at first, she stood and began walking around the room! The vertigo was gone, the knees were not grinding, and her feet hurt only slightly. Miss F. was so very thankful, almost to tears.

We continued treating Miss F. for almost a week, after which every symptom was gone, with the exception of periodic bouts of fatigue.

Without BRS to guide us and without the pure philosophy regarding what is required to facilitate healing, these types of rapid results could not be possible. Not every patient responds this rapidly, but in a review of 58 random patient files from the Hansa Center, it was found that virtually 100% patients are able to report at least one of their symptoms as 50% better after one treatment. The study found that on average, in 1.1 treatments almost 100% of the people were able to say that at least one of their symptoms was 75% better. In the 58 patients, 100% reported one of their symptoms was gone after daily treatments over a two-week period.

The educated reader will know that statistics can be tweaked to "prove" anything. Even these statistics are just what they are. They do not show whether or not these people were cured long-term; however, when questioned, almost all of these patients said, "Nothing that any other doctor has tried has improved any symptom!"

Case #2: Lyme Disease misdiagnosed as Multiple Sclerosis

For six and a half years, Mrs. L. was completely paralyzed in her left leg, with no muscle contractions from her hip all the way to her toes. She wore a leg brace that held her foot straight so she could walk by swinging her leg like a peg-leg. She had severe low back pain from the instability of the back and pelvis because of the muscle atrophy on the left side.

Mrs. L. suspected that she might have Lyme after having read the first edition of the *Beating Lyme Disease* book, which is now out of print and being replaced with this book. Her conventional medical doctors would not perform any blood test, stating that Lyme Disease is not present in her Midwest state, nor had she ever been to a state where Lyme Disease was a problem. Mrs. L took her health in her own hands and sought our care.

Subsequent BRS and blood tests performed by our clinic verified the presence of Borrelia burgdorferi infection.

Upon our initial physical examination at the Hansa Center, it was found that Mrs. L. definitely could not move any muscle in the leg or foot, nor could any twitching of a muscle be detected.

At the conclusion of her first one-hour treatment using BRS and the Biological Medicine processes of functional diagnosis and treatment, muscle twitching in the leg and feet could be felt when she would attempt to move the leg or toes. At the conclusion of her second one-hour treatment, she could wiggle her toes. By the fourth treatment, Mrs. L. could raise her knee off the table while laying on her back, lift her foot up to 90 degrees when laying on her stomach, roll her ankle around in a complete circle, and wiggle all of her toes! After just four days of treatment, she took off her leg brace and walked, with difficulty due to the severe muscle atrophy after the years of disuse, but without help!

It has now been years since Mrs. L. first came to our clinic. She has never needed the leg brace again. She still is working to rebuild her muscles with nutritional supplements, electrical muscle stimulation, and working out in a swimming pool.

This case is "medically impossible." From a conventional medical mindset, nerve conduction problems from a "demyelinating disease" cannot be restored in such a short time of four days! However, when the specific toxins of the Lyme are addressed, the organ circuit integrity restored, the crystalline matrix and electromagnetic field realigned, the structure and function of the body addressed, and the information needed by the body to resolve the microbial overgrowth provided, real miracles of restoration are possible.

Case #3: The power of the mind over illness

Ms. S. lived outside of the United States and was first seen in our clinic in 1999 after testing highly positive for Lyme Disease on blood tests. She was on disability and could not work. Ms. S. suffered from profound cognitive problems, severe headaches, short- and long-term memory loss, chronic fatigue with unrefreshing sleep, neck pain and stiffness with degeneration of the vertebrae, chronic low back pain, abnormal menstrual cycles, and right eye weakness. FACT testing revealed excessively high levels of neurotoxins affecting the

Step 5: Address all Structural Interferences

brain and nervous system (See Chapter 10 for more information on FACT tests).

The CRT tests confirmed that her vitality was that of an 84 year old woman instead of her actual 46 years. The CRT also revealed that every organ system was severely weakened from the strain of toxins clogging the machinery of her cells.

Ms. S. was treated aggressively on four different trips to our clinic over a five-year period. Each visit usually lasted two weeks, followed by continuing the recommended supplements and therapies at home with periodic phone consultations to monitor her progress.

Several of Ms. S.'s symptoms were at least 50% better within the first week of treatment. However, it took ongoing support for five years, especially since she didn't live close to the clinic and therefore couldn't be treated as often as needed, in order to realize the true wonderful health she so desperately sought.

As is the case in many Lyme sufferers, Ms. S. receive very little mental, emotional, or monetary support from her friends, family, or church. At one point of desperation she reached out for help from the elders in her church, only to be labeled as a "head-case" in need of a life! Ms. S. had a difficult time getting her conventional doctors to acknowledge anything was wrong, even with the positive Lyme tests. She was single and all alone to fight her battles, with the exception of occasional contact with our clinic. Lyme sufferers are often the most heroic and brave group of people, because unlike people with cancer, heart disease, HIV, and other well-recognized illnesses, Lyme sufferers must often bear their illness with no support whatsoever. There are lifesaving support groups now on the internet; my favorites are the Lyme Disease groups on www.healingwell.com and www.healthboards.com, both of which seem to be supportive of both conventional medicine and alternative medicine, unlike some other groups which seem to be very negative to anyone using alternative medicine.

I don't know of many other internet support groups, so my apologies to any truly open and positive group not listed.

After five years of up and down progress with our help, Ms. S. came to the clinic beaming! Every single symptom was at 75-100% better! She was once again enjoying life and very optimistic about her future. She requested a repeat lab test to "prove" to her doctors back home that the Lyme was indeed gone. Against my best wishes, she insisted on getting the test.

The blood test was performed, and to her immense dismay it was still positive! I had suspected it would be, due to my experience and the research that conclusively shows very few people ever test completely clear (though antibody tests and some of the others may test as negative because as one improves the free Lyme antibodies go virtually undetectable).

On the very same night of hearing that the test was positive still, Ms. S. took a nosedive in her symptoms! Every symptom came back with a vengeance.

It required treatment for the emotional crisis and counseling her before I could help pull her out of her nosedive. She quickly realized what her emotions had done to bring back her symptoms and by the next day was back to normal once more.

This case brings to light a saga that I have seen repeated time and again with people suffering from every conceivable illness. It also is a perfect place to tell you of some of the most compelling research ever written. Research reported about people with schizophrenia (multiple personalities) revealed that the MIND and SPIRIT are in complete control of the realities of the physical body! This research showed that in a person with two personalities, one personality may have insulin-dependent diabetes and perfect vision while the second personality would not need any insulin, yet required strong eyeglasses! If you never read another bit of research, if you never took another supplement, if you never had another blood test, see how YOU and the image you hold to be YOU in your HEART-OF-HEARTS really controls your physical reality!

Biological Medicine is the only healing philosophy that truly understands and has the tools and techniques to address the many aspects of the body, mind, and spirit. Biological Medicine recognizes that often the physical body needs to be treated before the mind and spirit can elevate, yet at the same time it recognizes that to truly heal the physical body we must also be addressing the incorrect "data" in the mind that is creating the disturbance in the body; at the same time, it addresses the spirit that is being held back from illumination by the body and mind. Can you see clearer now the error of thinking a better antibiotic or drug is going to give to you the health that only a truly coherent body, mind, and spirit can provide? Be careful not to fall prey to the testimonials that float around on the internet of someone "cured" with this or that drug cocktail, machine, vitamin, or supplement. YOU manifested this illness as part of your journey to a greater reality. Yes, the bacteria may have fueled the symptoms, but the weaknesses and need to learn from it all come from your own heart. I mean to offend no one here. I am not saying, "It is all in your head." I am saying that, with thoughtful help, you can shift from a disease-consciousness to a healthful-journey full of profound rewards. To find out more about how to change your reality, read the companion to this book, *Everyday Miracles by God's Design*.

Case #4: Not a Lyme patient, but this demonstrates the power of the mind and emotions in creating and perpetuating symptoms

Mr. B., a big man over 6'4", had been a compliant patient for almost a year, and although practicing some poor lifestyle choices such as smoking, presented consistently in good health overall. Recently, Mr. B. came in complaining of excessive weakness, pain, and decreased range of motion in the right arm and shoulder for the last four weeks. He stated that it was so weak he couldn't lift his lunch box. He had no idea what caused his problem. Normally with my training as a Doctor of Chiropractic, I would have focused in on the subluxations and the musculo-skeletal system, but instead I examined the shoulder using Bio-Resonance Scanning™. This exam revealed emotional upset as the primary cause of the problem.The pain and weakness in the shoulder was not coming from the shoulder, but instead it was referred from the liver due to emotional stress. Upon questioning Mr. B. regardingregarding excessive stress, I learned that he was in danger of losing his job of 20 years if a company merger took place. He had learned about the possibility six weeks earlier, and even though his job had been threatened this way before, it was definitely bothering him more this time than ever. He went on to describe his feelings as frustration, irritability, and resentment – all emotions that specifically affect the liver.

Further testing identified that the problem could be addressed by applying a specific essential oil blend over the liver. This was one of those moments when I wish there were a video camera in the treatment room. As soon as the oil blend was applied and he tried moving his arm and shoulder, all of the pain and weakness was gone, and he had complete restoration of his range of motion! His eyes wide, he exclaimed, "Even if I tell the guys at work about this, they will never believe it!"

Understand that without Bio-Resonance Scanning™ to identify not only the primary cause but the corrective remedy, one would be left ultimately treating the symptoms. Four weeks of suffering had been remedied in less than five minutes, possibly avoiding months and years of chronic arm and shoulder problems.

Before ending the office visit, I told Mr. B. that he could put the problem back again by continuing to carry negative emotions forward day after day. By controlling his thinking and by living only in the moment, he has remained symptom-free without any further treatments. Again, the *Everyday*

Miracles by God's Design book provides more detailed information on how to optimize every moment of every day.

Question: How did the essential oil get rid of an emotional problem in this case?

Answer: It is scientific fact that our thoughts are extra-low frequency waves found within the electromagnetic spectrum.[151] When one allows a negative thought process to be perpetuated overnight, and in Mr. B.'s case, for weeks, the frequency will get stuck in the crystalline matrix of the body, causing a physical disturbance. The essential oils all have their own electromagnetic frequency, based upon their unique molecular structure. The oils made by Young Living have some of the highest vibrational frequencies of any substance on the planet. The Bio-Resonance Scanning™ enabled the identification of the specific oil blend, which in this case was the inverse frequency that would cancel out or dissipate the negative emotional frequencies stuck in the liver (irritability, frustration, and resentment). Another way to look at this is that the emotions and the essential oil were like two identically sized waves on the ocean moving toward each other. When they collide, they cancel each other out and leave a peaceful calm.

Case #5: Remarkable ways illness can be from an obscure source

Mr. M., a 68-year-old suffered from heart arrhythmia, a condition where the heart does not beat with the correct rhythm. Although he took fistfuls of vitamins for years and prescription medicine for the condition, nothing was working. During our Bio-Resonance Scanning™ portion of his physical, the testing showed that the primary cause of his heart arrhythmia was heavy metals coming from his mouth. He laughed, thinking that he would show this form of testing to be bogus, and he informed me that he wore dentures top and bottom with no metal!

As it turns out, his dentures were hardened and colored with various metals. I had Mr. M. take out his dentures, which I set aside. I then checked his heart rate. It was perfect! Knowing his wife would never believe this, I called her to the room and placed a blood pressure cuff on Mr. M. so that she could watch the needle on the cuff jump crazily with his dentures in his mouth. Then I had him take out the dentures again, and the needle reflected the perfect rhythmical beating of his heart.

I can tell you for certain that dentures affecting the heart are not listed in medical pathology textbooks, nor had I ever heard of it before.

I then recommended that Mr. M. get a new set of dentures made without any metals. He smiled and said, "These are not expensive dentures, but they are the first ones that feel good. I'll just wear them when I eat, and for social occasions." That plan may sound good enough to some, but I informed him that it was unacceptable. Every organ circuit in the body has its time of highest energy, and each organ has two hours in every 24 when it gets the most energy to heal. The heart's time is between 11 a.m. and 1 p.m. -- lunch time. Mr. M. would be putting his dentures back in at lunch time, the time of highest stress on that organ, and, according to some, the time when most heart attacks occur.

No matter what I said, he insisted on keeping his dentures. He continued to not experience arrhythmia when he didn't have the dentures in; however, he would put them in to eat. Sadly, Mr. M. died of a heart attack at 12:30 p.m. a few months later, just a few weeks after he passed an electro-cardiogram test with flying colors, *without his dentures in his mouth*!

Step 5: Address all Structural Interferences

Case #6: How scars interfere with the body's ability to regulate itself

Mr. W., 65, a three-time kidney transplant recipient, presented with excessive pain, weakness, and occasional numbness in his shoulders, arms, and hands, threatening his ability to do his job. The case was complicated by the fact that he must remain on immune-suppressive drugs so that the transplanted kidneys would not be rejected. This causes difficulties since there is virtually nothing Biological Medicine could do that would not cause at least a secondary improvement in immune function. The risk was that the immune system might cause a rejection of the transplanted kidneys. However, it was agreed that doing nothing would leave Mr. W. to degenerate further and lose his livelihood and career.

The treatment plan agreed upon was to address the many large and long scars on Mr. W.'s abdomen, which was crisscrossed with scars from the kidney transplants, gallbladder surgery, and appendix removal.

Biological Medicine recognizes that scar tissue acts as a dam to the flow of photo-electric energy through the meridian system, and indeed as a dam to the communication through the crystalline matrix of the body.

Keep in mind, if a doctor truly cannot heal a simple paper cut, then if true healing is to occur, the doctor must work to remedy anything interfering with the body's ability to heal itself. Scar tissue is a definite interference!

Corrective scar therapy using a frequency-modulated, low-level, non-cutting type of therapeutic laser was used to reconnect and redirect the flow of bioenergetic information through the many scars. This procedure took about 45 minutes, after which Mr. W's individual arm muscles were strength tested. The before and after strength testing was remarkable! The previously-weak muscles were absolutely strong and firm when challenged, the numbness was gone, and the previous pain was gone with the exception of one specific movement.

Subsequent visits showed that the correction remained, much to the delight of Mr. W. Keep in mind, this is far from resolving all of Mr. W.'s health problems, but up to that point, nothing had helped this problem that had been worsening gradually over the previous 10 years.

Case #7: The beauty of the philosophy of Biological Medicine

Mrs. P., 39, had been suffering from viral-induced ulcers coating her tongue, gums, and inner cheeks. In this case, I want to show the logical path that training in Biological Medicine provided. With virtually no more information to go on as this was an initial phone consultation, I was able to determine the following predictable findings. Over the phone I asked her if her tongue was thin, red overall, but with a redder tip, and tooth-marks on the sides – she said it was. I asked her to gently put the tip of her tongue on the roof of her mouth and observe if there were big blackish-purple veins visible – there were. I told her that it was likely that she was a "chronic thinker", one who never relaxed her brain. She agreed and said she even dreamed that she was solving problems at work. I said, "It is likely that you are cold natured." She said all her friends even knew that her hands and feet were always "ice cold." I said it was likely that it hurt too much to get a massage and is difficult to stretch her muscles. She said, "My friends want to rub my shoulders just to be nice, but I can't even stand the pain." I then said that she is likely tired all the time, even after a good nights sleep. On the affirmative, I replied that it is also likely that you have taken a lot of antibiotics. She replied that she had been on many years of antibiotics and was sickly as a child. "How can you know all this about me?" she cried. "No one has ever been able to tell me anything about my condition. I've gargled with every essential oil and concoction friends have suggested, and the prescription drugs don't work either."

I knew these findings should be present because a chronic viral infection of this nature requires a certain internal environment -- a cold body temperature, which you may read more about in Chapter 27, Lyme and Low Body Temperature. The cold body leads to a devitalization of the blood, decreasing its ability to carry oxygen and nutrients, and leads to an acidic condition throughout the body. The cold, sluggish, devitalized blood is reflected in the swollen black-purple sublingual veins of the tongue.

Years of antibiotics often damage the fluid transformation and transportation of the body, leading to the tooth-marks on the tongue from the resulting systemic dehydration. She may drink a gallon of water every day, but she just urinates it out as the result of this fluid regulation problem. The tooth-marks often also reflect a person who never relaxes the mind, a condition that mirrors a person who is so physically tired all the time that they basically must live in their head; the body is just "along for the ride."

The dehydration further results in a hardening of the tissues and an overheating of the organs. The red tongue body reveals a condition of overheating throughout the body. The redder tip of the tongue reflects excessive heat in the heart circuit from a deficiency of fluids. This overheating of the body must be seen as a relative descriptive term only, as the body's core temperature remains low and completely dysregulated, even during this "overheating."

The heart is the body's electromagnetic generator, supplying the energy and vitality throughout. With the heart's energy production compromised, Mrs. P.'s energy levels were low, making her tired all the time.

Mrs. P. stated that she cannot tolerate meats or cheeses, high sources of protein. This is a given since protein must be carried by the lymph fluid, which is too congested in her body to perform this task efficiently. Testing found that Mrs. P. had a very poor response to color stimulation and could not generate any complementary (after-image) color. Excess protein disturbs the light metabolism of the body and can result in disturbances in the body's warmth organization. (We discuss more about light/photons as nutrients in Chapter 8.) The protein intolerance here simply verifies the overall condition of collapse of the body's crystalline matrix.

All of these problems must be reversed before the viral condition can be eliminated. All of these create a "happy home" environment for the viruses. This is why Mrs. P. got no relief from some really good treatments from famous hospitals and specialists. They all focused upon the virus instead of the body as a whole.

There is a happy ending to this story. The ulcers went away for good after these and many more problems were identified and corrected from the perspective of Biological Medicine and Bio-Resonance Scanning™. The types of treatment used are too numerous to list, as the entire body had to be restored. No single treatment can be pointed to as "the" treatment that did the total job.

---

[151] Oschman J, 2003, *Energy Medicine in Therapeutics and **Human** Performance*. Butterworth-Heinemann

Step 6
Align Lifestyle to Optimize Health

32

~

A Better Way to "Fight" Infectious Disease: Balanced Living

Prior to becoming ill, a person often senses that something is "out of balance" or "out of order" – simple but appropriate expressions since every illness provides its own unique signs of impending disease, sometimes hours, days, or weeks before the full-blown illness is made manifest. Paying attention to the changes in your body, mind, emotions, and spirit is the best way to recognize the preamble of infectious diseases.

Most people miss these early signs because our society has trained us from birth to live either in the past or the future. Rarely do people live in the exact moment they are in, therefore missing the earliest signs of imbalance and impending illness. We must all strive to live only in the moment we are in, no matter how busy our life. In truth, the busier you are, the more disciplined you must be to stay focused in the moment you are in to complete the tasks that lay before you. This does not mean that you live in the moment at the expense of your body, the so-called "burning the candle at both ends".

Living in the moment is a way of life; it is not a matter of time. It is focusing on whatever task needs doing at the moment, while remaining centered and alert to every change in your internal and external environment. The past is road kill, so don't go there. It is acceptable to plan for the future while living in the moment, but do not be worried or anxious about it. We will go into this topic in greater detail later.

The first symptoms of infectious processes arise once the population of microbes gets beyond the control of the body's growth-regulating mechanisms. Remember earlier we discussed that the only difference in a healthy person and a person experiencing symptoms of infectious disease is the increased number of the microbes in the sick person. It may seem that the obvious treatment is to take a prescription antibiotic and bring down the population of microbes, but is it truly?

What is the goal in the treatment of any infectious disease? This one question should be paramount in your mind when dealing with any symptoms of bacterial, fungal, mycoplasmal, or viral infection. If you understand the goal, the treatment selection becomes more logical.

If a perfectly balanced and healthy body is impervious to any infectious disease, then restoring the loss of balance from whatever cause should be the primary goal of treatment. Secondary to this is assisting the body in bringing down the populations of infectious microbes.

Often modern medicine spends a disproportionate emphasis on laboratory findings and diagnosis as compared to treatment. Objective findings, such as the numerical values of blood tests, perfectly support the prevalent symptom-based treatment style found in most hospitals and clinics in America. Critics speak of a "number-credulous laboratory medicine," estimating that 88% of all medications are of a symptomatic nature; moreover, the therapeutic value is asserted to be smaller than "we had assumed in the tumult of medicine's great and unquestioned victories."[152]

The majority of antibiotic usage in the United States falls within this 88% of symptomatic treatments. **If the microbes are not the cause of the illness, then they too are a symptom!** The cause is whatever caused the body to lose its ability to inhibit the unchecked growth of the microbes.

Many people will read all of this and still choose antibiotics as their primary treatment of choice because they may feel that the cost of balanced living is too high. These people live the way they do, and make the choices they do, because it fits their self-sabotaging goals, and most accurately fits the adaptation of their lives to their imbalanced choices. Balanced, healthy living requires one to want and do the right thing, to be self-disciplined, self-observant, and patient. Balanced life is a learned process. It requires lifelong effort to unlearn the past imbalanced living patterns and learn from the present-moment challenges. Each must learn to not be so disconnected from his/her internal and external environment.

Most of us do not even remotely live a balanced life. Thankfully, God designed our bodies to function very well within a range of relatively balanced living. Given half a chance, the body will be able to restore the semblance of normal symptom-free life. This said, supplementation with nontoxic medicines must be used to help the body halt the unchecked replication of microbes. This can be achieved by restoring the integrity of the body's energetic and crystalline-matrix properties and boosting the immune system, using frequency-matched natural medicines that work with the body's own energy to bring the microbe population back under control.

The foremost question in your mind should still be, "What changed in my life recently that weakened the body to the point of losing growth control of the microbes?" What stressful event were you not processing correctly? Who or what caused you to feel that you don't deserve only the best in life? Go through the previous list of potential causes of breaking down the body's defenses. Find the likely changes in your life that set you up for the infectious disease you are experiencing. Make changes to correct the situation. See that no one can *make* you angry. No one can *make* you depressed. Your reactions are solely *your* responsibility! Energy and the manifestations and realities in your life are fulfilled by your direct control.

Make a list of all of the things that you don't want ever in your life. List possibly that you don't want to have Lyme Disease or any symptom. You don't want to be sad. You don't want people to be mean to you. You may not want to live where you are living. Whatever you don't want in all of your life, write it down. Focus first on what you don't want. After completing that list, go back and in another column list the exact opposite of each thing you didn't want. You may say that you want perfect symptom-free life in all aspects. You want to be perpetually joyful in spite of what is going on around you. You want to surround yourself with supportive and loving individuals. You want to live in a tropical environment surrounded by palm trees. Once you have finished writing down all of the things you want, actively focus on knowing that you deserve and that you can really have each of these desires. Dr. Samantha Joseph tells patients to take their list and buy or go through old magazines and cut out pictures and words that represent their desires. Then make a collage by pasting the pictures and words on a poster board. Arrange the pictures in clever designs on the poster. Hang this in your house or place of work so that it will help you really be clear on what you DO want. When we focus on the disease, the symptoms, and the lack in our life, we send energy to those things and help those things grow in their power over us! The more you focus on what you do want, and the more you takes steps that will actually move towards what you DO want, the more energy is focused for those wants to grow into reality. You are not a disease. It is not your identity. You are not a victim! You are powerful and deserve to be whole in all of life!

Keep in mind that once you have allowed infectious disease of any kind to get a foothold in your body, the damaged tissues will take time to heal. But know that they will heal. In strep throat, once the membranes of the throat have been damaged, the throat will be scratchy, irritated, and sore. It is just like a blister on your hand – the damage is done and it is simply going to take time for the tissues to heal and stop hurting. When people experience pain in an illness like Strep throat, I've often seen them run to an antibiotic, not with the goal of killing all of the bacteria, but for what boils down simply to be pain relief. The event of painful Strep throat is interfering with their life, and instead of looking at it as a sign of imbalance, a message, and a chance to learn, they miss the entire point of the illness. Trust and really know that your body will naturally take control over the strep bacteria again with appropriate life-choice modifications and natural, nontoxic support. The pain can be eased through other natural methods and time. Learn to observe what changed just previous to the earliest signs of illness. You should be able to identify and modify, thereby averting illness altogether.

No matter what the plague, epidemic, or infectious disease, some people always remain untouched in the midst of it all. It matters not that you are bitten and infected by a mosquito, tick, or are sneezed on by a sick person and have the infectious microbes injected into your body. If your body is balanced, and therefore healthy, your body will respond correctly and you will stay healthy. **If you realized just how many potentially disease-causing microbes you breathe in, eat, or drink every single day of your life without getting sick, you would never worry about infectious disease again.**

Municipal water departments around the United States are warning people with specific illnesses not to drink the tap water because of the various microbes they cannot filter out and the chlorine cannot kill. Why do you think they don't warn everyone not to drink the water? They understand that while these microbes in the drinking water can cause disease, a generally healthy person will be able to drink it without harm.

This book will guide you through some of the processes of living a balanced life in body, mind, and spirit. You will learn to change the internal environment of your body so that disease from infectious overgrowth of Lyme spirochetes cannot continue to replicate at will. You will have no spirochete overgrowth when your body is no longer a happy home environment for growing these bacteria!

---

[152] Schaefer, H. *Plaedoyer fuer eine "neue Medizin."*

33

~

Redesigning Your Life to Overcome Illness

Chronic Lyme affects more than just the physical structures of cells and tissues. It disrupts the mind, body, and spirit.

To even hope to re-establish a state of wellness, your therapies must address the entire problem and not just attack the bacteria. One must immediately "clean house" – your internal physical, psychological, and spiritual house. A total lifestyle change is mandatory – the Lyme bacteria were allowed to grow unchecked in your body by the lifestyle and choices you have made! You must change the equation completely in every aspect of your life, constantly strengthening every area. Critical self-analysis will no doubt identify numerous weak links in your life, as well as many strong points. "You are only as strong as your weakest link." I see this in many chronic Lyme patients. Some of them have always eaten well, taken vitamins and herbs, and for all appearances lead a healthy life. What is not readily seen are the indulgences, intense chronic stress, bio-accumulative toxins from work or household sources, inherited traits, and hidden aspects that poison the body as a whole.

As long as we see the bacterial overgrowth as the cause rather than the condition of the organism's existence, chronic infections will remain a mystery. Lyme is no more a disease of bacteria than a traffic jam is a disease of cars. A lifetime study of the internal combustion engine would not help anyone to understand our traffic problems...A traffic jam is due to a failure of the normal relationship between driven cars and their environment and can occur whether they themselves are running normally or not. In the same way chronic Lyme is a disease of the human organism as a whole and not a disease of bacteria.

There are many ways to treat yourself as a "complete organism," most of which do not require that you now spend your children's inheritance. Lifestyle changes should be your primary focus, combined with the efforts of your doctors.

Always remember it is your body, the only one you have! It is your responsibility to protect it from harmful treatments. Don't trade one problem for another. Be sure your doctor is treating the "human organism" as a whole, and not just attempting to simply destroy Lyme spirochetes. More times than not, since the latter treatment does not treat the whole organism, Lyme infection reappears with a vengeance as soon as the antibiotics are removed.

New habits must be formed. The formation and process of developing new habits stimulates the regeneration of tissues. It is a known fact that the years of ingrained habits grind your inner being into a non-reactive sedentary mechanism. Forming new habits will re-awaken this healing force. Of course, forming good habits are going to benefit you the most. This awakening force allows your body to separate good healthy cells from dysfunctional cells and stimulates the reactive forces against the total illness.

Don't blow this off as being too odd! **Use your imagination** to come up with a list of things you want to make a habit out of. Make a list – write it down! This list may include anything at all -- change your handwriting, answer the phone with your other hand and ear than usual, hold your fork in the opposite hand to eat, stop eating junk food for snacks, stop smoking, develop new hobbies outside of your normal interests, read instead of watching TV, exercise whenever you feel like taking a nap, hang your clothes up every time, get up immediately without hitting the snooze button. It doesn't really matter what you decide to make into a new habit. <u>It is the process of doing it that wakes up an incredible healing inner force.</u> If you contemplate this issue, you may be able to recognize that part of you that has been asleep from being so comfortably in a rut. Too many of us work hard to achieve a comfortable life, so it will be difficult for some to even want to change. You want to know how to beat this diagnosis of Lyme; I'm telling you – change your life to increase your chances.

Focus and capture every thought before you think it! **Maintain a positive mindset**, no matter what the disease looks like or feels like, or how events and people want to depress or enrage you. To do this you will be required to activate the above described habit mechanism, since it is not normally a habit to always think positively. An inner peace in your spirit can be achieved only by exercising, and practicing with vigilance different ways to come into complete control of your spirit mind. There are several techniques geared to this end. Curative Eurhythmy is one method of expressing visual sound of your spirit through movement. A certified teacher is a must. Eurhythmy is a scientific method developed in Germany and Switzerland which is utilized in hospitals as a curative technique. As you progress in this therapy, you will be more centered and more aware of your connection to all of nature. In this process, you can focus more clearly and not be knocked about by events and negativity around you. It also activates strong healing within every nook and cranny of your being. If you cannot find a Eurhythmy class in your area, choose some form of movement therapy such as aqua aerobics or non-spiritualistic yoga classes that are offered in most health clubs.

Consider curative artistic therapy; profound healing forces lie hidden in art. The opening up and submission by a person into activities which are new and unfamiliar once again speak directly to the depths of one's being. The possibilities for artistic therapy include the entire spectrum of art – music, painting, sculpture, and dance. In general, our creative forces have been paralyzed by the advent of television, movies, and radio. Know how integrated every aspect of our existence is -- science has documented that a person purposely thinking depressing thoughts cause alterations of depressed function, reaching every cell and electrical signal in the body. It is easy to see (and it will become easier to see, with the more you distance yourself from these sedentary activities) that for hour upon hour we stare absent-mindedly at technology, exerting no effort at all, imaginatively or otherwise, laying waste to and atrophying the ego and formative forces in the body. An Artistic Therapist is highly trained in carefully guiding the ill patient to the realization of formative energies to be found here, so that the unfolding of personality can occur in a non-violating fashion. Deep acting healing can be found in the arts. These therapists are not just the Joe Public person who is good with a brush or musical instrument, but one trained specifically for therapy of ill people. If you cannot find an art therapist in your area, definitely find and participate in some form of art classes usually offered by various education centers.

Sunlight, regardless of how the information highway negatively reports on it, is vital to total health. Ultraviolet light stimulates the skeletal system and increases the formation of blood and bone. Up to a cumulative of one hour of sunbathing (allowing the sunlight to touch all of the body) has been demonstrated to enhance overall body function. Everyone has heard of "cabin fever." This is caused by lack of sunlight over prolonged periods, such as cloudy winter days. The sunlight on the skin activates metabolic processes that produce Vitamin

D. Depression and psychotic behavior, as well as a decrease in your body's metabolism, occurs from a lack of sunlight. There are varying degrees of this condition that one can see especially in people who are ill. It is vital to move even the bedridden into the sunlight, as it acts as a dimmer switch on the entire human organism to crank up the power.

Fill your house with live plants. Plants clean the air as they "breathe," especially broad, large-leafed plants. They permeate the air with healthy, negatively charged electrical ions, not to mention clean oxygen. The ion concentration in a house directly influences health, healing, and your sense of well-being.

We have all heard the saying, "It is an ill wind that blows no good;" this phrase refers to a phenomenon documented all over the world . When the winds blow from a certain direction in specific locations in the world, the number of accidents, deaths, suicides, and hospital admissions rise. Science has finally determined that these winds are predominantly positively charged electrical ions.[153] Positive ions promote disease. People enjoy waterfalls and feel happier and better near them because the water droplets in the air are negatively charged. Negative ions promote healing. Plants in your home will promote healing and an overall increased sense of well-being. Do not use pesticides, herbicides, or any chemical additive, as it will end up in the air you breathe as well.

One "no brainer" is **to follow the treatment protocol set up for you by your doctor**. It definitely won't work if you don't follow it correctly – be diligent. Believe in your doctor. If you cannot believe in your doctor, find a new one that you can believe in. There can be no room for doubt and negative energy between you and those trying to help you. Don't dabble with one doctor and another doctor. Therapies and treatments don't always mix. If you are the praying type, PRAY for your doctor! The doctor cannot heal you – he can only remove interferences and help awaken the healing power within your body. The pressure is somewhat on him, but it is really on you. YOU make it happen. YOU must perform. Most of healing occurs at the changing of your mind. YOU walk your healing out into manifestation every minute of every day. The doctor only sees you for a small amount of time in a day. The healing doesn't stop when you leave the doctor's office; the responsibility simply shifts completely back to you!

Deep breathing exercises are very important. One of the primary functions of blood is to supply over 50 trillion cells with oxygen, and yet the majority of Americans would be medically classified as "shallow breathers." The lungs are one of your body's primary pathways of getting rid of toxins and waste. As you breathe out, or exhale, you are eliminating cellular debris and toxic gases. If the Lyme is to ultimately die, the body must cleanse itself of the byproducts of these bacteria. Practice anywhere, but ideally out in the country where the air should be cleaner and you're surrounded by vegetation producing healing negative ions. Breathe deeply through your nose, and then allow the lungs to naturally release the air through your mouth, without forcing out.

Keep all parts of your body warm. Many people don't realize how poorly their body is regulating the temperature in the various parts of the body. This is a component of your body's overall vitality. Try to feel it yourself, or have a spouse or friend feel and compare the temperature from every part of your body. Don't be surprised by what you find. Lyme Disease dysregulates overall body temperature and makes it cooler. There are several external ways to combat this problem. There are also internal remedies to increase and vitalize these forces. Warmth is vital to healing.

Change your terminology. I see people with Lyme Disease that speak of the disease as "<u>my</u> Lyme." They have an intense intimate connection to the Lyme. It is not a part of you! Don't accept it, even verbally. Always refer to it as "the Lyme" or "it." Don't acknowledge negativity such as saying, "It's really getting the better of me today," or, "I feel like I'm fighting a losing battle." Negative thinking affects you as a total organism and drains away the healing energy every time. Measure successes in very small increments. Rejoice over them.Constantly guard your thinking and your tongue.

Visualize health and healing. Plan and keep times of quiet, uninterrupted meditative thought and visualize in your mind's eye, with great detail, what the disease looks like. Then visualize it in great detail being attacked, breaking apart, disintegrating, being carried away in dead pieces in the body fluids. See your body's immune system army hammering away at it. Then, with great attention to detail again, see yourself as totally well and physically fit, happy, and with a positive outlook on life. Do this as often as possible. Remember, your body is watching these visualizations also and will strive to achieve them.

---

[153] Walthers D, 2000, Applied Kinesiology, System DC.

34

~

50 THOUGHTS TO LIVE ON

1. In times of change, learners will inherit the earth, while the learned will find themselves beautifully prepared to deal with a world which no longer exists.
2. What you say, and what you think, is every cell's command – be sure the commands you are sending are not perpetuating the illness.
3. It's not "all in your head," but illness requires your head to be into and in line with your healing.
4. Determine and focus your mind on your body as you would have it be, and then never waver from that image. Your body will hear the command and make it so.
5. Focus on the illness and it will grow; focus on healing and it will be.
6. Doctors can help your body to heal, but only you can give your body the permission to heal totally.
7. What you need to learn is to never speak a negative. When you have a problem, never tell more people than necessary – your brain is listening.
8. This is a law of nature: That which I *greatly* fear (don't want) I draw to me faster. That which I *greatly* love (do want) I also draw to me faster.

9. Believe that you will be completely well again the way you believe that the letter you just mailed will actually reach its destination, or the way that you believe that the Statue of Liberty is in New York, even though you have personally never seen it.
10. In dealing with pressure, you have to realize that all pressure begins in the mind. You allow yourself to be pressured. Consciously choose to depressurize.
11. To speed healing, you must get the hurt and dirt out of your life.
12. Change involves work.
13. You will only get the answers to the questions you are asking. Ask a better question and you will get a better answer.
14. Truth is truth, come hell or high water.
15. We fear what we do not understand. The cure for fear is understanding the truth. Understanding comes from aquiring knowledge. Wisdom is gained through applied knowledge.
16. Where knowledge fails, heart sustains.
17. Negatives are like ticks on a blood hunt. They stick to you. Eliminate the negatives and accentuate the positives.
18. All strain is drain.
19. Positive thoughts combat negative thinking.
20. Thinking patterns determine your heart, and your heart determines your health.
21. Be patient with yourself.
22. Don't sacrifice your whole life because you have a wound in one area. Lyme Disease is not who you are.
23. You do your best. Trust God to do the rest.
24. Action cures fear. Non-action strengthens fear.
25. Be an active participant in your own healing.
26. What you are doing today will determine your tomorrow.
27. It's really not how long we live that counts, but the quality of our lives while we are living.

Step 6: Align Lifestyle to Optimize Health

28. The more healing you have to do, the more disciplined you have to be to get the desired healing done. The more sick you are, the more disciplined you must be to regain your health.
29. You are the sum total of the decisions your ancestors and you have made.
30. Wellness is not a state of being, but a state of mind.
31. The greatest part of education is learning to think for yourself.
32. I see my life far beyond today and tomorrow. I see my life from generation to generation, causing them to live a stronger heritage.
33. We plant the trees so that someone else may enjoy the privilege of sitting in the shade.
34. I wish I were the person I know to be; however, I always strive to do better.
35. Minds are like parachutes; they work best when they are open.
36. Why continue to go to the world for answers when it's the world that confused you in the first place?
37. One must be as willing to unlearn as to learn.
38. All life is dependent upon decision; accomplishment is attained by carrying out that decision.
39. Be assured of this – you never have a headache due to a deficiency of aspirin.
40. Looking back gives you a stiff neck.
41. Healing never occurs by accident; it is always the result of high intention, sincere effort, intelligent direction, and execution.
42. If you keep doing what you've always done, then you will keep getting the same results.
43. To change your life you must change your mind.
44. It's your body, and it's your decision on how to treat it. Don't allow a doctor to do anything you are truly not in alignment with.
45. Health in a bottle is a myth.

46. Practice every moment of every day to remain content and unchanged, by any internal or external circumstance.
47. Let go of yesterday. The past is roadkill. Live completely in the moment you are in.
48. "Many people wait for the feeling of fear to go away before undertaking something new, therefore they never do anything. Fear is just a feeling – get over it!" - T. Harv Eker
49. Traditionally, society has been concerned about four-letter words. Three-letter words are even more dis-empowering. Avoid saying "Try." Try gives you the permission not to succeed. Avoid saying "But." Anything that follows a "butt" always stinks. People often negate whatever positive words they say with whatever follows the "but" in their statement.
50. Certain statements have high energy when said or thought with feeling, due to the millions of times they have been said over the eons of time -- Thank you. Please forgive me. I am sorry. I love you.

35

~

Diet and Nutrition

The media is full of advertisements promoting this or that nutritional advancement or diet. To hear many of the leading experts talk, it seems that eating has become "rocket science." Testimonials are one of the favorite ways to promote and market (and ultimately sell you) books, tapes, supplements, and diet programs. The claims are often real; however, the results gained by one possibly enormous success overcoming some chronic illness are conspicuously absent when others attempt to do the same.

While eliminating poor dietary choices will always promote health, there is much to be said for the healing effects of proper diet and nutrition. Few disagree that eating nutritious foods is well within God's design of health and healing. Even the "process" of changing your dietary habits promotes healing in that we are creatures of habit, and the habits are what have created the reality you are now suffering if you are sick. Forming new and better habits will necessarily create a new and better reality.

Nourishment from natural foods raised and prepared in such a way as to preserve the inherent vitality will always provide more value to the human organism than any modern synthetically derived or processed "super-food." Only nature can provide food with the qualities of transformative energy. Only foods started from vital heritage seed, grown with respect for the timing of planting and harvesting, and maximized through the natural treatment of the soil have the ability to impact every level of the entire human physically, emotionally, energetically, and spiritually.

The quality of a food rests upon its content of formative forces. Formative forces are the inherent energy made possible only through the proper growing, harvesting, and preparing of the food. These formative forces are released from the food as it is chewed. Did you ever wonder why we must chew our foods? Birds don't chew at all. We chew the food because the teeth are an entry point into the electro-energetic organ circuits. If we had to wait for the digestion and absorption of nutrients, it could take up to six hours! Once released through chewing, the formative energy of food travels through specific teeth, as dictated by the type of food, at approximately half the speed of light -- roughly four times around the planet in one second. This enables the organ circuits to get the energy they need without having to wait for complete digestion. The formative energy of well-grown foods is enlivening and coherent energy. The nutrient content, enzyme activity, and bioavailability (how easily the nutrients are absorbed into the body) is greatly enhanced as well in these well-grown foods. High-quality natural foods ensure that the energy and the building blocks needed to heal are present.

What brings about the maximum benefit to the body from foods is the process of selection, preparation, intentionality, and transformation of the food you have chosen. The very process of changing your diet has its own healing consequences. It is important to recognize that all of the foods and all of the decisions you have made in your life have created your reality. If you seek a new and better reality, you must change everything you do. Denying yourself of habit foods (those comfort foods we all have emotional bonds to), and even the process of choosing and preparing your new foods, demands an exceptional amount of inner activity. This inner activity is very restorative and leads to the reshaping of the body. This concept can be seen in another way; the habits and ruts we have been living with for years have created the reality of today. Every process of changing and getting out of the ruts of your life will necessarily cause a whole new reality. Selecting more balanced and healthy food and lifestyle choices will breed only improvement in life quality.

While advancements in our knowledge of optimal diet and nutrition cannot be ignored, it must be said that our Creator did not make the task of eating to be "rocket science." When He created this universe, He had to have known that the Eskimos would not have a wide diversity of foods, nor would the nomads of the desert. God designed the body to function perfectly under a wide range of diets -- not to include dead junk foods, but the foods He provided, properly grown, harvested, and prepared.

At Hansa Center for Optimum Health, a blend of modern dietary science and natural foods is used to maximize healing. Foods are recommended based upon the phenomenal research of Dr. Thomas Rau, M.D., as presented in his book, *The Swiss Secret: Dr. Rau's Diet for Whole Body Healing.*

I personally trained under Dr. Rau. He is the founder and teacher of Biological Medicine, one of the most scientific and eloquent medical philosophies in the world. Over 6000 doctors from around the world have referred their toughest patients to his clinic, the Paracelsus Klinik in Switzerland.

As you read this book, keep in mind that it is written by a doctor. Therefore, it was written *specifically* for helping people to heal from serious illness. I think that people who are sick are often desperate to feel good and therefore are willing to drastically change their diets. However, it must be understood that one may suffer withdrawal effects of refraining from the foods to which they are addicted. These foods are often the foods that are consumed more than once in a three-day period.

I recommend that this book be used as part of the **Perfect-7 Treatment and Detox Protocol** to minimize any detoxification symptoms that one might experience by doing the diet by itself. It will help people with Lyme Disease by reducing the dietary protein sources of arginine, the amino acid that causes so much havoc in the brain by combining with Lyme-induced ammonia to cause the brain cells (astrocytes) to swell.

I respect Dr. Rau immensely and look forward to future advancements on this book. The unique two-part nutritional plan is highly effective in rejuvenating and healing a wide range of chronic systemic diseases. His diet for whole-body healing begins with the three-week "Swiss Detox Diet," which does the following:

- Eliminates hidden food allergies
- Purges old toxins
- Optimizes the pH of the body
- Boosts the body's natural immune system

The Swiss Secret also details an easy, anti-aging, and delicious way to eat for your health and vitality for the rest of your life. While effortless weight loss and renewed well-being is one benefit of this diet, the program is extremely effective at dealing with many autoimmune and inflammatory diseases. It includes menu plans and over 100 recipes.

In providing this new diet program, it is understood now that it will force you to change your dietary habits as discussed earlier. It may involve having to eat foods that you must learn to prepare, and to go outside your comfort zones in trying new recipes. I recognize this may be a huge challenge to those who have also have families to feed. My own children can be quite picky with what they will eat sometimes. You owe it to them and to yourself to get well quickly. I think that one of the most common things I have seen with my patients is that none of them realized that, 10 to 15 years after the first symptom, they would still be fighting for the quality of life they once had. Now is the time to blitz your body! This and the elimination of toxic processed foods and habit foods will go a long way to speeding you towards healing. Approach this dietary change with an open mind and a happy heart. Life is a journey, and we are not trying to complicate your journey, but make your way easier and more enjoyable. Does all this mean that you absolutely cannot partake of your favorite foods forever? Definitely not! This simply enables you to make better food choices.

Foods to Avoid

It is a great idea to always avoid these foods or consume in very limited amounts.

1. Foods high in saturated fats (pork, cream, lard, etc.)
2. Dairy products (except goat and natural, unprocessed cheeses)
3. Canned food and carbonated drinks
4. Iodized or regular table salt (Use only sun-evaporated sea salt)
5. Stimulants (coffee, black tea, alcohol, etc.)
6. Fried or roasted foods
7. All food preservatives, food colorings, flavor enhancers (MSG, NutraSweet, etc.)
8. Microwaved foods (Some L-form amino acids are converted over to the D-forms, which promote free-radical damage)
9. Refined sugar, cakes, jams, chocolate, and ice cream
10. Refined oils (non-cold pressed oils, even olive oils --sse only cold-pressed).
11. Foods cooked in aluminum cookware or with aluminum utensils

12. Tap water, or unpurified water. Use distilled water only under the advisement of your physician, since it can leach out helpful minerals from your body.

Supportive Dietary Measures

1. Maintain regular and consistent mealtimes.
2. Before eating relax momentarily for 10 seconds, then begin eating. (Bless your food in prayer – science has shown that this cleans the food, makes it more bio-available, more digestible, and consequently better tasting.)
3. Pay attention to what you are eating. Chew until each bite is smooth and easily swallowed. Seek to feel the energy and taste the subtle flavors of the food.
4. Force yourself to slow down -- this will aid digestion and appetite satisfaction. Eating should not be a chore. Many times food is eaten without much awareness of what is eaten, much like driving a car for miles and suddenly realizing you don't recall anything about the journey.
5. Eating by candlelight and with calming music can assist in setting a relaxing tone to the evening meal.
6. Avoid alternating between hot and cold foods on a frequent basis.
7. Eat most of your daily protein in the morning or at lunch time. (Stomach acid is highest early in the day, which allows for better digestion of proteins -- the bi-products of incomplete protein digestion are called nitrosamines and are very carcinogenic.)
8. Drink room temperature, purified water (a minimum of eight, eight-ounce glasses per day). Cold water requires more work by your body to bring it up to body temperature. This can be a problem when so many people today are suffering from low body temperature. Don't drink tap water as it often contains herbicides, pesticides, chlorine, fluoride, and other chemicals. Do not drink much

during the meal as this dilutes the stomach digestive juices. Do not drink over a gallon per day.

36

~

"No Brainer" Things To Do For Your Health

1. **Get off the Pill.** Ladies, if you are using a birth control pill or patch, you need to seriously think about finding an alternative contraceptive because of the intense strain birth control pills place on your body. Read *Taking Charge of Your Fertility* by Toni Weschler, MPH.

    Consider Natural Progesterone cream if you are having PMS, menstrual irregularities, menopausal symptoms, or energy and sleep problems. Proper hormone balance can make all the difference in your healing. Read *What Your Doctor May Not Tell You About Menopause* by John R. Lee, M.D. Even if you are a woman in your early twenties, you may benefit more than you could imagine from this book. Dr. Lee has recently written another book entitled *What Your Doctor May Not Tell You About Pre-menopause*. We recommend the Arbonne Prolief™ natural progesterone cream. It is in a pump dispenser that meters out the exact 20mg dose that is generally recommended.

Compared to other progesterone creams in jars and tubes that are on the market, the pump is better since I find that women will begin to ration the cream as they begin to run low, not getting the physiological dose that is generally needed. In jars, the cream is exposed to the air every time it is opened, often leading to increased oxidation and destroying the progesterone. Beware of some herbal wild yam creams, which, according to Dr. Lee, have little or no actual natural progesterone.[154] A pregnant woman produces about 800mg of progesterone every day, so this 20mg dose is considered very safe. The general recommendation is to rub one pump, two times per day (am and pm). Split the amount that comes out in one pump and rub half of it on one side of the body and the other half on the other side of the body. Rub it into thin skin areas, such as the sides of the breast, but not over the nipples, the inner arms, inner thighs, or groin.

2. Avoid MSG (monosodium glutamate). This is a flavor enhancer type food-additive. Read labels on foods and spice packs. This substance is known as a central nervous system excitotoxin. Glutamate crosses the blood-brain barrier, irritating brain function and peripheral nerve tissues. For more information, read *Excitotoxins*, by Russell L. Blaylock.

3. Avoid NutraSweet®, another excitotoxin to the brain and nervous system. A bi-product of NutraSweet is wood alcohol, which is widely known to be very toxic to the human body. (NutraSweet company has been in court fighting lawsuits due to the epidemic of problems being blamed on this sweetener. I recommend using a good quality Stevia, a natural sweetener that will not cause any adverse effects and will not affect diabetics.

4. Increase your water intake. Purified water is a must because of the documented impurities, parasites, and viruses known to permeate municipal water. Although drinking three

quarts of water per day will not flush out the Lyme bacteria, it will flush out many of the toxic byproducts that cause pain in the body. Keep in mind that water is required for every single chemical reaction in the body. Drinking coffee, teas, or juices cannot substitute for water because it requires all of the water in the coffee, tea, or juice to process those substances out of the body. Drinking these will actually create a water deficit, or dehydration, since many of these drinks have diuretic (stimulating urination) actions.

5. Absolutely no soda, pop, colas or whatever name you use for carbonated drinks. Most of these drinks have as much as **11 teaspoons** of sugar in a 12 ounce can. The sugar literally burns up the islets of Langerhan in the pancreas, the cells responsible for producing insulin. Eventually, enough of these cells are lost and hypoglycemia turns into diabetes. Many of you have chronic fatigue as a component of Lyme. Get off of the sugar roller coaster. Stevia is an herbal sweetener that can be found in many health food stores and is a much safer sugar substitute than the other artificial sweeteners. It is totally safe for diabetic people.

6. Eliminate all milk and dairy products. This may be too drastic for many of you, but you should be told anyway. "A sip of milk contains hundreds of different substances, each one having the potential to exert a powerful biological effect when taken independently of the others. Pus, blood, feces, allergenic proteins, naturally occurring powerful growth hormones, fat, cholesterol, pesticides with vitamin D added, viruses, bacteria (including bovine leukemia, bovine tuberculosis and bovine immuno-deficiency virus) all combine to produce a vast array of ailments in our society," according to researcher Robert Cohen. Lyme Disease is a war, and dairy products act as glue in your body's war machine. Dr. Julian Whitaker, M.D., is the founder and editor of the largest read health newsletter in the world. Dr.

Whitaker agrees that you should "knock off drinking milk altogether," and to "use all dairy products sparingly, and be sure to avoid products from hormone-treated cows." If you want to learn more concerning this matter, read the book, *Milk, The Deadly Poison*, by Robert Cohen.

7. If you are doing something obviously bad, STOP! These are things like smoking, chewing tobacco, drinking alcohol, taking recreational drugs, eating junk food and chemically dead foods, and guidelines most people know but choose to ignore.

---

[154] Lee, J., What Your Doctor May Not Tell You About Menopause. Grand Central Publishing, 1996.

Step 7
Identify and Address Emotional Triggers

37

~

German New Medicine®: Revelations Concerning Symptoms

I am delighted to write the first book in English that will introduce to the world the amazing scientific revelations of Dr. Ryke Geerd Hamer, M.D., and his concepts of what he now calls German New Medicine™ (GNM).

As with all new discoveries in medicine, the developer of the discovery is said to be a "pioneer," which is a historically accurate term. Pioneers can be easily recognized by the arrows and knives in their backs from the "Medical Establishment." In Hugh Riordan's two-volume set of books, *Medical Mavericks*, this same response and resistance to change within the Medical Establishment has been documented over and over.[155]

Historically, the Medical Establishment's response seems to be initially to ignore the research, then resist it, crucify or publicly denounce the pioneer as a "quack," take away the pioneer's medical license, and after years have passed, accept what the pioneer said as obvious and act as if the truth of it is self-evident. Often the pioneer is long since dead when this process is completed.

Thankfully, Dr. Hamer is not dead, although he is suffering from "Pioneer-itis." Like all people everywhere, even people considered to be spiritual gurus, all have their strong points as well as lesser points.

Regarding German New Medicine™, I only represent and am convinced of the science and the application thereof.

GNM provides a missing key, the scientific verification, of what many of the greatest voices in health sciences have been saying for years -- our emotional conflicts create the majority of our physical symptoms!

At its core, GNM simply demonstrates a predictable telltale sign of an unresolved emotion in the brain, visible only using a CT scan of the brain. Dr. Hamer and other researchers have documented and mapped which specific areas of the brain are affected by each specific type of emotional conflict! Over 40,000 CT scans have been analyzed and verified these findings.

What this means to you as a person, and to me as a doctor helping people heal, is that <u>many of the symptoms people are suffering can be corrected without a pill</u> when we recognize what event in our life likely started the brain "conflict." With this information, we can determine what daily thoughts and events we keep allowing to re-trigger that conflict, causing it to go back into the "Active Phase" instead of completing the very predictable "Healing Phase." The body was designed this way. If we play the game of life correctly, resolving our conflicts quickly, we realize that we (and only we) are in control of our own reactions and emotions! Nothing can make you mad, or make you sad, or disappoint you. More research into taking control of your life and resolving the emotional conflicts is in the companion to this book, *Everyday Miracles by God's Design*.

We create a visible trauma to the brain when WE don't handle our conflicts correctly.

Realizing this, and making the necessary changes in how we process our emotions and life challenges, means we can take control of our own symptoms. It ceases to mean that you haven't eaten enough vegetables, or that you haven't taken the right pill combination yet. That is often NOT the reason you are suffering, as you will see in the following article, written by one of the only certified GNM instructors, Caroline Markolin, Ph.D.

I have been trained in GNM and have used it with remarkable success in my own life and that of my family and patients. I could tell you many stories of people liberated from physical symptoms within minutes or days from making changes to their thoughts and emotions.

Earlier I mentioned that our emotions can be accurately called E-motions, or "Energy in Motion." Thoughts lead to feelings (emotional energy), which lead to actions, which create results -- either positive results or negative results.[156]

If you want to know how well you are resolving conflicts in your life? Just look at the "fruit." The signs and symptoms (dis-ease) are the fruit of your life. The roots control the fruits. The roots in your life are three things only:

1. Your Mind (thoughts),
2. Your emotions (energy behind what you thought), and
3. Your Spirit (your condition of perfect love and alignment with the Divine, yourself, and the people of the world).

Do you want better fruit? Then fix the roots![157]

Reading the Brain
...based on German New Medicine

By Caroline Markolin, Ph.D.
Reprinted with permission

Computer tomograms (CT) of the brain are commonly used as a means to look for brain tumors or other cerebral "disorders." But in 1981, Dr. med. Ryke Geerd Hamer, internist and originator of German New Medicine, made a startling discovery. By analyzing and comparing thousands of brain scans with his patients' history, Dr. Hamer established that every disease – from a cold to cancer - is initiated by an unexpected conflict shock.

Dr. Hamer found that such an unforeseeable conflict (unexpected anger or worry, an unexpected loss or separation, an unexpected insult, etc.) occurs not only in our psyche but simultaneously in the brain and on the corresponding organ. <u>The moment we suffer the conflict, the shock strikes a specific area in the brain causing a lesion that is clearly visible on a brain scan as a set of sharp target rings (see picture below).</u> With the impact the affected brain cells send a biochemical signal to the cells in the corresponding organ causing either a meltdown of tissue, a functional loss, or the growth of a tumor depending on which brain layer received the conflict shock.

The reason specific conflicts are irrefutably tied to specific areas in the brain is that during our historical evolution, each brain layer was programmed to respond instantly to conflicts that could threaten our survival. While the brain stem (the oldest part of the brain) is programmed with basic survival issues like breathing, reproduction and food, the cerebrum (the youngest part of the brain) is concerned with more advanced themes such as territorial conflicts, separation conflicts or self-devaluation conflicts.

After identifying the brain as the mediator between the psyche and the organ, Dr. Hamer found that the target configuration only remains sharp as long as the person was in conflict activity. Once the conflict is resolved, the brain lesion enters – along with the psyche and the organ - the phase of recovery. Like with any wound that is repaired, an edema develops that protects the brain tissue during the healing process. On the brain scan we can see the changes: the sharp target rings that submerge in the edema now appear blurry, indistinct and dark. These observations confirmed Dr. Hamer's findings that every disease runs in two phases: first, a conflict active phase, characterized by emotional stress, cold extremities, a lack of appetite, and sleeplessness, and then, provided we manage to resolve the conflict, a healing phase. The healing phase, commonly referred to as "disease." is often a difficult process with fatigue, fever, inflammations, infections, and pain.

At the height of the Healing Phase the brain edema reaches its maximum size, and exactly at this moment, the brain triggers a brief, strong push that presses the edema out of the brain. With German New Medicine, this crucial moment is called the Epileptoid Crisis (EK). Heart attacks, strokes, asthma attacks, bleeding tumors, migraine attacks, or epileptic seizures are just a few examples of this crisis. The severity of the resulting symptoms always depends upon the intensity, duration, and nature of the conflict and which brain layer is affected. After the brain edema is pressed out, neuroglia (brain connective tissue that provides structural support for the neurons) assembles at the site to restore the function of the nerve cells that were affected by the conflict shock. It is this harmless glia accumulation that is commonly called a **brain tumor**, even though it is actually a healing brain lesion from the initial conflict. Dr. Hamer already established in 1982 the link between these "brain tumors" and simultaneous disease manifestations on the corresponding organs.

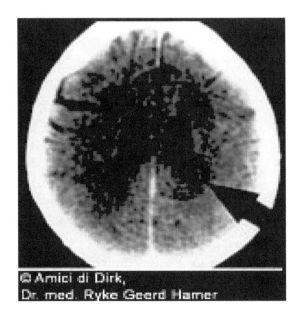

CT demonstrating the Target Ring of an Active Conflict

The above brain CT shows a target configuration (Hamer Focus, HH) in the right hemisphere of the sensory cortex of the cerebrum. The exact location indicates that the patient suffers from sensory loss in the left leg as a result of a separation conflict. Since the rings are sharp, we can conclude that the conflict has not yet been resolved. But why is the left leg affected rather than the right? Since the brain plays such an integral part in German New Medicine, laterality always has to be taken into account. The easiest way to establish our laterality is the clapping test. The hand on top is the leading hand and identifies whether we are right-handed or left-handed. This in turn determines on which side of the brain the conflict will impact and consequently which side of the body will be affected. There are two principles of laterality:

Step 7: Identify and Address Emotional Triggers

1) If we are right-handed we respond to a conflict with our mother or our children with the left side of the body, to a conflict with a partner (spouse) or (everybody except our mother or our children) with the right side. With left-handed people this is reversed
2) There is always a cross-over correlation from the brain to the organ. Since the person in our example is left handed we can conclude from the brain scan that the separation conflict must have been over a partner.

The <u>therapy of German New Medicine</u> focuses on identifying and most of all on resolving the conflict because only the resolution of the conflict allows healing to occur. The responsibility of the GNM practitioner is to assist the patient while the healing process runs its natural course. A <u>brain scan</u> together with a thorough medical history is vital to establish the duration of the healing phase as well as <u>complications</u> that might occur during the Healing Phase. Thus, reading brain scans according to German New Medicine is a highly responsible task that <u>requires extensive training</u>.

38

~

Childhood Stress and Lyme Disease

    Childhood Lyme infections can be somewhat easier to address, due to the pristine nature of most children's bodies, and usually minimal damage is done if it is caught early. At the same time, Lyme in children can be devastating, depending upon their health heritage and the degree of balance and stress in the child's life prior to becoming sick. These issues will dictate how well a child processes through the illness.

    In a child's life, stress comes from all directions. In children, as in adults, prolonged stress predisposes one to illness.

    Stress always affects organs. Every type of stress will target a specific organ. The liver is specifically targeted and damaged in the long run by intense and usually suppressed feelings of resentment, frustration, and irritability. Worry seems to preferentially affect the kidneys, and the list goes on. Again, imbalance creates illness. Restoring balance is the pure goal of Biological Medicine. Stress can start the domino effect that leads to the weakening of the body's ability to control microbes.

Even though most children have a high natural vitality, once a child is troubled by a chronic infection, the treatment decisions become crucial. All efforts must be made to support the body using biological methods to address the child at all levels: physically, mentally, emotionally, energetically, and spiritually. High-powered drugs and children do not mix well – the resulting imbalance is nearly impossible to reverse. Treatments must work with, never opposed to, God's natural design of the body.

Every direction a child turns, they encounter a barrier designed to force them to conform to a society-dictated norm. Parents should recognize that each child is unique in the world and has a unique path and strengths that should be nurtured. A child's life requires more balance than an adult, due to the fact that they are constantly evolving and developing who they will be as adults.

Did you know that at the time of birth, the nervous system is still developing? As the child grows, the number of nerve fibers will increase dramatically. Those certain neurological developmental stages must be realized, because before it is all completed, the child's nervous system will determine the best nerve pathways and will naturally reduce the number of nerve fibers by half. This is why it is important that a child learns to crawl before he/she walks. If the child learned to walk first, developmental problems would occur as the nervous system would not recognize the nerve pathways used for crawling as important and would eliminate them. Truly a situation of the cliché, "if you don't use it, you will lose it!" Developmental balance must be the goal of parents and teachers in every aspect of a child's life.

Parents and teachers must help children remain balanced and recognize the seven year, cyclical nature of childhood development. A discussion of the different cycles is beyond the scope of this writing. Many aspects of the Waldorf school educational philosophy are, in my opinion, superior to the prevalent educational philosophy which seems at times to

Step 7: Identify and Address Emotional Triggers

over-stimulate the intellect of a child. A good reference tool for parents and educators is the Association of Waldorf Schools of North America and their biannual publication, Renewal: Journal for Waldrof Education.

Children are often viewed by their parents as a bother to adult agendas. This view must change, and parents must take an active role in creating ways to bring balance to the lives of their children. A child with chronic Lyme has the greatest potential to almost spontaneously heal with the treatment protocol outlined in this book, when all conditions are brought to balance.

With proper guidance, creativity, handwork crafts, focus, eye-hand coordination, intellect, morality, independent thinking, social development, imagination, and intuitive thinking are but a few areas that can help establish the unique path each child must travel to reach a balanced adulthood. The hoops we force our children to jump through in our country's educational system do little to develop these areas. Doctors have been documenting for about 100 years that children who are driven to be over-achievers and who are over-stimulated mentally by the present educational methods become pale, pasty-faced, lackluster and easily fatigued. This clearly represents imbalance, when children raised and educated in a balanced manner are noticeably more full-blooded, with rosy cheeks and full of healthy vitality. Educational stressors that cause imbalance are part of the problem. Parents would be well-advised to look into Waldorf-style educational philosophy, even if it excludes your local schools and means home schooling.[158]

Parental emotional, verbal, and physical abuse warps the developmental shields of a child, setting them up for physical illness (such as chronic infectious diseases), as well as problems in spiritual, moral, and psychological development. (Remember, just having the bacteria in your body does not mean a child or adult will come down with a disease from that bacteria. Stress can break down anyone's ability to stave off disease.) Whether directed toward the child or between others in the family unit, words can wound the body, mind, and spirit, causing illness at each of these levels. In the same manner, loving words spoken from the heart can heal all levels. We have all heard and experienced the principle of "Actions speak louder than words:" don't simply speak the words, but be sure your actions in the future do not belie the words, for the wounds in this case strike deeper. You could be the actual cause of your child's illness.

It is definitely acceptable to admit to your child that you were wrong in how you handled a situation, and to ask forgiveness. This sets forth a standard for your children to follow throughout their entire lives.

Parents and teachers must also practice and maintain balance in their own life in order to respond correctly to the children in their care.

One more note concerning the sick child. Many cultures, though not as commonly in the United States, keep infants and young children in almost constant physical contact with the mother. In America, it seems at times that we are duty-bound from a social perspective to force our children to fight their illness alone -- to be tough, self-reliant, and seen but not heard. I highly recommend that especially young children be held often and even sleep in the same bed with the mother, or at least in the same room. This provides the ultimate healing energy of love. It also provides a sharing of body energy and warmth. A child should never have to deal with illness alone in their room. This will not spoil the child. Being there and holding them as they need it is often enough.

Keep in mind that children may not be able to tell you what is stressing them out. They may be afraid of your response, or it may be that they put much pressure on themselves, as in the case of the "perfectionist" child. It may also be that illness, household finances, school pressures, sibling rivalry, jealousy, or any number of things may be responsible. Your job as a parent is to provide a loving, nurturing home environment, as free from adult issues as is indicated for their age.

Detecting a child with stress problems

One of the best ways of determining an overstressed person, child or adult, is to use a penlight and shine the light in one of their eyes. Observe the pupil (the black part) of the eye; it should constrict, getting smaller. The eye is like a 35mm camera; the aperture of the camera needs to be smaller in bright light so that the film is not over-exposed. The pupil of the eye works the same to keep too much light from entering the eye. The pupil should normally be able to hold a steady size opening. In a child or adult suffering from long-term stress, the pupil will not be able to hold a steady constriction and will begin to pulse wider and wider as the light is held to it. This is testing the adrenal glands' ability to cope with stress of any kind. The adrenal glands are your stress organs, sitting on top of each kidney. Chronic stress fatigues the adrenal glands' ability to cope, resulting in an inability to deal correctly to even the light shone in the eyes. The worst cases are seen when the pupils are almost always very large and will only constrict slightly with the penlight. These children are usually very bothered by direct sunlight or strong lights.

Another method of finding out if a child is stressed is to shine a penlight in their eye from the side, illuminating the iris, the colored portion of the eye. This takes some patience, but what you are looking for are little rings on the surface of the iris that following the circular shape of the iris. These rings may be only in certain areas of the iris, or in extreme cases you may see as many as five layers of rings between the inner and outer edges of the iris. Any rings always indicate stress in the body and are actually formed by cramps in the four layers that make up the iris. We should never see any rings in children! Their young lives should be carefree and nurtured. Of course, we should never see these rings in an adult iris, either.

Dealing with childhood stress

The following are designed to address the body, mind, and spirit of the child.

- The above penlight tests reveal stress that has affected the adrenal glands, and therefore the child's ability to deal with stress correctly. The adrenal glands can be strengthened by taking half of a tablet in the morning, of DSF Formula (by Nutri-West). DSF was specifically designed as a De-Stress-Formula. At times it is somewhat impossible to completely remove all of the stressors in life, but this product helps in how one reacts to that stress.
- **Diffusing essential oils** in the home and in the child's bedroom can have not only a calming effect, but a healing effect as well. Anything you can smell is a chemical in the air that you breathe into the body. When you breathe in essential oils, they bring with them some of the world's strongest antioxidants and healing substances. You may remember how you used to feel when holiday potpourris set a festive mood in the house, or simply the smell of your favorite food being prepared. Some of our favorite oils for de-stressing are produced by Young Living Essential Oils: Peace and Calming oil blend, Lavender oil, Harmony oil blend, Frankincense oil, Valor oil blend, Forgiveness oil blend, and Surrender oil blend. You will find your own favorites after trying a few, but let your child pick the oil for each day. These oils are usually well-tolerated even by the chemically sensitive and asthmatic children.
- The homeopathic **Rescue Remedy** was specifically designed to remedy all forms of stress, especially the acute stressors like a death in the family, auto or other

accidents, or any stress that threatens the integrity of the body -- real, perceived, or otherwise.
- Increase family and house organization. Children need some semblance of order even in the midst of their disorder. Consistency of house routines, chores, and expectations should be the rule. A disorderly house breeds stress and chaos, while a spotless house creates its own stress for children. There must be a flexible balance maintained in the household.
- Read and teach the principles presented in *Everyday Miracles by God's Design* and in this book: keeping a quiet mind, controlling your thinking, taking your authority, and practicing color therapy at home. All of these principles are wonderful to teach your children. My children are far advanced in balanced life from where I was at their ages. They keep me in line now, when I stray!
- Make the difficult decisions that will eliminate stress in your child's life. This may be anything -- moving to a better neighborhood, deciding to home school, getting a different job that will allow you to be around more or one that will be less stressful for you and the family, change babysitters if you have a bad one, separate siblings into their own bedrooms or bring them together -- do whatever it takes to eliminate stress.
- Change your priorities so that your family is the most important part of your life. Find ways to spend quality time with each child, drawing and coloring together, reading stories and books together, take art classes together, buy models and assemble them together, ride bikes, purchase bird books or nature books and go for nature walks with them identifying birds and flowers together, or think of your own child-specific hobbies. Whatever it is, it really does matter that you DO it with them, consistently and often.

- If you have not started video games with your children, don't even let them in the house. Children get lost in the "cool" worlds of these games, and their real world cannot compete, leading them to discontentment and resentment towards you and the issues of the real world. These train your child to live in his/her head only.

---

[155] Riordan, H, *Medical Mavericks*, Vol. 1 and 2, Bio Communications (September 1989)

[156] Eker, T. Harv, *Secrets of the Millionaire Mind: Mastering the Inner Game of Wealth*, 2005 Harper/Collins, New York.

[157] Eker T, *Secrets of the Millionaire Mind: Mastering the Inner Game of Wealth*, 2005 Harper/Collins, New York.

[158] Association of Waldorf Schools of North America (www.awsna.org) 3911 Bannister Road, Fair Oaks, CA 95628-6805 call or write for information 916-961-0715 or for a subscription to their biannual journal: *Renewal: Journal for Waldrof Education*.

39

~

Adult Stress and Lyme Disease

Chronic Lyme infections affecting adults should be viewed as a sign of imbalance and is usually the result of excessive or prolonged stress in life.

Infections can begin with the following possible scenario: Life is out of control, you haven't exercised in years, you work such long hours that you are too tired to eat right, the children need your attention but you can't handle it, and you yell at them, wishing you could have a vacation away from everything. You are worn down to the point that no matter how long you sleep, you still are tired all day. The television news announces that a flu epidemic is sweeping the city -- through suggestion and weakness, you find yourself feeling a scratchy throat coming on, your neck is beginning to ache, and you think you may have a fever. The rest is history, as your body forces you to sleep, take a break, and removes your appetite as it attempts to catch up and repair.

Another such scenario might be this: You have a very important meeting coming up, at which you have to give a presentation. Rumor has it that if you mess it up, the boss is going to fire you. In your fear, you feel your throat tighten up and begin to get scratchy. You then think, "A bout of strep throat is the last thing I need," but it gets worse and you can barely speak.

Many people feel, somewhat subconsciously, that illness has liberated them from responsibility, and others find it is "just one more thing that is screwed up" in their life. You must not be a victim of your life.

I have had many people tell me that they get sick in cycles. They suffer infections in cycles of every three weeks, or every so many months, or even a certain season of the year. If you keep making the same mistakes, you will continue to suffer the same consequences.

Make a list of all of the aspects of your life that you know are out of balance. Draw up a step-by-step plan for each to restore balance. Reduce stress. If you don't like your life, then you are way out of balance and should make a list of reasonable changes that you would like to see in your life. Draw up a step-by-step plan to achieve each item. Stop doing what doesn't work. Many times we hold tightly to a way of life because it is easier to stay in the rut than it is to get out of the rut. Choose today to take a different path. Change yourself. If you are in torment about your life, change the way you respond to the stressors in your life. Sometimes you cannot change the things that stress you out, but you can change the way you respond to that stress.

We all choose how we respond to stress. To some degree, the way you respond to stress is a learned process. Without realizing it, you may be influenced in your response to stress by the people you socialize with. The people you surround yourself with may be lewd, crude, and generally angry people, while other people in your peer group may be quite the opposite, suppressing their true feelings, inwardly bitter, and believe they are basically victims of the unfairness of life. Maybe when growing up, your family members were yellers and verbally sarcastic and abusive. It is easy to see that stress can seem like a normal way of life to you.

Television programs of family violence, lawsuits, and juvenile delinquent representations also seem to be attempting to represent "normal" life. I recommend that you turn off the television, or get rid of it all together, since it is the absolute worst teacher of your mind and morality. The adage "garbage in, garbage out" is most appropriate here.

We should strive to walk in light, love, and wisdom. Choose to change in spite of your environment or upbringing. Replace hate, fear, and negativity with optimism, love, and a positive outlook. You will be surprised at how good you will begin to feel and how your environment will change in response to your light and balance.

If your job is a stressor, then ask yourself, "What job would I like to do where I would be the most fulfilled and the happiest?" Write it down, and make a step-wise list of how you can make it come true.

If what you have been doing has created the reality of today, then if you want a new reality, you must change what you're doing to get that new reality. I'm not proposing that "the grass is always green on the other side," but I am telling you that you must change, and change for the better, in order to get a better reality tomorrow.

Admit your mistakes, seek forgiveness for your part in all conflict, and move ahead. You must get out of simply surviving your day.

Often adults with chronic disease suffer from depression. The doctor says, "Well, Mr. Smith, you are deficient in happy hormones; take this psychedelic drug, and you won't feel anything anymore." Don't even go there! Read the book, *Prozac; Panacea or Pandora,* by Dr. Ann Blake Tracy, Ph.D. These drugs are a trap that lead to years of declining health, as well as mental and emotional disturbances. They also lead to an average of 50-60 pounds of increased weight and diabetes, not to mention the fact that one cannot simply stop them once started due to the severe withdrawal effects. Dr. Tracy reports that experts say that they are "slow-fuse LSD," which was also a prescription medicine for psychosis until banned for its adverse effects.

Prescription drugs are not the way to deal with adult stress! Read Dr. Tracy's book mentioned above to find out why they are terrible and how to get off of them.

40

~

Miasms: Predispositions to Illness

Have you ever wondered why you act the way you do, or why you suffer with certain types of illnesses? How you act and the things you suffer from may have more to do with your ancestors than with your lifestyle. The theory of miasms may explain some of what makes you operate. This is not "new age" and is not genetic aberrations, but it is more of an energetic phenomenon.

A miasm, by definition, is a predisposition, or tendency, of certain psychological and physical problems that you either inherited or acquired within your own lifetime.[159,160] Miasms are not to be confused with genetic abnormalities, such as missing or mutated genes. Miasms are more of an energetic abnormality. John Davidson, a researcher and author on bioenergetics, states that, "miasms are essentially an energy disharmony, disease pattern or imbalance."[161]

Research dating back over 200 years documents the reality of these energetic problems.[162] Miasms are usually started by improperly treated illnesses that can go back as far as seven generations of your family tree. In other words, some of the tendencies you have could be the result of illnesses your parents had, or medications they took before you were born, or even by your great, great grandparents' illnesses.[163]

For over two hundred years, scientists have been tracking the miasms caused by specific illnesses. Today we have immense collections of data outlining what kinds of problems future generations may experience due to different illnesses. Gonorrhea, syphilis, tuberculosis, cancer, and many more, all will generate a specific set of problems unique to the illness when suppressive therapies are used to treat them. Antibiotics are a suppressive therapy and, some agree, the major culprit to creating miasms. The antibiotics do kill the bacteria that cause these different illnesses, but they do nothing to address the damage already done by the bacteria on a physical and bio-electrical level in the patient's body. The same example from Chapter 2 applies here. If you find that you have termites in your house, you can call an exterminator to kill the termites. By killing the termites, you have eliminated any worsening of the problem; however, you have done nothing to correct the myriad of tunnels through the woodwork of your house. To make matters worse, you now have a very toxic chemical insecticide in your house. These tunnels and toxins, in a nutshell, are what cause miasms to occur.

How are miasms passed from generation to generation?

When a girl or boy is born, they carry the family blueprints in their eggs and sperm. These blueprints are being constantly modified. You might say it is an ongoing project that is passed on to each new generation. The husband's sperm carry the blueprints unique to his family. When combined with the wife's blueprints, each generation puts in their "two cent's worth" on how the child should be made. Throughout both sets of blueprints, there are energetic flaws (miasms), which went uncorrected out of the ignorance of past doctors. The union of these blueprints results in a child. This child came to this world created with his or her unique set of blueprints. Let us assume for the sake of demonstration that this is a boy child whose parents properly treated their health and passed on no miasms. His blueprints have no flaws. The years go by, and he gets an ear infection, which the parents have treated with antibiotics due to social pressures. Instantly, the blueprints in the little boy's sperm are modified. His sperm will now create offspring that may have tendencies to similar problems (i.e. ear infections) and the psychological problems unique to the miasm. The boy will live through these minor illnesses.

The boy grows up, and we'll say he is sexually promiscuous before he is married and catches gonorrhea. Gonorrhea has been identified as the cause of a major type of miasm. Gonorrhea infection, along with the standard treatments, causes major modifications to the blueprints in his the sperm. He later settles down and marries a nice girl. This is where it really gets interesting – keep in mind that the blueprint in the sperm is being modified bio-electrically (or energetically).

Can a Miasm be sexually transmitted?

When the above couple has sexual intercourse, the man's sperm is deposited within the woman. Research has verified that the sperm are viable from three to five days, so during days the woman is likely forced to integrate some of the miasmic energy of the sperm! In a bizarre way, the woman becomes linked to that man energetically. This may be some primeval mechanism to ensure the procreation of the species, much like the way many birds and animals mate for life. It may also ensure that miasmic corruption of blueprints is kept to a minimum (for example, reducing inbreeding problems seen in the breeding of purebred dogs). It is theorized that this may also be one reason why some wives continue to stay with a husband who excessively abuses them physically and emotionally.

Even if this couple never has children, the woman will suffer primarily on a psychological level because of the miasmic transfer from the husband's sperm. It is on the psychological level since it is the most vulnerable to energetic change; however, over the course of many years, the woman may experience physical symptoms as well, caused purely by the miasm.

If this couple were to have children, the father's miasm-damaged blueprint would be passed on to the child, predisposing the child to similar problems and tendencies which, if left untreated, will be passed on for another five generations.

What if a woman has had multiple sex partners?

In theory, each man's sperm can adversely affect the woman on a miasmic level. Besides the fact that the Holy Bible teaches against premarital or extramarital sex, this may be the scientific reason behind God's preference for monogamous marriage. Having multiple sex partners means that potentially each of the woman's partners imprinted their miasmatic "garbage" upon the woman and may impact her and her offspring.

Like father, like son!

The Bible even mentions that the iniquities of the father are passed on through the blood up to four generations.[164] So the next time you hear someone say, "I'm just like my Mom, a worrier," or, "I have my Dad's hot temper," or, "Everyone in my family has diabetes," or, "Everyone in my family dies of cancer," you can recognize it for what it really is – a miasm running through the family up to seven generations.

Marriage Concerns

I know it is not romantic, but you should be concerned about your potential spouse's family health history. If nothing else, you and your significant other should be tested and treated for miasms before you start a family.

How are miasms corrected?

The only recognized way to effectively eliminate existing miasms is with the proper homeopathic remedy. In the above gonorrhea scenario, the homeopathic nosode called Medorrhinum would be the appropriate remedy. Normally only one to three doses is necessary to remove the miasm from the blueprint. "Energy is never lost, only transformed or relocated and homeopathic cure attempts, therefore, to smooth out the disharmony of the miasm, as the basic cause of disease...The release of the entire miasmatic trait would result in a complete cure... If therefore, a miasm is successfully treated, the energy field is re-polarized."[165]

The best way to avoid acquiring new miasms is to combine the proper homeopathic remedies with whatever other treatments you choose. Only a doctor trained in homeopathy, or a professional homeopath trained in the treatment of miasms, should address these types of issues.

---

[159] Murphy, R., Lotus Materia Medica, Lotus Star Academy Publishing, 1995.
[160] Davidson, J., Subtle Energy, p. 222-28, C W Daniel Co, 1993.
[161] Davidson J, 2004, *Subtle Energy*. Random House UK.
[162] Hahnemann S, 2007, *Organon of Medicine*. Kessinger Publishing.
[163] Davidson, J. 1993.
[164] Exodus 20: 5-6, Biblegateway.com.
[165] Davidson, J. 1993.

Section 4
Remedy Suggestions and Emotional Conflicts

41

~

Remedy Suggestions and the Associated Emotional Conflicts for Specific Symptoms

The following are general treatment considerations based upon clinical experience. The assumption is that one is already doing the standard Lyme protocol recommended in this book. For every symptom listed below, there are literally dozens of very good possible remedies and therapies that could be listed, so only a few of my favorites are listed. An entire book could be written on each symptom and how to best deal with it.

These remedy recommendations are generally recognized as safe for the lay person to apply, unless otherwise noted with *, which indicates it requires a health professional to provide it. All **highlighted** products are available to order through Jernigan Nutraceuticals (www.jnutra.com), or the Hansa Center for Optimum Health (www.hansacenter.com), or you may ask your healthcare provider to contact the individual companies and obtain the remedies for you.

How to Best Use this Section:
1. Start the Perfect-7 Treatment and Detox Protocol, and you should also be doing the protocols for correcting low body temperature (if indicated, see Chapters 27-29).
2. Instead of taking a different remedy for each and every symptom you have (something that would, for some people, lead to 40-50 different remedies), strategize by making a list of the top 3 symptoms and work on these first. Often when one addresses the "big fires," many of the little ones will go out on their own. I am not a fan of protocols that end up requiring 12-60 different remedies at the same time. Our bodies are designed to heal themselves. A person should not feel like they must run their body on pills -- "I take this to fall asleep, this to wake up, this to digest my food, this to eliminate, this to have energy ...." The idea should be to assist your body in returning again to the point where you don't have to take anything in order to feel good!
3. Work on the emotional conflicts for every symptom you have. Make a list of where in your life you have unresolved conflicts, and beside each conflict, note what people, places, situations, music, sounds, smells, sights, etc. might trigger the conflict. Remember, it isn't the occurrence of a "bad" thought, emotion, or situation that causes disharmony in the body. It is important how rapidly you recognize the thoughts are "triggering" you and your symptom, and how rapidly you bring yourself to send energy (E-motion) to the inner and outer condition of being the personification of love. The symptom will fade and often disappear within five seconds for a person in a state of love. When a symptom suddenly flares up, stop at that instant and investigate what is triggering the brain conflict by looking at the GNM conflict that is listed for that type of symptom. The target ring patterns of conflicts in the brain tissues will run their course and fade away only if you don't continue to reactivate them by repeatedly re-triggering them. The associated emotional sconflicts listed are noted either from Louise Hay's book, *You Can Heal Your*

Life,[166] (Hay) Karol K. Truman's book, *Feelings Buried Alive Never Die...*[167] (Truman), or have been determined by Dr. Ryke Geerd Hamer as presented by Caroline Markolin, Ph.D., as German New Medicine[168] (GNM).

Fatigue, tiredness, poor stamina

- Fatigue plagues almost every Lyme sufferer. As difficult as it may seem, fatigue can be purely a brain perception only or it can be a true biochemical depletion of the body. When there are neurotoxins like ammonia affecting the brain, the resulting swelling of the brain tissues (astrocytes) causes a brain energy metabolism deficit. When this happens, simply talking or having to concentrate mentally can cause a profound sensation of global fatigue, even though no physical activity was actually performed. The **Perfect-7 Treament and Detox Protocol** should be diligently followed for a few months beyond the disappearance of the fatigue.
- The energy output of the body will be choked off by the overcooling of the temperature of the body. You might find the oral temperature is within the normal range, but the arms and legs are cold. If the arms and hands are tiring out after a short burst of activity, you may be hypothermic and actually depleted of oxygen as a result of coldness. This is the same reason that even a muscular person cannot tread water for more than a few minutes in very cold water. The phenomenal product **Core Warmth**™ by Jernigan Nutraceuticals is the chief remedy for raising the core temperature of the body. **Low-Body Temperature Protocol** will go a long way to restoring circulation and the blood's ability to deliver a sustained supply of oxygen and nutrients to the muscles. As with all of physics, the higher the temperature, the higher the energy potential.
- Mitochondria fatigue is made evident by the progressive weakening of muscles as they are used in repetitive activities. Mitochondria are the energy

factories that produce adenosine triphosphate (ATP), the fuel of every cell. ATP is needed for muscles, brain, and every other tissue in the body to work and avoid fatigue. Muscle fibers are filled with mitochondria. As you put increased and sustained demands for more energy upon the body, it responds by building more mitochondria per muscle fiber. The more mitochondria per muscle fiber, the bigger the muscle gets, and the more endurance you will experience. Body builders with large muscles actually do not have more muscle fibers than other people; they have just pumped up their fibers with more mitochondria. If you are sedentary and don't require much energy in the form of exercise, the body responds by saying, "If you are not going to ask me for much energy, then I will have to close down some of the mitochondria energy factories." If you want more energy and endurance, you will have to consistently require more energy through daily exercise. Even doing repetitions of lifting with canned beans or bottled water is fine if you are too tired to do much. For the first time ever, there is an oral supplement that provides you with the actual ATP molecules! This product is called **Peak ATP®** (made by Life Extension) and should be called the Best New Remedy of the Century! Never before could you literally take ATP orally and over-the-counter. Many people have a difficulty that this product can solve. They know they need to exercise, but they are too tired to do so, due to the depletion of ATP. I recommend taking 1 tablet, 2 times a day, and then work at increasing your exercise in any way possible. The Peak ATP is the same molecule that every cell in your body uses for energy, so there should be no limit to how long you can take this product. Keep in mind that this is not a caffeine-like stimulant kind of rush. What you will likely notice is a gradual improvement cognitively and in your endurance. There is also an instant boost you can take to "turn on" the mitochondria factories which are still working while you take the Peak ATP. The

product **Total Mitochondria®**, produced by Nutri-West, is phenomenal in how it can instantly improve your ability to produce sustained energy with repetitious activities. A normal dosage is 1 tablet, 2-3 times per day.
- Many people can be said to have "lost heart." This is a term describing an actual physiological event of weakening of the heart muscle. Direct heart support that is very safe for most people to use without a prescription is best supplied by Dr. John Brimhall, D.C.'s perfectly-formulated product, **Total Heart**, by Nutri-West.
- The heart is the electromagnetic generator for the entire body. If you are consistently tired, the generator is likely running on reserve energy only. You have previously read in this book that the heart takes the core beliefs and thoughts as a direct command and sends laser-like emissions to the entire DNA in your body, with the information necessary to make the thought commands become reality. You will never find energy in life as long as the dominant belief is that the world is deficient and your life is broken-down. **Homeopathic Aurum 30c** as well as **Homeopathic Cactus grandiflorus 30c** can go a long way in facilitating the elimination of the residual frequencies of emotional traumas, such as lost love, death of loved ones, and broken hearts from whatever cause. These may be available in your local health food store or alternative doctor's office.
- The "tired heart syndrome" can be aggravated by elevated homocystiene, an amino-acid that is a normal breakdown product of protein. The newest and possible best nutraceutical for helping restore normal processing of homocystiene is **Silphitrin**, a product developed by Jernigan Nutraceuticals. According to BRS testing, Silphitrin also helps eliminate heavy metals and breaks up mucus/phlegm in the chest. Normal dosage is 1-2 droppers, 3 times per day.

- Adrenal gland fatigue is almost universal in chronic illness and people under chronic stress. Alexis Carol won the Nobel Prize in Medicine by demonstrating that a person given a glandular product from bovine or other source would stimulate vitality in the corresponding gland in the human body. There are many different adrenal support products on the market. A beautiful product, developed by Dr. John Brimhall, D.C., called **DSF Formula**, produced by Nutri-West, is the first-line product I have used for years with outstanding results, and it is safe enough to be used by just about anyone. A normal dose would be from 1 tablet split in half 2 times per day, up to 1 tablet 3 times per day. I do not recommend taking DSF near bedtime, as you may find yourself too alert, even though there are no stimulants (such as caffeine) in this product.
- The **BIOPRO Home Harmonizer** is a must in every home, not just for those who suffer from fatigue and exhaustion! This BIOPRO company and products have been impressively substantiated at prominent research institutions and testing facilities around the world. I also recommend the **BIOPRO Cell Chip** on all cell phones and Bluetooth headsets. Have you ever noticed the cell phone gets hotter the longer you use it? The cell phone uses microwave technology! It is not a good idea to use cell phones without protection.
- **Potential Emotional Conflicts**:
    - Hay: Resistance, boredom, Lack of love for what one does.
    - Truman: Not enjoying your place in life. Experiencing burnout in your job or relationship.

HemiSync® CDs can assist in restoring one's ability to release old emotional conflicts during quiet meditation. The CD *Opening the Heart to Love* can help tremendously.

Exhaustion upon awakening, disturbed sleep
(too much, too little, early awakening)

- Much of your perception of wakefulness and vitality upon awakening is a matter of the biochemistry of the brain. Different brainwaves and neurotransmitters are secreted when you are asleep than when you wake up. To help your brain and body relax and achieve the optimum brainwaves and brain chemistry in order to fall asleep, I recommend getting a iPod or MP3 player system with two external speakers – arranged on either side of the bed. This way you can play one song when going to sleep but set the player's alarm clock to play another song. Alarm clocks jar you awake. Often the brain chemistry and brainwaves are not able to make the shift to the waking state so quickly, which leads to the "grogginess" that can last through half the day. To combat this problem, scientists developed a process called Hemispheric Synchronization (HemiSync). HemiSync music enables the brainwaves to become balanced and active in both the left and right brain at the same time. When you lie down to go to sleep I recommend you play the HemiSync CD called **Deep 10 Relaxation**. This, I almost guarantee you will get you to sleep! To assist with avoiding morning fatigue, I recommend setting your iPod alarm clock to wake you with the HemiSync® CD called **Morning Exercise™**. Having two speakers on either side of the bed enables the HemiSync music to emit different frequencies to each side of the brain to gradually shift you from a sleeping state to being wide awake and feeling positive about your day. Use these CD every evening and morning to help get your brainwaves and brain chemistry into the rhythm of restful sleep and awakening refreshed. Hemi-Sync produces CDs that can help with other areas of health as well.
- Get rid of all computers, electric blankets, and any other similar devices from your bedroom. Don't use laptop computers on your lap or while laying in bed without

protecting against electromagnetic pollution. The **BIOPRO Home Harmonizer** is a must in every home, not just for those who suffer from fatigue and exhaustion! The motors of all electrical devices and appliances, not to mention the wiring in the walls surrounding you when you are indoors, emit 60 cycle alternating frequencies, which interfere with the normal functioning of your nervous system, and therefore they alter the secretion of brain chemicals.[169] You should hit various sleep stages (REM sleep is one of them). If you are being awakened to go to the bathroom or for other needs, it will interrupt the sleep chemicals of the brain, especially if you turn a light on or there is a street light, night light or other light source used while getting up. The light tells the pineal gland to reduce the levels of melatonin to almost zero, which potentially will not return to sleep levels for hours later, therefore impairing sleep and making it almost impossible to awaken rested. Supplemental melatonin, in combination with 5-Hydroxy-Tryptophan (available in a great Nutri-West product called **Total 5-HTP**), can be used before bedtime to help adjust the body clock to realize it is time to go to bed. Most people and even doctors are not aware that melatonin requires insulin to carry it up the brain. To correctly use melatonin, eat a handful of fruit (like a few grapes) five minutes before taking the melatonin and Total 5-HTP. The sugar in the fruit will cause a bit of insulin to be released by the pancreas. The insulin will grab onto the melatonin and Total 5-HTP and rush it up to the brain. If melatonin causes aggravation, such as wakefulness, and you find it difficult to fall asleep, the body's clock may be completely set wrong. In this case, take the melatonin in the morning for a week or so, and then try it closer to bedtime again until you are sleeping well.

- Keep your bedroom as dark as possible, but still be able to wake up to the sunrise. The sunlight will be detected by your pineal gland even with your eyes closed, which will then awaken you through the release of waking

chemicals. If you wake abruptly from an alarm clock, the pineal does not have time to secrete "waking up" chemicals so that you will wake rested and feeling refreshed.
- Showering with a hot shower often causes increased fatigue; the chlorinated water of most cities, when super-heated in the water heater, comes out in the steam of the shower as chloroform gas! A shower head filter or whole-house filtration system to remove the chlorine will eliminate this source of exhaustion and grogginess in the morning.
- For both men and women, **Progesterone Cream** applied 1-2 times per day can be helpful for balancing the emotional reactions. For menstruating women, a general dose is 20mg, morning and evening, skipping the week of your period. Men and menopausal women can benefit from 20mg applied 1-2 times per day. My favorite Progesterone creams are those with pump bottles that measure out exactly 20mg per pump and last a month or so.
- High dose **Vitamin B-6** can improve sleep patterns. Use the activated form of B-6 called Pyrodoxyl-5-Phosphate. One symptom of a need for B-6 is failure to remember your dreams or a feeling that you don't dream. This has nothing to do with interpreting dreams; if you don't dream, your body is indicating a B-6 deficiency. B-6 is also needed for proper hormone function and energy production in the body. A good starting dosage is one 200mg pill, 1-3 times per day. Discontinue or cut back if you experience tingling sensations, which would indicate you are getting too much.

Neuralgia / Neuritis

- These conditions are due to the Lyme toxins, as well as other environmental toxins and/or structural aggravations.
- The **Perfect-7 Treatment and Detox Protocol** is imperative to remove the source of nerve irritation.

- **Neuro-Antitox II CNS/PNS** is tailored to deal with toxins in the Central and Peripheral Nervous System.
- **Chiropractic care*** can be the pivotal treatment to often permanently correct nerve irritation and nerve pains. So often patients get into the erroneous mindset that everything should be fixed with a pill. If there is a structural interference or nerve compression, no pill will correct it, and only physical correction will relieve it. See your local Doctor of Chiropractic.
- Homeopathic **Rhus Toxicodendron 30c** can provide virtually instantaneous relief of joint and nerve pain. In that it is homeopathic, you cannot have an allergic reaction to it. It has been used for over 100 years for easing nerve and joint pains.
- **Acontite Nerve Oil** blend, from Wala, is specially formulated for such pain and used in hospitals in Europe to ease neuritis/neuralgia.
- **Potential Emotional Conflicts**:
    - Hay: Anguish over communication, guilt.
    - Truman: Feeling of being irritated without your consent. Your power is negated through being irritated.

Neck creaks and cracks, neck stiffness, neck pain

- **Valor Oil** has been called the "Chiropractor in a bottle." Rub this oil from the base of the skull to the sacrum. It is very soothing and works with the electromagnetic fields of the spine and spinal muscles to align the spine and ease pain.
- Obviously, proper spinal alignment is important. See your Doctor of Chiropractic.
- **Borrelogen** has been reported by many people with Lyme disease to have cleared this problem up in just a few weeks.
- **Potential Emotional Conflicts:**
    - Truman: Want to let feelings out but don't dare: Inflexible state of mind; Not wanting to yield to opinions you feel are wrong.

- o Hay: Refusing to see the other sides of a problem; stubbornness.
- o GNM: An intellectual self-devaluation conflict; any insult against our intellect can trigger this conflict.

Very nervous, laughs or weeps without cause, mood swings, depression

- Using the bi-temporal ceramic MRBT (Magnetic Resonance Bio-Oxidative Therapy) magnets (**Soother 1**) during periods of emotional upsets will normally calm and restore balance.
- The homeopathic Bach flower **Rescue Remedy** is a tried-and-true remedy for balancing your emotions in stressful situations. It is absolutely safe and can be used as often as needed without fear of addiction or toxicity.
- Homeopathic **Palladium Cord** is most indicated for depression, where one holds up brightly in public and crashes when alone. Palladium is a metal that is a component in catalytic converters of cars. It is being sprayed out in car exhaust – we all breathe it in. Palladium is known as "the depressive metal." Is it any wonder the world is suffering from epidemic depression? Homeopathic Palladium Cord will cause the stored palladium in your body to be released and also calm the depression.
- For both men and women, **Progesterone Cream** applied 1-2 times per day can be helpful for balancing the emotional reactions. For menstruating women, a general dose is 20mg, morning and evening, skipping the week of your period. Men and menopausal women can benefit from 20mg applied 1-2 times per day. My favorite Progesterone creams are those with pump bottles that measure out exactly 20mg per pump and last a month or so.
- Often when one can't seem to respond to stress or stimuli appropriately, causing laughter at the wrong

time or weeping at every trifle, the first thing to consider is adrenal fatigue, which can be a result of the prolonged stress of Lyme Disease and life in general. **DSF Formula** (Nutri-West) is the first-line product I have used for years with outstanding results, and it is safe enough to be used by just about anyone. A normal dose would be from 1 tablet split in half 2 times per day, up to 1 tablet 3 times per day. I do not recommend taking DSF near bedtime, as you may find yourself too alert, even though there are no stimulants (such as caffeine) in this product.

Joint pain or swelling

- From the nutraceutical perspective, the product **Joint-Aide**, by Ancient Formulas, Inc., has been a best-results winner with my patients. It contains Glucosamine hydrochloride (the best form of glucosamine), which is one of the first known substances to actually repair and regenerate the worn-out cartilage of joints! It also contains high-yield bromelain, a proteolytic enzyme from pineapples, which research shows goes right to any area of inflammation in the body, instead of just circulating around aimlessly in your bloodstream. Bromelain stimulates increased healing, is anti-inflammatory, and relieves pain. If that were not enough, Joint-Aide contains Boswellia, Sea Cucumber, and many synergistic joint support nutrients and minerals.
- Homeopathic **Rhus Toxicodendron Cord** is actually Latin for Poison Ivy. Don't be alarmed -- it contains no actual poison ivy, just the homeopathic dilution/potentization of poison ivy. It has been used for over 100 years for easing nerve and joint pains. It is my absolute "silver bullet" for carpal tunnel types of wrist pain and unstable joints.
- A great oil blend from Germany is the **Solum Uliginosum oil** (made by Wala), which is possibly the best remedy for those whose joints hurt due to

variations in the barometric pressure associated with weather changes and storm fronts moving in. It seems I have used gallons of this oil with my patients. Whenever you have swelling in the tissues and joints of your body, it hurts. However, when the barometric pressure outside falls, there is not as much atmospheric pressure on the outside of your cells, so the already-swollen cells in your muscles and joints will swell even more, causing you to know it is going to rain before the weather man. No other remedy assists with this problem better. It also improves joint pain associated with reactions to chemicals, perfumes, exhaust fumes, etc. **Homeopathic Solum Uliginosum** is also available as an internal-use product for those seeking extra benefit.

- **Potential Emotional Conflicts:** The specific emotional conflicts are different depending upon which joints are involved.
    - **Shoulder/Head of the humerus**
        - GNM: Loss of self-respect
        - Hay: Shoulders represent our ability to carry out experiences in life joyously. We make life a burden by our attitude.
        - Truman: Bearing burdens that don't belong to you; Lacking in courage; Carrying stressful responsibilities.
    - **Hand and fingers**
        - GNM: A self-devaluaton regarding dexterity or clumsiness conflict, such as failing to perform a manual task.
        - Truman: Severe self-criticism and criticism of others; Rigid, perfectionist or controlling personality.
    - **Spine**
        - GNM: A centralized self-devaluation when a person feels devalued as a whole.
        - Truman: Has to do with the ego; Feelings of inferiority; feelings of shyness; Ego getting carried away in pride.

- **Lumbar/Low Back**
  - GNM: Self-devaluation from feeling unsupported by your spouse, friends, colleagues, or boss.
  - Truman/Hay: Feeling unsupported financially; Wanting to back out of something; Running away from something.
- **Pelvis/Pubic Bone**
  - GNM: Self-devaluation from a sexual conflict; Feeling devalued below the waist.
- **Femoral Neck and Head**
  - GNM: A self-devaluation when person is unable to endure; I can't carry on; I can't handle this.
  - Hay: Fear of going forward in major decisions; Nothing to move forward to.
  - Truman: Not wanting to accept major decisions; Lack of emotional and physical self-support.
- **Knee**
  - GNM: A physical-performance self-devaluation, such as in sports or endurance.
  - I have found that the knees are affected whenever the head and the heart are not in alignment when undertaking a physical task, even walking further than you desire out of peer pressure can cause this self-devaluation.
  - Truman: Unable to be flexible; Not wanting to bend, usually to authority; Stubborn: wanting own way.
- **Ankle Joints and Toes**
  - GNM: A self-devaluation conflict from not being able to walk, run, dance, or to balance.

- Truman: Fears falling or failing; Instability in present situation.

Muscle pain or cramps (Fibromyalgia)

- Like so many of the symptoms of Lyme Disease, the primary relief will be realized when the toxins are removed from the tissues. The **Perfect-7 Treatment and Detox Protocol** achieves this best of any protocol I have seen.
- The low temperature of the body must be corrected in order for the locked up and semi-solidified muscle tissues to be eased. The primary nutraceutical for a Lyme patient suffering from painful muscles is **Core Warmth™** by Jernigan Nutraceuticals. This remedy will provide dramatic relief from pain while also helping to correct the core temperature problems and therefore assisting with chronic fatigue.
- **Marjoram oil** (Young Living) rubbed into painful muscles is warming to the body and has been used for all types of muscle problems for centuries. Interestingly, it is known to be anti-bacterial, and while it works on your muscles it is very calming to the nervous system; it helps with constipation, asthma, bronchitis, insomnia, neuralgias, migraine headaches, and is anti-viral.
- **Potential Emotional Conflicts:** The muscles are affected by the same emotional conflicts as the nearest joint; however, the emotional conflict is not as intense.

Difficulty processing auditory or visual information

- As with most every brain or nerve-related symptom in Lyme Disease, the interference of neurotoxins in the brain are the primary cause. The **Perfect-7 Treatment and Detox Protocol** is the primary treatment. However, there are many things that can be do to enhance brain function and promote the healing of brain cognition.
- At the Hansa Center, we would definitely perform **NeuroPhotonic Therapy** with the addition of a

brainwave, binaural hemispheric synchronization challenge to re-integrate the normal processing of visual, cognitive, and auditory processing pathways.

- It should make sense to everyone that the data processing ability of the brain will be aggravated by sticking your head in a microwave, or by living next to a huge electrical power plant! Of course this is the extreme situation, but the electricity in your house and the microwaves from cell phones and cell phone microwave towers still can cause problems. The **BIOPRO Home Harmonizer** is a must in every home! The BIOPRO company and products have been impressively substantiated at prominent research institutions and testing facilities around the world. I also recommend the **BIOPRO Cell Chip** on all cell phones and Bluetooth headsets. The cell phone's microwave technology should be avoided or protected against.

- In any Central Nervous System disturbance, all efforts must be made to oxygenate the brain, control the brain waves, stimulate normal communication between the right and left hemispheres, and eliminate irritations to the brain and nervous system. There are no better ways to hyper-oxygenate the brain than through Hyperbaric Oxygen Therapy (HBOT). Almost 90-95% of all brain disturbances are caused by irritation, low oxygen, the Cytomegalovirus Epstein-Barr virus, and the Human Herpes virus-6. To date, there are very few safe medicines that will cross the blood-brain barrier. HBOT is the safest and most restorative therapy of the brain known to man. Both HBOT and the Super Magnetic Head Unit will increase the levels of oxygen all the way to the core of the brain, both will kill viruses, and both will stimulate regeneration of the neurons. HBOT is a one-hour treatment several times per week.

- From a nutritional perspective, the product **Neuro-Plus** (by Integrative Therapeutics) is beneficial in supporting normal brain function and contains Bacopa, an herb

Section 4: Remedy Suggestions and Emotional Conflicts

from India which is known to increase one's ability to learn new information.
- The frequency modulated, low-level "cold" lasers are being used with remarkable results in restoring cognitive disturbances. Many Doctors of Chiropractic, as well as Neurologists, are using this high-tech device. When it comes to the nervous system, these doctors handle it best.
- **Eyelights™** are some of the most amazing brain treatments to come along. These are specially designed glasses with four small red lights that can be set to flash with different intensities in the various fields of vision. They are easy to use and work by stimulating specific parts of the nerves of the eye, which will thereby stimulate the part of the brain responsible for various tasks. They can be used to re-educate and strengthen the muscles of the entire body, improve coordination, improve reading comprehension, improve learning time, and more. I have tested timed mathematics exams on my own children before and after using the eyelights, and the results are phenomenal. The children were able to cut the amount of time needed to do the tests in almost half! These glasses are a must for anyone with cognitive difficulties and should be used in rehabilitating the brain and musculo-skeletal system.

Upset stomach/Pain

- An upset stomach in Lyme Disease can often be associated with lowered acidity of the stomach. A favorite of mine is a product by Thorne Research called **Formula SF-734,** which contains, among other ingredients, Betaine Hydrochloride, bentonite, bismuth, and deglycerinized licorice, all of which are regulating and normalizing to the stomach.
- Antibiotic usage is almost always shown to have damaged the stomach's ability to transform and transport fluids out to the tissues. The only way your tissues get fluid is through what you drink. Many Lyme

patients have "beef jerky" for muscles, due to chronic dehydration of the tissues. This damage to the stomach leads to what the Chinese call a Spleen Qi deficiency, and ultimately a state of dehydration of the blood and tissues. This is evidenced by tooth marks along the edges of a dehydrated tongue. Being over-mental, or experiencing otherwise too much mental stimulation (never turning off the brain activity), will also cause this stomach/spleen problem and often an upset stomach. For this condition, an herbal product by Kan Herb Company called **Gather Vitality** is my favorite for stopping the continued progression.
- An often-overlooked aid for stomach pain is simply to drink purified water -- not juice, coffee, or other liquids, but just water, 8-10 glasses per day. See product list for my favorite water purifier.
- You may also have a hiatal hernia where the stomach portrudes up through the hole in the diaphragm where the esophagus comes through. This can cause terrible stomach pain, or no pain at all, heart burn, and acid reflux, not to mention the fact that it can lead to chronic "walking pneumonia" or recurrent bronchitis from the aspiration of stomach gases into the lungs. This does not require surgery! Your Doctor of Chiropractic can usually correct this in two minutes! It can be almost miraculous how this correction can instantly end the pain, acid, heartburn, and chronic pneumonia through simply pulling the stomach back down, resetting the muscular tone of the diaphragm, and correcting the fascia restrictions usually aggravating it.
- **Potential Emotional Conflicts:**
    - GNM: A territorial anger concerning someone or a circumstance (home or place of work, one's territory).
    - Hay: Fear of the new; Dread; Inability to assimilate the new.
    - Truman: Condemning the success of other people.

Section 4: Remedy Suggestions and Emotional Conflicts

Heart palpitations, pulse skips, heart block, heart murmur or valve prolapse

- Since the 1970's, scientists have known that cholesterol is not the enemy. It is a symptom of poor liver/gallbladder function, as well as poor digestion. Even though this has been known, the cholesterol industry that has been built cannot just be shut down. It is becoming widely known that elevated Homocystiene is the primary cause of heart disease. Homocystiene, an amino-acid, is a normal breakdown product of protein from your diet. The problem lies in the inability to break down homocystiene into other amino acids, so it builds up in your body, wreaking havoc. If you were to inject the tiniest amount of homocystiene into a lab animal, the blood vessels would become inflamed, sticky, and clog up with plaque. The newest, and possibly the best, nutraceutical for helping restore normal processing of homocystiene is **Silphitrin**, created by Jernigan Nutraceuticals. According to BRS testing, Silphitrin also helps eliminate heavy metals and break up mucus/phlegm in the chest. Normal dosage is 1-3 droppers, 3 times a day. Nutrititional support for breaking down homocystiene is found in the product **Homocystiene Redux.**, by Nutri-West.
- Direct heart support is best supplied by **Total Heart**, also by Nutri-West.

Sore throat

- Rub **R.C. oil blend** or **ImmuPower** (by Young Living Essential Oils) over the sore throat, using a stroking and gliding motion starting at the back and base of the ears and moving down the neck towards the heart.
- Gargle with about 3 drops of pure **Melaleuca oil** (Tea tree oil, by Melaleuca) in a mouthful of water.
- **Lemon Wheel Throat Wrap** -- this unusual treatment is one I picked up from the medical doctors in Germany. It sounds odd, but works like a charm, and the best

thing about it for you is that it doesn't cost much and you can get the supplies from the grocery store. (See Appendix C.)
- Another tried-and-true remedy is a hot tea you can buy in just about every health food and grocery store, called **Throat Coat Tea**, by Traditional Medicinals.
- Low-level "cold" laser therapy for 5 minutes can at times completely take the pain away. Clinical research seems to show it also may "kill" viruses and bacteria, but it most definitely promotes healing and restores balance to the tissues.
- **Potential Emotional Conflicts:**
    o Hay: Holding in angry words; Feeling unable to express oneself.
    o Truman: Feelings of anger or other feelings going unexpressed.
    o GNM: Unable to swallow this.

Ears/Hearing: buzzing, ringing, ear pain, sound sensitivity

- **Helichrysum oil** rubbed around the external ears has restored the deaf to hear, as well as taken away the ringing of the ears in some of my patients.
- **Juniper oil** rubbed around the external ears is also very good for ringing and sensitivity of the hearing.
- **Homeopathic Aconite napelis 30c** and **Levisticum 30c** both are renowned for their healing of neuritis and neuropathies.
- The ears are controlled or affected by the kidneys, so supporting the kidneys may help with normal ear function. For this I like to use a product from Kan Herb Company called **Strengthen Kidneys**, and another one called **Quiet Contemplative**. The latter is more indicated for people with a fast lifestyle or busy, stressful life.
- Some people report that the complete elimination of pork, dairy, and refined sugar from the diet for three

months completely relieved the ear ringing, even when they reintroduced these foods back into their diet later.
- Often ringing in the ears and sound sensitivity is from the hyper-stimulated sympathetic nervous system due to prolonged mental and emotional stress. Meditation techniques are important to calm the mind and nervous system; ultimately one should not rely upon a pill or remedy to relieve what is basically a symptom of your choices. However, after years of stress on the system, you may need a temporary boost to relieve the chemical loop feeding your tendencies to hold a lot of stress in order to "feel normal." **DSF Formula** by Nutri-West is my "go to" remedy for facilitating balance in the stress-management systems of the body.
- Lymphatic drainage treatments with the ST-8 device outlined elsewhere can be of primary importance in these ear problems. Seek out a doctor using this therapy.
- **Potential Emotional Conflicts:**
    o GNM: Don't want to hear this.
    o Truman: Trying to force someone to hear it your way; Ringing: Refusing to hear one's inner voice; Not wanting to listen to higher laws.

Difficulty with concentration, reading

- The ability to concentrate is directly related to oxygenation of the brain and the degree of coherence in the brainwaves. The QEEG (Quantitative Electro-Encephalogram) of Lyme sufferers often shows cold or low energy in the frontal lobe of the brain. This can be caused by the presence and interference of Lyme toxins. The **Perfect-7 Treatment and Detox Protocol** is imperative to remove the source of brain irritation.
- For adults and children with severe disabilities in concentration, there is a wonderful computer program called **Journey into the Wild Divine™**, which uses biofeedback to retrain the brain pathways.

- **Neuro-Antitox II CNS/PNS** is specially tailored to deal with toxins in the Central and Peripheral Nervous System. See Chapter 10 on Lyme toxins for research on Neuro-Antitox II's ability to facilitate the removal of toxins from the brain, verified by FACT testing.
- One of the most important things to remember when you find you cannot concentrate while reading is that you must never read past a word that you do not understand. You must look it up in a dictionary and write it in at least three sentences or until you feel you have mastered the word. If you go past even a simple word without understanding it, you will not be able to go on with any reading comprehension and you will find it difficult to concentrate.
- **Eyelights™** are some of the most amazing brain treatments to come along. These are specially designed glasses with four small red lights that can be set to flash with different intensities in the various fields of vision. They are easy to use and work by stimulating specific parts of the nerves of the eye, which will thereby stimulate the part of the brain responsible for various tasks. They can be used to re-educate and strengthen the muscles of the entire body, improve coordination, improve reading comprehension, improve learning time, and more. I have tested timed mathematics exams on my own children before and after using the eyelights, and the results are phenomenal. The children were able to cut the amount of time needed to do the tests in almost half! These glasses are a must for anyone with cognitive difficulties and should be used in rehabilitating the brain and musculo-skeletal system.
- Nutritional supplementation ("Brain Food") is contained in **Beyond Chelation Improved** by Longevity Plus. Beyond Chelation Improved is part of the **Perfect-7 Treatment and Detox Protocol**, so if you are using the Perfect-7, you are covering many aspects of restoring the body and the mind. Beyond Chelation Improved contains ginkgo biloba as well as Lecithin (Phosphatidyl-serine/choline), Omega-3 Marine Lipids

(EPA), Evening Primrose Oil (high in GLA), and many more nutrients that boost brain function and have been shown in research to help improve cognition and memory.
- Many, if not most, of chronic Lyme sufferers have thick (viscous) blood. Your doctor can check for hyper-viscosity with a simple blood test. With this condition the blood is devitalized, so it stands very little chance of providing nutrients and oxygen to the brain even if you take the best nutritional supplements on the planet. A simple way to check for thick blood is to look in the mirror and gently lift your tongue up so that you can see underneath it. Look to see if you have blue/black veins visible at the base of the tongue or on the bottom surface of the tongue. If you see little clusters of tiny grape-like dilations on the veins, this indicates more advanced blood stagnation. To help facilitate the correction of this condition, use a non-prescription product with millions of dollars of research to back it up -- **Endozym** by Longevity Plus is the best, safest remedy. Watch the veins under the tongue for improvement over the course of several months. In a healthy person, the veins should not be visible under the tongue.

Twitching of muscles

- Twitching is caused by physical or chemical irritation and hypersensitivity of the nerves supplying the muscles. In Lyme Disease, this is most often the result of toxins and the malabsorption and utilization of nutrients in the body. Detoxification is a must. The **Perfect-7 Treatment and Detox Protocol** is imperative to remove the source of nerve irritation that is usually located at the junction where the nerve contacts the muscle.
- **Neuro-Antitox II CNS/PNS** is tailored to deal with toxins in the Central and Peripheral Nervous System.

- **Vitamin B-complex** is also needed for normal nerve function and can be an easy solution at times.
- **Vitamin B12** plays an important role in nerve function and energy production. There are different forms of B12, though. The classic, but less effective, form is called cyanocobalamin. For Lyme Disease, the most ideal form of B12 is called Methyl-cobalamin or Methyl-B12, as a sublingual pill or liquid that is held under the tongue to increase its absorption. One pill per day is ideal. My present favorite is **Beyond B12** by Longevity Plus. It has the methyl-B12 with folic acid and tastes great.
- **Marjoram oil** and **Aconite Nerve oil** both work well rubbed into any muscle problem area as often as needed.
- For severe twitching of large muscles, your doctor may want to test you for homeopathic Drosera 30c.
- If the twitching of muscles is constant and visibly "worming around," it may be what is called muscle fasiculations. Fasiculations are now understood to be connected to accumulations of ammonia in the extremities, a condition that is rarer since ammonia in the extremities is usually instantly converted into nitric oxide. It appears that the ammonia plays an important part in causing fasiculations. This is more important to report to your doctor as it may indicate a more serious condition. These fasiculations have been dramatically improved by soaking in a warm bath containing 2 fluid ounces of **Neuro-Antitox II Basic** for 30 minutes.
- **Potential Emotional Conflicts:** GNM: Not being able to escape; not being able to get away, to flee; The muscles affected are in direct correlation to the exact nature of the emotional conflict.

Sciatica

- Use **Aconite Nerve Oil** applied topically over the lower back, sacrum, and along the leg wherever the pain radiates.

- Chiropractic adjustments and ST-8 Lymphatic Drainage treatments of the entire pelvic and kidney regions will also help. Ask the doctor to check for fallen arches, rolling of the ankles, or an anatomical short leg.
- Recent research has demonstrated viral infection in the sciatic nerve in most cases of sciatica, so keep in mind this may not be purely a structural problem. **Microbojen** and/or **Monolaurin**, both by Jernigan Nutraceuticals, are the best at facilitating the correction of viral neuritis, especially when combined with homeopathic **Aconite 30c** and homeopathic **Rhus Toxicodendron 30c**.
- **Potential Emotional Conflicts:**
    - Truman: Mental anxieties regarding creative abilities; Sexual abnormality or frustration; Over-concerned with money issues.
    - Hay: Being hypocritical; Fear of money and of the future.

Headaches

- Headaches come from several causes -- structural, chemical, stress, and bio-electrical problems. No one treatment will be a true cure-all. All four of these potential causes should be addressed at the same time. It is a definite truth that you are not fixing anything by taking aspirin or Tylenol types of pain relievers.
- The **Perfect-7 Treatment and Detox Protocol** is imperative to remove the source of nerve irritation.
- **Neuro-Antitox II CNS/PNS** is tailored to deal with toxins in the Central and Peripheral Nervous System.
- The trace mineral **Molybdenum** is a long-time favorite of many of my patients to relieve the toxins responsible for many headaches.
- The **Mustard Foot bath** can really help with headaches that do not respond to even narcotic-type painkillers.
- **Peppermint oil** applied to the temples, base of the skull, and in the soft spot behind the ears can often provide virtually instant relief of headaches.

- Chiropractic alignment of the entire spine is also beneficial.
- **Potential Emotional Conflicts:**
  - GNM: Often headaches are the midway point (epicrisis) of the Healing Phase for every type of emotional conflict. They are caused by the pressing out of edema where the initial emotional conflict target rings were. However, if one continues to allow their emotions to re-trigger the emotional conflict, it will repeat the cycle and force the experience of the headache as the Healing Phase hits the midway point again.
  - Hay: Emotional triggers may be: "Invalidating the self; Self-criticism; Fear.
  - Truman: Hurt feelings going unexpressed; Feelings of fear and anxiety getting the best of you; Inability to resolve emotional upsets.

Vertigo, dizziness, poor balance

- Homeopathic **Cocculus comp.** has been a "silver bullet" for many of my patients with these problems for years.
- Often dizziness and balance problems are an inner ear problem. The essential oil blend **ImmuPower** (from Young Living) has at times corrected dizziness and vertigo overnight when applied topically around the ear at bedtime and upon awakening.
- Therapeutic-grade **Juniper oil** and **Helichrysum oil** applied topically around the ears can also work wonders when ImmuPower oil doesn't work.
- Here is a simple test you can do with a friend. Stand with your feet together. With your friend standing close to catch you if you begin to fall, close your eyes. If you sway or begin to fall, open your eyes immediately. If you can stand with your eyes closed pretty well, with your friend still close lift either foot and stand on one foot. If you have to put your foot down to maintain your balance or start to fall, you likely have a problem with equilibrium from the cerebellum. This problem

can be often easily corrected with a non-prescription nutritional supplement called **Core Level RNA** by Nutri-West. Chew 3 pills to start and rinse your mouth with a bit of water. Retest yourself standing on one foot. If you still cannot do it, chew 3 more. Retest and repeat until you can stand better on one foot. Chew the same amount you found necessary to stand steady every morning until you can stand steady on one foot without the remedy.

- A Doctor of Chiropractic or Doctor of Osteopathy who is trained in Sacro-Occipital Technique (SOT) can often correct these problems in just a few office visits.
- Lymphatic drainage of the head, neck, and upper thoracic region using the **ST-8 Lymphatic Drainage Machine** is a must as these problems are often related to fluid accumulation in the inner ear and cranium. These machines can be purchased or leased from ELF Laboratories at 618-948-2393. The company can also direct you to a practitioner in your area that uses the ST-8 machine.
- **Potential Emotional Conflicts:**
    - Hay: Flighty, scattered thinking; A refusal to look.
    - Truman: Feeling overloaded; Feeling you don't want to cope anymore; Not wanting to accept things as they are.

Eyes/Vision: double, blurry, increased floaters, light sensitivity

- Eye function is heavily influenced by the liver. When the liver is toxic and straining to keep up with its role in detoxifying, the toxins begin to lodge in other areas of the body. The liver is the primary organ of detoxification, so cleansing the liver and supporting the liver nutritionally will go a long way to benefiting eye dysfunction. The **Perfect-7 Treatment and Detox Protocol** in this book will detoxify the liver, and by using the **Infrared Sauna** in this protocol, the largest

- organ of elimination (the skin) will also be purged. I have had many people tell me their floaters and vision dramatically improved with just doing this protocol.
- My favorite blend of oils for the Lyme patients with toxic livers is **Juvaflex oil** with **Ledum oil** applied on top. Place a hot (but not scalding) wet towel folded on top of the oils over the liver. The moist heat is an age-old liver treatment. The oils penetrate with marvelous effect.
- Nutritional support for the eyes is found in a product called **Total Eyebright-C** by Nutri-West. The eyes can take a while to respond to supplementation, so I recommend that if the eyes are one of your primary concerns, take 3 tablets, 3 times per day for up to a year.
- Freshly prepared carrot juice at the rate of two 8-ounce glasses per day is healing to the eyes as well as the body. I recommend a macerating juicer, such as a **Champion Juicer**, due to the fact that most of the nutrients in carrots and other vebetables are inside the plant cells, which must be broken in order for you to fully benefit. For a bit of increased action add celery, parsley, and apples to the carrot juice.
- **Potential Emotional Conflicts:** Hay: Represents the capacity to see clearly – past, present, and future.

Facial paralysis (Bell's Palsy)

- **Helichrysum Oil** (by Young Living) applied topically over the affected area, as well as the front and back of the external ear, has been shown to apparently cause the nerve fibers to regenerate and restore normal function.
- **Primula Oil** (by Wala) is applied topically and is used in cases of muscle atrophy from disuse, which is the case in palsy.
- Low-level cold laser therapy is also beneficial.
- **Potential Emotional Conflicts:**
    - GNM: Having lost face; Having been made out a fool.

- o Hay: Unwillingness to express feelings; Extreme control over anger.
- o Truman: Feeling stagnant in life.

Forgetfulness, poor short-term memory

- Nutritional supplementation ("Brain Food") is contained in **Beyond Chelation Improved** by Longevity Plus. Beyond Chelation Improved is part of the **Perfect-7 Treatment and Detox Protocol**, so if you are using the Perfect-7, you are covering many aspects of restoring the body and the mind. Beyond Chelation Improved contains ginkgo biloba as well as Lecithin (Phosphatidyl-serine/choline), Omega-3 Marine Lipids (EPA), Evening Primrose Oil (high in GLA), and many more nutrients that boost brain function and have been shown in research to help improve cognition and memory.
- Many, if not most, of chronic Lyme sufferers have thick (viscous) blood. Your doctor can check for hyper-viscosity with a simple blood test. With this condition the blood is devitalized, so it stands very little chance of providing nutrients and oxygen to the brain even if you take the best nutritional supplements on the planet. A simple way to check for thick blood is to look in the mirror and gently lift your tongue up so that you can see underneath it. Look to see if you have blue/black veins visible at the base of the tongue or on the bottom surface of the tongue. If you see little clusters of tiny grape-like dilations on the veins, this indicates more advanced blood stagnation. To help facilitate the correction of this condition, use a non-prescription product with millions of dollars of research to back it up -- **Endozyme** by Longevity Plus is the best, safest remedy. Watch the veins under the tongue for improvement over the course of several months. In a healthy person, the veins should not be visible under the tongue.

- Of all of the technology and advances made by medicine, not many medicines are known to cross the blood-brain barrier. The oils in the blend called **Brain Power** contain high levels of sesquiterpenes and sesquiterpones, which have actually been shown to cross the blood-brain barrier! These oils are highly oxygenating and healing to the brain. Rub Brain Power into the base of the skull, behind the ears and earlobes. Some have found benefit by placing a drop on the roof of the mouth, which seems to benefit the pituitary and pineal gland. Apply 2-4 times per day, or as needed.
- **Eyelights** are outlined above and would be beneficial in retraining the areas of the brain responsible for memory retention.
- Reading, meditating, and just listening to slow Baroque music has been shown to enhance memory. According to Janalea Hoffman, an acclaimed expert in Rhythmic Medicine, this has to do with the body's entrainment to the frequency of the music and the way most "slow Baroque music affects body rhythms and facilitates both the relaxation process and improved intellectual functioning."[170] To learn more about using music in your healing journey, her book *Rhythmic Medicine* is a must-read.
- **Potential Emotional Conflicts:**
    - Hay: Inability to stand up for the self.
    - Truman: Feelings of helplessness, hopelessness; Wanting to escape life's problems/running from life; Feels unable to be in control of own life.

Chronic asthma worse at night

- **Silphitrin liquid extract** is made from Silphium laciniatum plants, which are historically known to break up mucus and be beneficial in cases of asthma. Take 1-3 droppers, 2-3 times per day.
- Ozone Air Purifiers eliminate much of the particulate and chemicals in the air that may aggravate asthma.

Section 4: Remedy Suggestions and Emotional Conflicts

- **F-Complex** (by Nutri-West) contains many of the essential fatty acids, such as Omega 3, 6, and 9's. A key essential fatty acid needed in asthma is gamma-linolenic acid which is in F-Complex, but is found in various plants, such as black current seed, borage oil, and evening primrose oil. The recommended dosage is 1-4 softgels, 3-4 times per day.
- Chiropractic care has a long history and much research documenting the necessity of proper spinal alignment in all cases of asthma.
- BRADE allergy desensitization treatments work to eliminate the hypersensitivity reactions from continuing.
- The four-day Rotation Diet (Chapter 35, Diet and Nutrition) will go a long way toward eliminating the food maladaptive syndrome found in every case of asthma.
- **Potential Emotional Conflicts:**
    - Truman: Reliving childhood fears; chronic anxiety and fear; Feeling dominated by a parent; Unconscious dependency wishes.
    - Hay: Suppressed crying; *Smother* love; Feeling stifled.

Unexplained fevers

- <u>**The Gradual Onset Fever:**</u> To a certain degree, fevers should be encouraged in the body for necessary healing. At the early onset of fever (around 99.0° F), support the fever process with a general goal of reaching about 102.0° F. Initial treatment of 6-10 drops or pellets of homeopathic **Belladonna 6x** should be given every half hour. The Belladonna supports and directs the efforts of the body without allowing the fever reaction to progress out of control. The head and torso will be warm and dry to the touch, while the arms and legs will remain cool during this stage, due to the fact that the body is focusing its healing efforts where most needed. Do not attempt to bring the fever down with compresses or baths during this phase, as the fever should continue to rise -- this is a good thing. (There are some people who advocate the use of saunas and hot baths early in the beginning stages of illness, to "bypass" the need for the fever entirely -- do not do this! In light of the prevalent low core body temperatures experienced by most children and adults today, it is of great importance to support and allow the body's own efforts to go through the process of generating the heat necessary for the condition.)

- If the fever continues to progress beyond 102.5° F, then homeopathic **Silver 30x (Argentum)** should be used to restrain the excessive fever process. Use 6-10 drops or pellets every 15 minutes until the fever breaks or stops rising. (Note that homeopathic Silver is not the same as colloidal silver; the latter will not achieve the same results, nor is the homeopathic silver being used to "kill" bacteria in this situation.) Although fevers <u>much higher than this</u> present no great danger in children, they generally indicate that the organizational and restructuring efforts of the body are somewhat in need of greater control of the situation. In this excessive fever condition, measures to assist in bringing down the body temperature can be used. Lemon water compresses on the abdomen and calves, as well as tepid water enemas, can help to disperse excessive heat.

- If the fever is only weakly manifested, around 99.0° to 100.5° F, then support and strengthen the body's efforts. Actually promote a stronger fever response so that the goal of the inflammation is reached. Support the weak fever by using 6-10 drops or pellets of homeopathic **Sulphur 6x** or **Hepar sulphuris 6x** at the same time as adding external warmth through warm baths (no warmer than 100° F). Ensure that the sick room is warm. It can be comforting and warming to the spirit to have the room lit with candlelight. Rub the body with peat-based oils, such as **Solum Uliginosum oil** (by Wala), and wrap the body warmly in peat/wool blend bedding, if available.

Section 4: Remedy Suggestions and Emotional Conflicts

- When the fever breaks and begins to fall, it is time to support the formative forces working with the purpose of the rebuilding and restructuring of the body. It is at this stage that the heat of the fever will be felt in the arms and legs, and the patient may break out in perspiration as the heat is no longer needed and the body is attempting to vent it in the extremities. Lemon water compresses can be used on the abdomen and calves to help the cooling process. Herbal extract of **Echinacea augustafolia,** along with homeopathic **Quartz 3x,** are beneficial for supporting the formative process well beyond the end of the illness event. Refer to specific illness protocols for how to proceed after the fever breaks. Remember, the fever is just the first stage of the body dealing with the problem.

- <u>The Sudden onset Fever:</u> See protocols for individual illnesses for more specific treatment recommendations.
- When dealing with a sudden onset rapidly increasing fever, as opposed to a gradual onset fever, it usually indicates virus-associated inflammation. In that it is likely viral, the initial supporting measures will be different than for bacterial infections.
- Viruses can cause a sudden and rapidly rising fever, and no remedy is more indicated than homeopathic **Aconite napellus**. The optimum dosage is **Aconite 6c to 30c** potency, 6 to 10 drops every 15-30 minutes, increasing time between doses as the fever begins to slow its incline. Aconite has strong anti-viral actions but is used all the way to the breaking of the fever. Aconite puts a restraining action on the rapidly-progressing fever process of the body. Remember that viruses do not replicate well in a hot body, so once again the point of this remedy is not to bring the fever down, but to harness the fever and drive its attack. Be patient; do not use anti-viral medicines until the fever begins to fall. We want the body to achieve the degree of fever it needs and trust its wisdom.

- If the fever continues to progress beyond 102.5° F, then homeopathic **Silver 30x (Argentum)** should be used to restrain the excessive fever process. Use 6-10 drops or pellets every 15 minutes until the fever breaks or stops rising. (Note that homeopathic Silver is not the same as colloidal silver; the latter will not achieve the same results, nor is the homeopathic silver being used to "kill" bacteria in this situation.) Although fevers <u>much higher than this</u> present no great danger in children, they generally indicate that the organizational and restructuring efforts of the body are somewhat in need of greater control of the situation. In this excessive fever condition, measures to assist in bringing down the body temperature can be used. Lemon water compresses on the abdomen and calves, as well as tepid water enemas, can help to disperse excessive heat.

- When the fever breaks and begins to fall, discontinue the homeopathic Aconite. It is time to support the formative forces working with the purpose of the rebuilding and restructuring of the body. It is at this stage that the heat of the fever will be felt in the arms and legs, and the patient will break out in perspiration as the heat is no longer needed and the body is attempting to vent it in the extremities. Lemon water compresses can be used on the abdomen and calves to help the cooling process. Herbal extract of **Echinacea augustafolia,** along with homeopathic **Quartz 3x,** are beneficial for supporting the formative process well beyond the end of the illness event.

- **<u>Febrile Convulsions in Children</u>:** The possibility of a convulsion is remote and is not necessarily due to an excessively high temperature. The convulsion might manifest as shaking of the whole body, biting the tongue, wild, rolling eyes, and may even include loss of consciousness. Dr. Otto Wolf, M.D. says it best in his book, *Home Remedies,* "In rare instances there can be febrile convulsions. While this looks dramatic, in most cases they have passed by the time medical help has been sought. Such convulsions can happen during the time of the increase of the fever, but not at the time of its maximum. For this reason, anti-fever drugs are inappropriate. However, if the convulsions last for longer periods, or are repeated, the doctor should be consulted."[171]

Unexplained weight change (loss or gain)

- Digestive Enzymes will help take the strain off of the pancreas and digestive system. Digestive enzymes, such as protease, lipase, amylase, cellulase, and peptidase work to break down your food into smaller, more easily digestible molecules, releasing the nutrients. They help eliminate food allergies caused by foods passing into the colon incompletely digested. By improving digestion, weight loss and gain should be improved. **Total Enzymes** (by Nutri-West) are strongly supported by clinical evidence of improvement seen in darkfield live-blood analysis as well as the improved digestion.
- Never eat the same food more than two times in a four-day period. This will help eliminate maladaption and poor digestion of foods. This will also speed the utilization of your food into energy instead of it being stored as fat.
- While Lyme Disease can cause unexplained weight loss, so can cancer. Have your doctor rule out the possibility before assuming it is due to Lyme infection. In the case of "Cell-Replication Problems," our favorite remedy is **Pomifetrin** (from Jernigan Nutraceuticals). This works phenomenally in combination with **TPP Protease** (from Transformation Enzymes) and **Iscar** (injections that must be supplied by a Doctor) to help restore the body's control and regulation of any cell-replication problems.
- Although viewed by some as too controversial, Kevin Trudeau wrote *The Weight Loss Cure*, a book based upon sound research by Dr. Simeon. If I hadn't seen it with my own eyes and witnessed the consistent effectiveness of this program, I would be highly skeptical. You will

need the participation of your medical doctor before starting. The majority of people I have seen on this program have literally lost 1- 2 pounds per day, every day, and their hypothalamus was reset to normal over the course of the program, resulting in better sex drive, higher motivation levels, and raised core temperature.
- **Potential Emotional Conflicts:**
    o **Under-weight** -- Truman: Feeling extreme tension; worries, fears; Distrusting life.
    o **Overweight** -- Hay: Fear, need for protection; Running away from feelings; Insecurity; Self-rejection; Seeking fulfillment. Truman: Feeling are being stuffed inside; Unexpressed misperceived and inappropriate feelings.

---

[166] Hay L, 1999, *You Can Heal Your Life*. Hay House Publishing.
[167] Truman K, 1991 *Feelings Buried Alive Never Die…*,, Olympus Publishing.
[168] Hamer, Dr. Ryke Geerd, as presented by Caroline Markolin, Ph.D. 2007 Seminars of German New Medicine, Vancouver, B.C.
[169] Becker R, 1998, The Body Electric: Electromagnetism and the Foundation of Life. Harper Paperbacks.
[170] Hoffman J, 1995, *Rhythmic Medicine: Music With a Purpose*. Rhythmic Medicine Publishing.
[171] Wolf, O. Home Remedies, Herbal and homeopathic treatment for use at home. Antroposophical Press 1991.

Section 5
Advanced Techniques for Doctors

42

~

Advanced Techniques for Doctors of Lyme Patients

Research often indicates that many individuals having Lyme Disease are misdiagnosed due to the similarities to Multiple Sclerosis, ALS, Systemic Lupus, and other supposed autoimmune diseases. I have seen tremendous improvement in patients in all of the above illnesses using this basic Lyme treatment protocol, many of which tested positive to Borrelia burgdorferi in blood and urine tests. In light of the recent research by Dr. Lida Mattman, Ph.D., et al. identifying a newly found strain of Borrelia spirochete in all cases of MS and ALS, we are beginning to see why we were finding "Lyme Borrelia" frequencies in patients with these illnesses.[172]

These Borrelia bacteria are unique in that they thrive in the same environment most conducive to viruses -- a cold, low body temperature. The usual antagonism of bacteria and viruses is missing; they are working in a terrible synergism. This is why Lyme Disease affects the nervous system and joints in a majority of cases.

Normally, bacteria thrive best in a warm-blooded environment, which is in direct polarity to the preferred cold blooded environment preferred by viruses. Here we find the two microbes living in harmony with devastating results.

Borrelia burgdorferi are anaerobic organisms, bacteria that do not survive well in a high-oxygen environment. They are, like all bacteria, viruses, and fungi, predominantly positively charged electromagnetically and need the body to bring down its predominantly negative polarity before the microbes can replicate and thrive. When a tissue is cold, as in a body with low temperature, the metabolic rate (chemical reactions that normally create heat) is slowed. As the metabolic rate slows, all of the body fluids cool as well. The oxygen supply to the tissues becomes depleted as the blood supply feeding the tissue with oxygen also cools down. As the blood cools, it becomes more viscous (syrupy) in consistency, which decreases its oxygen-carrying capability. The body become hypoxic, hyper-acidic, and only weakly negatively charged at the cellular level – all of this creates a wonderful environment for Lyme spirochetes to grow and thrive.

Any effective fight against Lyme Disease would necessarily need to include therapies and lifestyle changes that would increase the core body temperature, increase the body's alkalinity, and strengthen the body's normal electromagnetic negative polarity.

Immediate improvement in symptoms should follow the increase in body temperature, as the body fluids begin to liquefy from their cold, syrupy state and the oxygen-carrying ability returns to normal. As you increase oxygen in the tissues, you decrease acidity, increase negative polarity, and kill Lyme bacteria!

Lyme Disease requires a very multi-faceted treatment approach. It is a systemic infection and is poorly understood by most doctors. Chronic infections lasting years are common, due to the prevalent mentality of the germ theory. As in all infectious diseases, it is erroneous to think, "I will be well when my doctor figures out how to kill all of these bacteria." You will be well when your body is no longer a happy home

Section 5: Advanced Techniques for Doctors

environment for the bacteria and viruses, and when the balance is restored in the tissues and the entire organism that is you! You would have never manifested the disease, even if a tick injected you with a giant load of Borrelia burgdorferi spirochetes, unless your body as a whole was far out of balance to start with.

Most people who have recovered from chronic Lyme Disease are terrified of getting bitten again and contracting the disease again. These people need never be afraid if they and their healthcare team will take the time to understand and implement the principles presented in this book.

Advanced Techniques for Using Borrelogen™, Lymogen™, or Microbojen™
For Healthcare Professionals Only

<u>Advanced Technique #1</u>: In that Borrelogen, Lymogen, and Microbojen are liquid supplements, it is easy to add low-potency homeopathic sarcodes (homeopathically potentized body tissues) into the bottle of Borrelogen or Microbojen to help direct or drive it specifically to the affected areas of the body. In that Borrelogen, Lymogen, and Microbojen are primarily frequency-based formulas, they will not be as restricted in where they will go in the body. Their energetic information works within the body's own communication network and seems to not be as restricted by cell membranes and absorption issues as conventional medicines. However, in difficult cases, I like to use sarcodes to further open the communication pathways specifically being affected by Lyme, as the disease process itself seems to interfere with the communication and self-regulation efforts of the body.

The lower potency sarcodes (3x or 6x) will bring up the vitality of weak, hypo-functional tissue, while higher potencies like 30x sarcodes can help the body bring down a hyper-stimulated tissue of the body. Between these potencies, a 12x will have a more balancing effect when the tissue is not under- or over-active and simply needs support.

Careful monitoring of the continued need of this sarcode-imprinted Borrelogen must be maintained during the use of this technique to ensure that hyper- or hypo-stimulation of the body tissues does not occur. If one feels the need to balance the tissue, finish the treatment with a middle potency of a 12x sarcode given by itself for as long as is needed.

<u>Advanced technique #2</u>: Borrelogen, Lymogen, and Microbojen are complex botanical formulas with resonance signatures unique to the interaction of their combined ingredients. Healthcare professionals can therefore use one of the many "homeo-bioenergetic" imprinting devices on the market to take an energetic "potentized" imprint of Borrelogen and imprint it into various essential oils which are high in sesquiterpones and sesquiterpenes. These substances in the following oils are known to cross the blood-brain barrier. Once imprinted with the energetic signature of Borrelogen, the oils appear to carry it across the blood-brain barrier, naturally oxygenating the brain tissues and glands, and also delivering the corrective healing energy of Borrelogen to affected brain tissues. Essential oils high in sesquiterpenes and sesquiterpones are frankincense, sandalwood, helichrysum, and lavender (all made by Young Living). I often use the Brain Power blend by Young Living for this purpose and apply it over the brainstem, scalp, and reflex points to the brain on the foot, hand, ears, and teeth 2-3 times per day. (Of interesting note: "Research has shown that sesquiterpenes play a role in dissolving petrochemicals along the receptor sites near the pituitary gland and increase the amount of oxygen in those areas."[173]

<u>Advanced technique #3</u>: Call any microbial specimen supply house for microscopic specimen on slides, and obtain a microscope slide of each of the Lyme microbes. Using the

principle of "direct resonance" testing, one can hold the slide over parts of the patient's body while performing a muscle test. To do this, with the patient laying supine, use the arm extended perpendicular to the body and the palm of the hand facing out away from the body. Grasp the arm just below the wrist (not over the carpal bones) and instruct the patient to "hold strong" while you gently, but firmly pull the arm in the direction of the patient's feet. You don't have to pull hard. You are simply looking to see that the patient's arm muscle "locks" immediately, demonstrating good integrity of the energy supply to that muscle. Now with the strong muscle identified, move the slide over the patient's problem areas, such as the liver, colon, joints, small intestines, spine, shoulders, or wherever needed. Each time you move the slide over an area, test the muscle strength. If the previously strong muscle goes weak, you have identified an area containing Lyme spirochetes, or whatever the microbe is on the slide. Basically, you are frequency-matching the molecular structure of the death microbe on the slide, which is "fixed" on the slide (and therefore its molecular structure is not degraded or disintegrated), to the same frequency of the molecular structure of the live microbes in that area of the body. Having identified the specific spot in the body, using a pen or marker, draw the zone on the patient so they know precisely where it is. The following is a technique taught to me by one of the top Lyme-literate doctors in America, Dr. Marah Cannon, D.C., of California. She realized the powerful benefits that could be gained by using Borrelogen, Microbojen, or the Neuro-Antitox II Formulas as transdermal medicines. After identifying the problem areas, use the Borrelogen, Microbojen, or combination of the two, and saturate the gauss pad of a 4x6" bandage and cover the area indicated by the resonance test. This bandage should be replaced two times per day, and at the very least be worn to bed at night. This type of treatment works like the medicinal transdermal patches that are currently very popular.

Of course, the patient should continue taking the remedies internally as well.

Advanced Understanding about the Recommended Treatments:

- **Neuro-Antitox II Formulas™** may be one of the most important supplements in any effective Lyme protocol. In theory, a person could have Lyme bacteria and yet have no symptoms if the toxins alone were addressed. This product should be considered especially in patients who have severe symptoms. Although Lyme spirochete toxins are known to be neurotoxins, their effect is not limited to neurological symptoms. As research has demonstrated, virtually all of the symptoms are in fact due to these toxins, making the bacteria only the indirect cause.
  - While the true gem in this formula is the Silphium laciniatum, the sarcobioenergetic potencies are the components that get the Silphium and other ingredients to the affected tissues. This is a state of the science technology working in the embryonic field of biophysics. One can have the world's best antitoxin, but if it cannot reach the area of the body containing the toxins, it will not work. Besides serving as a driving agent, these sarcobioenergetic potencies have a harmonizing effect of the corresponding tissues of the body.
  - Clinical findings demonstrate these sarcobioenergetic potencies follow closely the anticipated effect of true isopathic sarcodes. That being, a low potency of D6 myocardium tissue will increase the function of the corresponding tissue in the patient, while a D12 potency will balance and harmonize the tissue, and a D30 will bring down a hyper- or over-active tissue. The effect of all three potencies added together, as in this formula, results in an increased overall healing and

Section 5: Advanced Techniques for Doctors

harmonizing effect of the tissues involved, while eliminating much of the single potency potential for energetic injury to the tissues of the patient. In that these sarcobioenergetic potencies are not true homeopathic sarcodes (homeopathic being manufactured from repeated dilution and succussion of a mother substance), the designation P6, P12, and P30 are used to indicate a similar anticipated effect.

- **TPP Protease®** (from Transformation Enzymes) seems to help remove interference to the movement of healing energy and medicines in the tissues. Volumes of research over many years and millions of success stories bring strong confidence in this well-known systemic enzyme. Its many benefits include immune system support, anti-inflammatory activity, and acceleration of the rate of healing. In my experience, TPP Protease also helps restore the body's warmth organization through breaking up the accumulation of antigen/antibody complexes and by freeing the metabolic processes from their cold, sclerotic, low output. It seems that in Lyme Disease, as in many cold/sclerotic illnesses, the body's chemical reactions (metabolism) are being held captive and the energy-producing mechanisms of the cellular factories have wrenches in all of their gears. TPP Protease seems to remove these wrenches over time by directly and indirectly breaking up excessive protein accumulations in the intracellular spaces. Excessive protein, as we have said, promotes darkness and cold, and therefore TPP Protease should break up the darkness, allowing the light and warmth metabolism to be restored by the other treatments specifically designed to do so. Dosage is large due to the fact that these enzymes are used up as they work their way through to the farthest reaches of the body. Generally start with 11 pills, 3 times per day, on a completely empty stomach. An empty stomach is at least 2 hours after eating and 45 minutes before eating. This is not a digestive enzyme, it is a systemic enzyme. This dosage should be maintained for 1 month, then reduced to 6-8 pills, 2-3 times per day thereafter for six months to a year, or as directed by your doctor.

- **Hyperbaric Oxygen Therapy** (HBOT) is highly beneficial. No other therapy can saturate every nook and cranny of the body. Within the first 30 minutes of HBOT, every tissue of the body (even the brain and nerve tissue) is saturated with oxygen. In that a cold body does not carry oxygen efficiently, external assistance is essential. Cells begin to degenerate and die in direct proportion to oxygen deficiency. All of the chemical reactions in the body require oxygen. With the saturation of the tissues with oxygen, the cellular energy goes up and the warmth organization of the body can finally get busy with its job. There are various HBOT protocols for Lyme Disease, but I recommend hitting it hard and fast to start with. One hour sessions, two times per day, should be performed in the first five days. Neurological Lyme symptoms seem to respond best at 2.5 atmospheres, while joint and muscular symptoms seem to respond better at 3-3.5 atmospheres. Depending upon the advancement of the condition to start with, and the response to care, HBOT sessions should continue from there, one hour every other day, such as Monday, Wednesday, and Friday, for about a total of 48 sessions, or as directed by the doctor.

---

[172] Per phone conversation with Dr. Lida Mattman, Ph.D. 2003.
[173] Higley C, Higley A, Reference Guide for Essential Oils 2001 Abundant Health Publishing.

43

~

Two-Person Energy Balancing For Stress Resolution

Energy Clearing of Two People

Any time two people come into contact, there is an intermixing of their energies. It does not matter if they live together or simply come into casual contact with a handshake. The potential for residual and harmful effects is greatest for people who are in frequent close contact, such as married couples.

Whether you are holding hands, hugging, loving, or spending hours sleeping together, your energetic fields are repeatedly coming together. It would be good to know that you are not "blowing" each other's electrical circuits just being near each other! Even the best of marriages would benefit from Two-Person Energy Balancing.

Have you ever gone to an amusement park and stood in front of one of those funny mirrors that distort your image? The mirror stretches your image or squashes it and distorts it in all kinds of ways. That is the way I see the couple's bodies when they are together as a condensed cloud of energy that gets distorted when they are near each other.

Energy distortion occurs any time there are disruptive events inside and outside the body. In truth, the electromagnetic fields emitted by the wiring in your house, electric blankets, and even the alignment of the planets and solar flares cause distortion of the body energy fields, just as these events alter the growth of the plants and the level of the ocean tides.

Following this same line of thought, when two people come together, distortion can occur even if they are madly in love with each other. The distortion of the energy fields causes imbalances physically, mentally, and emotionally. The removal of all distortion between two people is the goal of Two-Person Energy Balancing.

This is the whole point of the mind/body movement. It is not "New Age;" it is a new scientific realization that every aspect of the human being is interconnected, interdependent, and inseparably interwoven. Imbalances anywhere will necessarily imbalance the whole mind, body, and spirit.

Two-Person Energy Balancing was developed to specifically address imbalances that occur when two people's fields are causing energetic distortion.

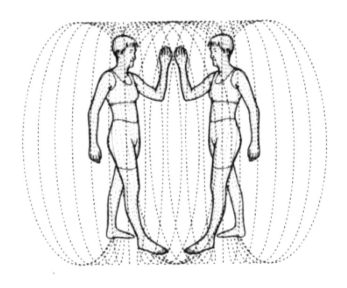

The Scientific Basis of Two Person Energy Balancing

Energy Balancing is a new concept to most people. Therefore, I hope this brief explanation will help bring it out of the 'shadows' and into the light for you.

Any time people touch or come into each other's space, there is an energy transfer. The human body is widely documented as being electrical, electronic, and otherwise electromagnetic.[174] Thanks to advances in technology, these "energy forces" of the body are no longer considered "mystical," or as in the past, "unworthy of true scientific study."[175]

We now recognize that the boundary of a human being does not stop at the skin. It is a scientific fact that energy fields are unbounded by physical matter, and indeed physical matter is at its very matrix simply energy.[176]

The body at all levels is by nature an intricate, coherent, dynamic, energy organism. The energetic fields of the body determine the shape, form, and function of the body, mind, and spirit.[177]

Understanding the energetic nature of the body, one can begin to see how there can be potentially beneficial or harmful changes when one mixes energies by coming in contact with someone else. It is a scientific fact that the body's fields change from moment to moment in relation to events inside the body or outside of the body, such as when two people's fields come in contact.[178]

It is interesting that research has determined that the heart produces the strongest electromagnetic energy.[179] The heart's electrical output is distributed throughout the body via the circulatory system.[180] You might say it is the 'power generator' for the entire body. The magnetic fields of the heart reach out 15 feet from the body.[181] The next time you hug someone, you may want to hug them left side to left side, so that your strong heart fields can really say hello. All of this is not to say electrical and magnetic fields are the only types of fields the body emits. There are other fields, such as infrared and photonic emissions, and it is likely that there are still other fields of energy yet to be discovered.[182]

Our understanding of human physiology and pathology has taken leaps forward through the development of sensitive superconductors, SQUID magnetometers, galvanometers, electrocardiograms (ECG), and many other types of electromagnetic devices.

Potential Benefits of Two Person Energy Balancing

- Improved rate of healing
- Better sleep
- Smoothing out of emotional ups and downs
- Improved energy
- Disappearance of mysterious aches and pains
- Better mental clarity
- Improved interpersonal relationships
- Improved communication
- Improvement of chronic symptoms

An energetic irritation can occur between two people which can almost be viewed as an allergic reaction. This "irritation" is a unique form of stress caused by the imbalances within the two bodies. One's resistance to the effects of stress is weakened in any chronic illness such as chronic Lyme Disease. Never before has science realized the full potential that one person may exert over another by just being in the same vicinity.

The information contained herein is provided to improve your understanding of the nature of this problem in this type of energy medicine. The treatments outlined are not stand-alone treatments, but are only part of a well-rounded wellness program of care. Two-Person Energy Balancing is not intended to cure disease in the classic sense of the term, but it is designed to help remove any interference stressor hindering the body from functioning correctly.

The Treatment

How do we go about treating energy fields? We must treat energy with energy. And since everything is made up of the same thing, vibrational energy, potentially every type of treatment or therapy can be used.

Clinical Neurology research has determined that the more sensory input the body receives for the purpose of energy balancing, the better and deeper the effect. Therefore, the doctor will use as many vibrational tools as possible all at the same time. These tools may include low-level laser therapy, medical tuning forks, meridian stimulation, colored glasses, music/sound therapy, chiropractic adjustments, essential oils, homeopathy, and nutritional supplementation.

The original treatment protocol to balance two people was developed by Dr. John W. Brimhall, D.C., and was presented in his "Health Paths" post-graduate lecture series.[183] Two-Person Energy Balancing is not a cookbook process that treats everyone the same. Each doctor performing this treatment tests and treats as directed by Bio-Resonance Scanning, or other sensitive testing method, and therefore the actual treatments and tools utilized may vary from session to session.

It must be first determined if the two individuals are truly "blowing" each other's electrical circuits. Each person is tested to see how well his or her body is working, without the addition of the other person's energy. Then the two are asked to hold hands and are retested to see if any electrical circuits are disrupted that previously were working well. Clinical testing has shown that almost everyone blows out in some way during this test. It has nothing to do with liking or disliking the other person; it is simply how your energy fields blend.

The doctor, through Bio-Resonance Scanning or another sensitive testing technique, will determine the therapies needed to balance the two people, using as many different therapeutic sensory inputs as possible, while they continue holding hands. At the end of the treatment, no energy circuits in either person should "blow out" when retested. Periodical repeat treatments may be needed because so many external influences can affect a person on a daily basis.

How soon will you notice a difference? Only time will tell in regard to noticing change. The treatment itself is dealing with subtle energy, and the effect may be subtle, revealing itself only through introspection over the course of time. We have had couples report that after Two-Person Energy Balancing, they were able to finally talk out and resolve their differences, thereby improving their relationships. Others just felt a greater comfort and well-being around their spouse. I know of at least one couple who came in determined to get a divorce, and after this treatment they returned the next day hand in hand with great smiles of renewed love and thanking me profusely. The effect for this couple seems to have been long-lasting, as at last contact they were still reportedly happily married.

Some co-workers who work in close cooperation with each other have noticed greater synchronicity after receiving this treatment.

There is the possibility of improvement in some chronic symptoms, such as fatigue, depression, pain, and hormonal imbalances, after this treatment. The actual potential for benefits is limitless. In chronic Lyme Disease, this treatment aids in removing any interference to the body's ability to heal.

[174] Morton MA, Doulhy C 1989 Energy Fields in Medicine. John E. Fetzer Foundation, Kalamazoo MI
[175] Oschman JL, 2000 Energy Medicine, The Scientific Basis, Churchill Livingstone
[176] Chien CH, Tseui JJ, et al. 1991 Effect of emitted bioenergy on biochemical function of cells. American Journal of Chinese Medicine 19:285-292
[177] Adolf EF, 1982 Physiological Integrations in Action. Physiologist 25 (2) (April) Supplement.
[178] Kobayashi A, Kirschvink JL 1995 Magnetoreception and electromagnetic field effects: sensory perception of the geomagnetic fields in animals and humans. In Blank M (ed) Electromagnetic fields: biological American Chemical Society, Washington DC pp 367-394.
[179] Baule GM, McFee R 1963 Detection of the magnetic field of the heart. American Heart Journal 66: 95-96.
[180] Cohen D 1967 Magnetic fields around the torso: production by electrical activity of the human heart. Science 156:652-654 Marinellli R, van der Furst, 1995 The heart is not a pump: a refutation of the pressure propulsion premise of heart function. Frontier Perspectives 5:15-24.
[181] Oschman JL, 2000 Energy Medicine, The Scientific Basis, Churchill Livingstone.
[182] Oschman JL, 2000 Energy Medicine, The Scientific Basis, Churchill Livingstone.
[183] Brimhall, Dr. John W., D.C. *Health Paths* lecture series. Kansas City-Atlanta, June 2002.

44

~

ST-8 Lymphatic Drainage Therapy

"This is the medicine of the future," was the response I got when I asked one of the best doctors in the country, Dr. John Thompson, D.O., about the ST-8 Lymphatic therapy machine before I bought mine. He was not kidding, as I soon found out. Once I started using my new ST-8, I found that the ST-8 makes a great treatment protocol even better.

Doctors have known for years that before effective detoxification of the body can occur, the lymphatic system must be able to flush out the toxins. Many therapies I have used for years have worked to pull, drag, or sweat out the heavy metals and chemical toxins stored inside the cells and from around the cells. But until now, stimulating the movement of lymph fluid and opening the primary lymphatic drainage ducts was next to impossible to do quickly.

One treatment with the ST-8, according to some experts with 15,000+ hours of manual lymph work completed, is equal to 6-8 manual lymphatic massages! Because the ST-8 works so quickly on the lymphatic system, I have witnessed the true role that the lymphatic system plays in healing. By relieving the lymphatic congestion, we have seen near-miraculous disappearance of acute and chronic pain and symptoms of all kinds greatly improved. This convinces me and every patient I have used it on that it truly is the "medicine of the future."

Now finally, when we use detoxification dietary supplements and detoxification therapies such as the IonCleanse, Infrared Sauna, and dry skin brushing, we have the confidence of knowing the cleansing lymph fluid is flowing and effectively washing out from around all of the cells and tissues of the body. This is important because if the lymphatic system is not circulating efficiently, then there is no supplement that will be able to reach the toxins locked far in the nooks and crannies of the body.

Every illness will benefit from the ST-8 therapy. Every doctor involved with Lyme Disease should be using an ST-8 to limit Herxheimer reactions, which are the bane of every Lyme patient. Remember, these Herxheimer reactions are toxins dumping into an already toxin-overloaded body from simply living in this time.

The ST-8 utilizes the latest technology of electro-medicine, non-invasive scalar waves, low current, cold gas photon therapy, ozone therapy, and resonance frequency technology, all wrapped into one painless, highly effective device.

Cells in the body can become clumped and stuck together, bonding electrically and leading to swelling or abnormal growths. The cells are either held together or held apart as determined by their electromagnetic charge (polarity). One can think of it as two magnets with either north pole facing north pole repelling each other, or north pole of one magnet facing the south pole of the other magnet, which attracts the magnets to stick together. It is this "stuck together" situation that the ST-8 corrects by rebalancing the polarity of the cells so that the cells separate from each other. Once apart, the energetic frequencies, photons, and ozone of the ST-8 boost the immune system.

Besides being beneficial in Lyme Disease, the ST-8 has accumulated quite a reputation in the realm of cancer. In truth,

Section 5: Advanced Techniques for Doctors

I and doctors I associate with have such a long list of illnesses benefited by the ST-8 that it would be futile to try to list each one.

More research and testimonials can be viewed at, www.elflab.com or www.lightbeamgenerator.com. The Light Beam Generator is the predecessor to ST-8 technology.

45

~

IonCleanse® Detoxification

We live in the most toxic time in the history of the planet! This is not hype, but it is a scientifically documented fact. Every person in America is breathing, eating, and absorbing chemical toxins or poisons in micro to large amounts on a daily basis.

Toxins that find their way into the body should be excreted through the organs of elimination. These organs are the lungs, liver, kidneys, colon, and skin. The problem lies in the fact that these organs can become overwhelmed by the constant bio-accumulation of toxins. When toxins cannot be excreted through the body's normal elimination processes, the body must store the toxins somewhere in the body. Toxins enter the body three ways: by absorption through the skin, by being breathed into the lungs, or by ingestion through the mouth.

The IonCleanse device appears to pull the toxins out of the tissues where they have been stored. One of the greatest advances in chemical and heavy metal toxin removal, the IonCleanse has become one of the primary detoxification methods in many of America's most elite doctor's offices.

In an IonCleanse session, the feet are immersed in a footbath of warm water. An array is placed in the water with the feet. This array generates electrical ions in the water. Ions are electrically charged particles, either negative (-) ions, or positive (+) ions. Because the human body is approximately 70% water, we will interact electrically with the ionic field set up by the IonCleanse.

With the feet in the ionized water there will be virtually no sensation, although some people may experience mild tingling of the skin.

The IonCleanse works by causing the neutralization and pulling out of toxins from all over the body and out through the pores of the feet, via electrical osmosis. Electrical osmosis is the movement of electrically charged particles (ions) across a membrane from a lower concentration of ions towards a higher concentration. In this case, the higher concentration is set up by the array in the water. The array in the water receives a small direct current that causes the metal of the array, the water, and the salt, to generate positively and negatively charged ions by separating the water into hydrogen and oxygen.

Detoxification occurs as these ions travel through the body, attaching themselves to toxins. Once attached, the toxin's own electrical charge becomes neutral, which allows the toxin to be drawn out of the tissue where it was stored. The toxin can then be excreted via the organs of elimination; however, many of the toxins seem to travel great distances through the osmotic attraction of the higher ionic field within the water of the footbath.

You will see the accumulation of particles in the previously clear water of the footbath. Over the course of a 30 minute session, the IonCleanse water will have quite a bit of toxic material of various colors floating around. This is desirable and represents the toxins that have been aggravating or potentially causing dysfunction in the body.

Approximately 20-40% of the toxic residues in the water represent toxins and heavy metals already present in municipal water. The toxins in the water have been tested using EAV (Electro-Acupuncture by Voll) testing. Based on this testing the following chart shows what the different colors found in the water may represent:

Yellow-Green	Detoxifying from kidney, bladder, urinary tract, female/prostate area
Orange	Detoxifying from joints
Brown	Detoxifying from liver, tobacco, cellular debris
Black	Detoxifying from liver
Dark Green	Detoxifying from gallbladder
White Foam	Mucous from lymph
White Cheese-like particles	Most likely yeast
Black Flecks	Heavy metals

By design, the IonCleanse causes an exhalation of sorts as heavy metals, minerals, and chemical toxins are drawn downward and out through the feet. I have discovered that the electromagnetic fields of the body often get "stuck" in a downward pull from the charge of ions in the footbath. To restore the normal electromagnetic condition of the body, I always recommend spraying the feet with Dr. Hauschka®'s Rosemary Leg and Arm Toner™. This process is designed to leave your body energized and feeling lighter. Once I implemented the Rosemary spray in the clinic, patients no longer experience fatigue or worsening of symptoms because of the heavy detoxification taking place.

While the Ion-Cleanse is not expected to "cure" any disease, the detoxification of the body will remove the sludge that has been clogging the tissues and hindering the proper healing of the body. Many people have reported improvement in a wide range of symptoms.

IonCleanse EPA Study

The following chart reflects the results of two before and after tests performed on six randomly selected patients of Dr. David Shiflet, a Phoenix based chiropractor, at the EPA laboratory in Phoenix, Arizona, August 1, 2001.

Each patient was tested twice with his/her feet in Phoenix tap water. The "Before %" numbers represent the average mineral content of twelve water samples before each IonCleanse session. The "After %" numbers reflect the average mineral content after the IonCleanse sessions.

METAL	SYMBOL	BEFORE % (mg)	AFTER % (mg)	CHANGE (mg)	% + OR -
Aluminum	Al	.2659	.8538	.5979	225% +
Antimony	Sb	.0054	.0248	.0194	359% +
Arsenic	As	.0051	.0056	.0005	9% +
Barium	Ba	.1026	.2573	.1547	150% +
Beryllium	Be	.00008	.00015	.00007	87% +
Boron	B	.3608	.5878	.2269	63% +
Cadmium	Cd	.00042	.00295	.00253	602% +
Calcium	Ce	.38	.59	.21	55% +
Chromium	Cr	.682	.701	.019	3% +
Cobalt	Co	.0947	.5190	.4243	448% +
Copper	Cu	.395	10.13	9.735	246% +
Iron	Fe	.81	.9	.09	11% +
Lead	Pb	.0015	.005	.0035	233% +
Selenium	Se	.0063	.0074	.0011	17% +
Magnesium	Mg	.23	.93	.7	304% +
Molybdenum	Mo	.840	.66	- .18	21% -
Nickel	Ni	.339	.68	.321	95% +
Potassium	K	.037	.39	.02	5% +
Silicon	Si	.458	.722	.264	58% +
Silver	Ag	.0001	.0014	.0013	1300% +
Sodium	Na	.3	.9	.6	200% +
Thalium	Tl	.0092	.0102	.001	11% +
Tin	Sn	.0082	.0272	.2638	321% +
Vanadium	V	.0401	.2314	.1913	477% +
Zinc	Zn	.1346	.1579	.0233	17% +

Section 5: Advanced Techniques for Doctors

46

~

Valve Corrections for Colon Problems

This correction can be very beneficial when you are suffering from constipation or even diarrhea. In fact, abdominal bloating and pain can often be relieved using this maneuver. Keep in mind that many people have heard of increasing fiber for intestinal problems, but many times what is really needed is more water. You should be consuming at least 64 ounces of purified water per day.

Ilio-cecal Valve (ICV)/Valve of Houston (VOH) Rebound Activation:
- Using your fingers, locate your hip bones at each side of your upper groin area. You should feel a bony point just below the waistband of your pants.
- Using the bony point as one point of reference, your ICV correction point is right between the bony point and your belly button.
- Press straight inward at the soft fleshy point between these two reference points on both sides of the groin. Quickly rebound or release off of the point so that the flesh fairly bounces. Repeat this rebound activation of

the valves three times on each side. The ICV is on the right side and the VOH is on the left.
- These valves are sphincter muscles, much like the anus muscle, which partition off the colon into three general zones. This rebound activation helps re-establish the peristalsis, or in other words, helps reset the musculature that lines the colon for the wavelike movement of fecal material out of the body.
- Without proper peristalsis, the fecal material collects, putrefies, and ferments causing gas, constipation or diarrhea, and promotes the habitat for harmful bacteria and parasites to grow. It can also lead to Irritable Bowel Syndrome or Leaky Gut Syndrome which can lead to the reabsorption of toxins from the fecal material back into the bloodstream.
- Chronic constipation can lead to cancer, liver problems, and a whole host of other problems for the body, including psychosis.
- Ideally, you should have at least two bowel movements per day.
- Constipation, gas, bad breath, and diarrhea are all signs of dysfunction in your digestive tract, which may include your stomach, liver, small and large intestines, gallbladder, and pancreas. If your problems persist after performing the ICV/VOH Rebound Activation Maneuver, then something else needs to be done. See a doctor of Biological Medicine for testing. Many times, chronic diseases and chronic problems originate in the intestines and are best dealt with early.

Section 6
Advanced Diagnostic Considerations

47

~

Computerized Regulation Thermograpy™

Through powerful computerized thermodiagnostics, your physician can finally see the multiple functional problems that lead to disease. When we realize that Lyme Disease is an infection affecting multiple organ systems and even the teeth, then we can understand how computerized regulation thermodiagnostics can help physicians stop the treatment of symptoms.

Chronic Lyme Disease indicates a total dysregulation of every organ circuit and tissue in the body. Multiple areas of dysfunction in predictable patterns can be easily seen using Computerized Regulation Thermography, giving the physician a way to see the body beyond the symptoms.

There is a reason for society's poor treatment record in chronic Lyme Disease, cancer, and other chronic illness; a doctor cannot fix what he does not know is broken. Doctors rely on blood tests to monitor illness. Many people suffering from Lyme, cancer, and other chronic degenerative illnesses will attest to the fact that blood testing can be a very poor way of identifying illness and tracking progress. Often people are diagnosed with Lyme Disease and/or cancer only after exhaustive lab testing, which generally showed no dysfunction in the body.

Computerized Regulation Thermodiagnostics is not to be confused with the colorful imaging thermographic devices, which are also coming of age after three decades of research. CRT displays multiple graphs, revealing to a certified thermologist or trained physician specific information regarding how 15 different organs and related systems regulate themselves in response to a cold stimulus.

With over 1500 CRT units in hospitals and physicians' offices in Europe, and over 20 years of correlative research, it is about time the people in the U.S. benefit from this technology.

CRT is a relative newcomer to the United States, as it only received FDA approval in the last 10 years as a Class 1, adjunctive diagnostic device. The CRT is scientifically reliable, provides reproducible results, is totally non-invasive, and is completely safe, with absolutely no side-effects. It truly is the "ultimate early warning system" and premier preventive and Longevity Medicine tool of this century.

Does the CRT negate the need for conventional lab testing? No, your physician will still need to use other tests that can monitor specific aspects of your health, but it is amazing the amount of information the physician can see even on totally asymptomatic patients.

The CRT is an amazing tool for the early diagnosis of dysfunctional aspects of a person. It also may provide the doctors with the following information:

- Where the primary problem resides.
- It enables the doctor to give tailored-made protocols for individual patients instead of the same treatment plan for the same diagnosis for each patient.
- The CRT clearly shows a patient if they can handle an aggressive treatment, since an aggressive treatment may kill them before the illness kills them.

- The CRT also shows the physician and the patient if the treatment protocols are working and improving the functional capacity of the patient's body, and if the prescribed protocols are actually creating more problems and doing more harm than good.

Who is Using the CRT?

Primary care physicians, Oncologists, Radiologists, Biological Dentists, and the full spectrum of healthcare professionals are beginning to use this effective new tool. When a CRT test is performed, your physician will provide the you with a computer-generated graph of the test. This allows easy tracking of any progress. This is not to be confused with the Electrodermal computerized testing devices.

The CRT supports what is called Functional Medicine, or Biological Medicine, whose philosophy is that if every tissue were functioning correctly, your body would have no disease. These doctors seek to remove any interference and provide your body with the building blocks it needs to heal completely. From this functional perspective, patient quality of life and lifespan is maximized.

As of yet it is not cleared to be a primary diagnostic device, but does that matter? History has proven that putting a label on a disease does nothing to help us see the disease outside of its symptoms. For example, fibromyalgia, chronic fatigue syndrome, multiple sclerosis, and even cancer are all basically a non-diagnosis. These terms all simply describe a set of symptoms. A true diagnosis identifies the cause of a disease. Since we can't identify the cause of these diseases, your physician will treat the only thing he can see: the symptoms. Even in cancer, the tumor is truly nothing more than the symptom created by dysfunction in multiple tissues of the body. The CRT provides the doctor with so much relevant information that he can finally stop the "cookbook" doctoring and start treating with a sense of where the primary causes lie and how to strategically tailor a treatment plan, from a total body functional perspective. Why wait for testing until you have an irreversible problem?

Who Should be Tested with the CRT?

Every person over 5 years of age should be CRT tested annually, at the minimum. Prevention of serious illness is made more realistic via periodic CRT testing and subsequent preventive medicine.

The Centers for Disease Control's (CDC) tracking of diseases reveals ever-increasing occurrence of childhood and adult asthma, ADD, dermatitis, cancer, chronic fatigue, fibromyalgia and other chronic illnesses. There is no one who shouldn't be tested. We all know that prevention is best, but how do you prevent what you do not know is about to happen? Should everyone be taking fistfuls of remedies to prevent every conceivable illness? Or, should you strategically support those areas you know need help? Definitely the latter.

Occasionally people will say, "I'm afraid of what it may find." It should be recognized that this comment stems from fear created by the poor treatment record of most serious diseases. Doing nothing will not change the future. The CRT is not about "putting nails in people's coffins" as some people like to think. It is actually all about "taking nails out of their coffin" and prolonging their quality of life.

The CRT offers <u>reproducible</u> and scientifically valid information that can be crucial to the development and tracking of a successful treatment strategy.

What to Expect in a CRT Exam

A professional Thermodiagnostic technician will perform the CRT testing. You will be asked to sit in a fairly cool, but not uncomfortable room for 10 to 15 minutes.

We will then take the first skin temperature measurements of the head, teeth, and neck. This is performed by a gentle touch of the probe to the surface of the skin. You are then asked to remove your clothes to your underwear, thereby subjecting your whole body to a controlled cold air "stress." The room is not excessively cold, only about 68° F. The remaining measurements on the chest, breast, abdomen and back are made rather quickly.

You will be asked to sit as you are, exposed to the room air for 10 minutes to complete the stress effect. According to clinical research, it takes 10 minutes for your body to stabilize and acclimate to the regulatory changes from the internal organs onto the skin. After this period, all measurements are then repeated and the test is concluded.

The results are shown by a computerized printout, which reveals the reactions of the body and the functional health of various organs and their associated systems.

How does the Skin Temperature Reveal Organ Dysfunction in a CRT Test?

How well the body maintains an optimum skin temperature is determined by the integrity or health of the organ or tissue directly beneath the point of the skin being measured by the CRT temperature probe.

A healthy body, in reaction to cold weather, will cause a constriction of the superficial blood vessels of the skin and organs. This constriction shunts blood away from the skin and organs and sends it to the head to keep the brain from getting too cold. The diverting of blood from the skin causes the skin to cool in the absence of the warm circulating blood. The normal amount of blood left in the skin in response to the 68 degree cold stimulus of a CRT test is enough blood to maintain a 0.3-1.0 degree cooler temperature after ten minutes of exposure.

When the organ underlying the point being tested is not functioning correctly, your skin temperature will show the type of dysfunction by the difference in the first and second CRT temperature readings. Correlations can then be made to all of the other temperature readings. Your CRT test will reveal much about your state of health.

48

~

Lyme Disease Meets Biological Dentistry

Biological Dentists are all previously conventional dentists who became aware that the teeth play an important role in the overall health of the body. One of the leaders in Biological Medicine, Dr. Thomas Rau, M.D., stated that if he could have only one other doctor to work with him, it would be a biological dentist. This is because of increasing amount of research showing a connection between cancer, degenerative diseases, and infectious diseases, with the heavy metals and toxins leaching out of dental materials, appliances, and root canals.

You will or have read in this book about Circuit Healing. These circuits are electrical/energetic organ circuits in the body that have been identified through thousands of years of research and only recently verified by technology. Each tooth has been determined to share the same electrical pathway as a specific organ, gland, spinal segment, joint, and muscle group. If anything goes wrong in the circuit, all parts share the same fate. The entire circuit can be poisoned by toxins leaking into the circuit. For example, a "silver" (or more accurately, mercury) amalgam in a wisdom tooth will steadily release small amounts of the mercury, tin, silver, and nickel that the amalgam is made up of into the heart and brain specifically, because the wisdom teeth and these organs share the same circuitry. Hidden infections and cavitations in the jawbones will leak bacterial toxins throughout the entire circuit, wreaking havoc as well.

Teeth are hiding places for Lyme spirochetes that must be resolved, because they are a major interference to the body's efforts to heal. Research reported in the book, Root Canal Cover-Up Exposed, by Dr. George E. Meinig, D.D.S., F.A.C.D., stated that Dr. Weston Price, a renowned dental researcher, performed thousands of tests on people with chronic degenerative diseases, those that did not respond to treatment.[184] He found root canals harbored bacteria inside the microscopic dental tubules of the dead tooth. Most often the bacteria was pleomorphic, as described earlier, and most often the bacteria were streptococcus, staphylococcus, and spirochetes! How important is it to recognize that Lyme spirochetes can be hiding in your old root canals and jaw infections?

The next finding of Dr. Price's is monumental – he found that even when the root canalled tooth is extracted and heat sterilized, it did not stay sterile. Dr. Price found that within 24-48 hours, the disinfecting medications lost their disinfecting ability. This is only trying to kill all the bacteria specifically in the teeth, not like typical Lyme Disease antibiotic treatments, which attempt to kill bacteria everywhere in the body! So, one can see further evidence of the extreme limitations of antibiotics against most microbes.

In some amazing research, Dr. Price also found that he could surgically implant the old root canal tooth under the skin of a rabbit and the rabbit would develop the same disease as the person the tooth belonged to! Very often, once the root canal tooth was removed, a large percentage of the patients recovered.

Even though many dentists believe the methods they are using to seal and sterilize root canals are efficient, Dr. Price found that the bacteria remain within the microscopic tubules of the teeth; even in the rare occasion where they cannot escape from these tubules, their toxins can still leach out through the cementum sealers. Most often, however, he found a disturbing fact, that these bacteria are almost always found in the first few millimeters of the adjacent bone in the jaw.

Dr. Price's findings have been confirmed by many bacteriologists. What this means to you is that if heat sterilization does not ensure the killing of the Lyme spirochetes inside of your teeth, that antibiotics, which you now understand are not that effective in the first place, have little chance of reaching these hiding places. This may be why so many people seem to mysteriously get "reinfected" or suffer a relapse of Lyme Disease.

"Dental factors have been associated not only with the cause but also with the cure of chronic disease."[185] Also, research has demonstrated that "factors contributing to chronic degenerative diseases include energy blockages and toxicity from mercury amalgam dental fillings. Symptoms ascribed to mercury toxicity include fatigue, depression, anorexia, insomnia, arthritis, moodiness, irritability, memory loss, nausea, diarrhea, gum disease, swollen glands, and headaches, among others."[186] Published studies have reported reversal of illness in such cases as Multiple Sclerosis, Alzheimer's, Cancer, Arthritis, and Parkinson's Disease.[187]

Research performed by Dr. Harold Hawkins, D.D.S., Melvin Page, D.D.S., and Emanuel Cheraskin, M.D., D.M.D., and many others found that people with tooth decay are more susceptible to degenerative disease. Understand now that each tooth effects every tissue and organ on its electro-energetic circuit, so decay from the tooth could be from poor dental hygiene, but it could also be that the tooth is having problems due to problems in the organ, gland, muscle, or joints that share the same circuit with that tooth. One begins to see even more clearly why doctors must specialize in addressing the entire body, including the teeth, instead of specializing in "pieces and parts" doctoring.

Search the internet using the keywords "Biological Dentistry" to find a local doctor. Only a dentist who has been trained this way will know what to do for you and have the correct tools and knowledge to undo the damage.

The political environment is such that, at this time, no claims for treating organic disturbances can be made by a Biological Dentist. Please respect this and come to him having already done your homework (reading the above book and others). Knowing this, you can simply request a Biological Dental Assessment and removal of potentially harmful filling materials for cosmetic reasons.

---

[184] Meinig, Dr. George E., D.D.S., F.A.C.D. Root Canal Cover-Up Exposed.
[185] Hodgson-Brown, E. and Richard T. Hansen, DDS. *The Key to Ultimate Health*. Writerservice Publishing. First edition. 2000.
[186] Hodgson-Brown 2000.
[187] Hodgson-Brown 2000.

Appendix A

Questions and Answers for Dealing with Alcohol in the Remedies

Question: I cannot tolerate even minute amounts of alcohol. I want to take the Jernigan Nutraceutical products. What can I do?

Answer: There are a few options for people who cannot physically tolerate alcohol. First of all, there are different forms of this intolerance as outlined below:

> **Group 1** - People who may drink alcohol, possibly a little wine every now then, but who know they feel the effects of the alcohol after the first sip and get brain-fog and fatigue.
>
> **Group 2** - People who never drink but know that remedies containing alcohol mildly aggravate their symptoms.
>
> **Group 3** - People who are recovering alcoholics and don't want to risk tasting even the small amount of alcohol in the remedy.
>
> **Group 4** - People with severe chemical sensitivities, including alcohol and cannot bear even the least amount of alcohol.

First of all, it must be understood that the Jernigan Nutraceutical liquid herbal remedies contain 20% alcohol by volume. To put this in perspective, an average dropperful (a dropperful is considered to be one good squeeze of the bulb even though the dropper only looks half full) will hold approximately 32 drops of liquid remedy. At 20% alcohol, a dropper contains about 6 ½ drops of alcohol.

The alcohol is present in the remedy to serve very necessary purposes. Distilled water and alcohol are used in the extraction process of the plants. The distilled water will extract, or pull out, certain types of medicinal substances from the plant material, while alcohol will extract or pull out other types of medicinal substances from the plants which would otherwise not be extracted by the water process. By using a hydro-alcoholic extraction process such as this, more of the various types of active ingredients can be obtained from plants, resulting in a broader-acting supplement.

Alcohol in a remedy serves another purpose. Alcohol preserves the final remedy and keeps microbes and fungi from growing in the remedy, once the bottle has been opened and the dropper is exposed to open air -- accidental contamination could occur if you breathed on or touched the glass portion of the dropper to your mouth or tongue.

Possible Solutions

Group 1 and 2 - The liver is the primary organ responsible for detoxifying alcohol and its breakdown component, aldehyde. Often the people in Group 1 have a systemic overgrowth of Candida yeast, due mostly to antibiotic usage disrupting the friendly bacterial flora in the gut that normally kill and keep Candida from growing out of control. As you may know, yeast consumes sugar and converts it into alcohol (as is the case when making champagne). The yeast in your body is also fermenting the sugars from your diet, even if you are not consuming refined sugar! Even if you have no obvious signs of yeast infection, like thrush or vaginal yeast symptoms, if drinking a few sips of wine effects you negatively, then it is likely you are on the verge of being "hung over" with the resulting brain fog and fatigue from the micro-brewery in your gut!

Because so many people suffering with Lyme have been on massive amounts of antibiotics and have yeast overgrowth, one must assume that yeast is a problem. I have used and clinically tested many of the best herbal and nutraceutical solutions for treating people with yeast overgrowth and found them to either be too weak or to be too strong. While Oregano or Olive Leaf Extracts are powerful, most of the people I have tested were allergic to them or they also kill off friendly bacteria. High-Allicin Garlic and Capryllic acid supplements are excellent, though they can be slow to act and seem to have difficulty finishing the job in the long run. There are a few good homeopathic combination remedies for yeast infections available at your local health food store. Because even conventional medicine has very few safe and effective anti-yeast medicines, I sought out (and found growing wild in Kansas) what many consider now to be the most effect anti-fungal and anti-yeast herb to date. It is now available only through Jernigan Nutraceuticals as the proprietary formula **Yeast Ease™**. It is the most effective, yet the most gentle, remedy found out of thousands of herbs clinically tested.

Once the process of helping the body kill the Candida yeast is under way, then it is time to reintroduce friendly bacteria back into the gut. These products are readily available from your health food store or doctor and are globally referred to as *probiotics*. Get a probiotic supplement that contains as many types of different friendly bacteria as possible. Many women know that eating cultured yogurt is a good way to replenish friendly bacteria; however, this only supplies the body with one or two different types of bacteria, such as Acidophilus species.

No matter what, you must give the liver the trace mineral Molybdenum (Ma-lib-denum). Molybdenum is a necessary component for the liver enzymes that break down alcohol and its byproduct aldehyde. As a matter of fact, if you take three of the Jernigan Nutraceutical **Molybdenum™** capsules (300 mcg/vege capsule) 10-15 minutes before taking your liquid remedies or before drinking a bit of wine, no side-effects of the alcohol would be experienced. Taking Molybdenum before drinking alcohol is so effective that it renders one virtually impervious to becoming drunk or even getting a "buzz." Molybdenum should be taken to manage the die-off toxins of bacteria and yeast no matter what anti-yeast medicine you take. As an added benefit, Molybdenum has been used for over 12 years to antidote the potential toxicity and allergic tendencies for virtually every type of pharmaceutical or natural medicine.

Group 1 and 2 Summary:
- Help the body naturally bring down the population of yeast, the source of your alcohol sensitivity. Take **Yeast Ease™** (General Recommendation: 1-4 droppers, 2-4 times per day for 1-3 months). One dropper is one good squeeze of the eyedropper bulb, even though the dropper will look only about half full.
- Re-inoculate the gut with friendly bacteria with a broad-spectrum probiotic. **Total Probiotics™** by Nutri-West is a favorite. (General Recommendation: 1-2 capsules, 1-2 times per day for as long as you are taking antibiotics, or if not taking antibiotics, take probiotics for at least 2 months).
- Detoxify the alcohol and aldehyde using **Molybdenum™**. (General Recommendation: 1-3 capsules (300 mcg each capsule), 1-3 times per day for 1 month, or as directed by your healthcare professional).

Appendix

Group 3 -- Recovering alcoholics have a difficult time because even the taste or smell of alcohol in a remedy can trigger addictive cravings. All of the recommendations for Groups 1 and 2 should be followed, with the exception of the Yeast Ease, which contains alcohol. The best way to be able to still use the Yeast Ease and other Jernigan Nutraceutical liquid supplements is to do one or more of the following:

1. **Dissipate the alcohol by water bath.** Put the required dosage of the liquid remedy in a small glass and warm the glass gently by placing it in a small pot of water that is only hot enough to be comfortable to keep your finger in. Many plant substances are heat sensitive, and some can be destroyed by as little as 110°, just slightly hotter than a high fever, so more heat is not recommended. Allow the glass to sit in this water bath for 10-15 minutes, after which no alcohol should be remaining. This technique is much like cooking with wine. The alcohol in the wine cooks off, but the taste of the wine remains, so if necessary to avoid a taste reminiscent of alcohol, the dosage should be mixed with a healthy juice with a strong enough flavor to effectively mask the taste. Mixing the dosage in a small amount of fruit yogurt can be effective as well.

2. **Dissipate the alcohol by open air.** Put the required dosage of the liquid remedy over the surface of a non-flavored rice cake (available in most grocery or health food stores) and let the remedy to sit for 15-20 minutes to allow the alcohol to evaporate. This process can be sped up by placing the remedy-saturated rice cake on the open door of a toaster oven or conventional oven so that only gentle, warm heat can pass over the cake without damaging the ingredients of the remedy. Eat the cake as is, or if taste masking is important, a light amount of an organic fruit spread can be put on top.

Group 4 -- People who are highly chemically sensitive (very little of a medicine can be taken orally) need to follow all of the recommendations they feel are possible as listed for Groups 1-3. The sensitivities can be minimized by first taking care to balance the Sympathetic Nervous System, primarily the adrenal gland function. This is best done by taking the oral tablet **DSF-Formula**™ by Nutri-West, and available only through a doctor. DSF-Formula is important because it will help gently reduce the hypersensitivity of your body. Taking **Molybdenum**™ is especially important, since chemical sensitivities often are caused by the liver's inability to effectively deal with any chemical, natural source or otherwise.

Another very effective way to be able to take a liquid remedy is to use it transdermally. To do this, follow the instructions for Group 3 water bath dissipation of alcohol to get the alcohol out of the remedy. Take the resulting dosage and saturate a 3"x3" gauze of a bandage and place it over the affected area of the body. Some people can tolerate this better than taking the remedies orally. Transdermally applied liquid remedies are just as powerful if not more so, and therefore caution is advised. The bandage should be replaced two times per day, and at the very least be worn to bed at night. This type of treatment works like the medicinal transdermal patches that are popular today.

A general rule of thumb is that anything you would eat or ingest can be used in an enema. Though unpleasant to some to consider, some find that it is beneficial to inject a post-water bath liquid remedy into the rectum in a retention enema. A retention enema is done by putting a small amount of liquid into the rectum with the intent that it be held there without releasing it in an immediate bowel movement. This is so that it can be absorbed into the body through the colon. Use the same amount as you would normally use if the remedy were to be taken orally. A small amount of water can be added to the dosage to aide in its delivery.

Appendix

Question: I am allergic to wheat, rye, barley and oats (gluten) and other things like soy and corn. Isn't the alcohol you use a "Grain Alcohol," and if so, will I be allergic to the alcohol?

Answer: All of the formulas which I developed used "Pharmaceutical-Grade 190 proof Alcohol," which means it is at least 95% pure alcohol and the remaining 5% is water. If you look at the molecular formula for alcohol, it is CH3-CH-OH. Gluten is a generic term when discussing "gluten intolerance." The actual molecule is a class of Gluten Exophines, whose basic molecular structure is $C_{25}H_{30}N_4O_7$. It is quite impossible to have a grain-type allergic reaction to Pharmaceutical-grade alcohol, even though it was distilled from various grains. Periodically, you may read that a remedy is made from Potato Alcohol and is therefore "superior." As you can see from the above molecular formula for alcohol, every alcohol is CH3-CH-OH, and one is no more or less superior if it is 190 proof. Also, if a remedy were made with less than 190 proof alcohol, such as 90 proof alcohol, there is the possibility of grain molecules remaining in the alcohol. In this case, there is a slight possibility of an allergic reaction in a highly sensitive person.

Question: My doctor says I should not use alcohol if I am taking Rocephin®, Flagyl® (generic name: metronidazole), and other antibiotics. I want to take the Jernigan Nutraceutical remedies, but they have alcohol. What do I do?

Answer: First of all, it must be understood that alcohol in the body is broken down into aldehyde, specifically acetadehyde. It is the acetaldehyde, not the alcohol itself, that causes the hangover and antibiotic/drug interference and adverse reactions. Acetaldehyde itself also is a mutagenic and carcinogenic chemical.[188] Acetaldehyde is easily detoxified by taking the trace mineral Molybdenum prior to using a product containing alcohol.[189]

The next consideration about antibiotics and remedies containing alcohol is that very small amounts of alcohol are actually consumed in the normal dosage of most remedies. Most liquid remedies contain a standard of 20% alcohol. This means that in 30 drops of a remedy, only 6 drops are alcohol. While the potential for any adverse effects is minimal, especially when compared to a glass of an alcoholic beverage, simple precautions to take your remedies away from your drugs and take the inexpensive mineral Molybdenum will likely be enough to avoid any problems. Of course, check with your doctor first if you have any concerns regarding this issue. Your doctor may not be aware of Molybdenum, so it may help to have him/her read this Q+A.

Appendix B

The Secret to Proper Tick Removal

There are many theories as to how to remove a tick that has become imbedded in the skin. We now know that most of them are incorrect, since the majority of ideas actually cause the tick to regurgitate (vomit) more bacteria into your body as you try to extract them.

Some of these erroneous tick removal methods:

- Putting essential oils, nail polish or remover, or any other substance on the tick to agitate it and cause it to pull itself out, all of which cause the tick to vomit before backing itself out of the skin.
- Using tweezers or the fingers, gripping as close to the head as possible. This sounds good until you attempt to do it without crushing the head, which often leaves the ticks mouth piece still embedded in the skin and still squeezes more juices into the your body.
- Holding a match over the back of the tick is an obvious mistake as it definitely causes the tick to vomit from the agitation.

Here is the best way to remove a tick and why it works the best. To understand why this works the best, study the structure of the mouth portion, called the hypostome and pictured here, generously provided by the Trix® Tick Remover company. The serrated teeth will hold tight with virtually any pulling action. However, they will literally fold flat if they are rotated in either direction. If you ever wondered how the tick removes itself after it has finished feeding, now you know -- it twists the teeth flat!

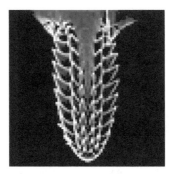

The serrated mouth portion of a tick.

I recommend only one type of tick remover, the patented TRIX Tick Removal System®, made in Sweden by InnoTech. This device is available through various distributors worldwide (www.tickremover.com) or through Jernigan Nutraceuticals (www.jnutra.com), or the clinic general store (www.hansacenter.com). I like to keep the TRIX® in several places so that I can use it as soon as I find a tick on myself, others, or on a pet. You may want to buy several to keep in your backpack, kitchen drawer, auto glove compartments, boat, RV, fishing tackle box, hunting jacket, barn/horse stable/kennel, and where you work. Obviously, it is best to have a TRIX® handy when you first notice a tick embedded in the skin.

Appendix

Here is the premise of the TRIX® tick remover:

- The Tick Remover is working by the **lasso principle**. It is very **fast to adapt** and therefore **easy to use** on children and pets, who sometimes find it difficult to hold still.

- The design makes it easy to use in ears, thick fur and other **difficult places**. The remover also works very well even if fur or hair comes into the loop.

- The removed tick is always stuck at the tip of the remover and can be disposed of easily. The loop is made of special fiber which has a pull strength of more than 20 pounds. The loop is big enough to take care of most tick species in the world.

The following is from the User Manual for the revolutionary TRIX® tick remover:

TRIX is a very effective remover which **easily and safely** can remove the **whole tick**, big or small. Even the smallest tick nymph is easy to remove with this tool.

1) Press down the loop and put it over the tick, as close to the skin as possible.

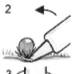
2) Let go of the button and tilt the tick remover perpendicularly against the skin.

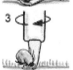
3) Keep the green point against the skin and turn it one round between your fingers. Lift away.

If it is a very small tick: Place the green point close to the tick and press the point down a little into the skin to angle up the loop. Release the button, twist and lift away.

1. Twist the tick away

If you look at the photomicrograph of the ticks sting- and suction organ (hypostome) you can easily see that if you **pull straight out** the barbs grip and get **even more stuck** in the skin (that's what barbs are for). The **risk of pulling** the tick **apart increases**.

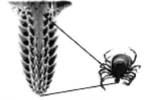

Mouthparts of Tick
Photo: G.Wife & T.G.T. Jaenson

If you **twist instead** the barbs will **release their grip easier** and all of the front part together with the **head** can **come along**. Tests have shown that it does not matter what direction you twist, clockwise or counterclockwise gives the same good results.

2. Twisting also reduces pain

When you **pull a tick away**, it causes some **pain** in the skin which may cause some pets to really dislike the treatment. But if **you twist it away with a tick remover** which keeps the mouthpart in a firm grip, the removal will be painless and the **pet** usually do **not even notice** because the bite area is stunned by the tick.

3. Always twist the tick away when using TRIX TickLasso

- It's faster.
- Gives less pain.
- Safer complete removal of whole tick.
- Decreases the risk of infections.

Appendix C

Lemon Wheel Throat Wrap

This is a therapy I learned in Germany from Medical Doctors who treat every type of illness using natural medicines and treatments such as this one. I like this treatment because it is something that kids like to do, its inexpensive and above all it works. It supports the body's normal healing process and can dramatically relieve the pain of a sore throat. It can also help when there are swollen glands in the neck.

You will need:
- 1-2 Lemons (Preferably organically grown, but go ahead and use any lemon you have)
- Medium size mixing bowl (preferably glass or ceramic)
- Purified hot water
- Cotton linen napkin
- Wool or Wool/Silk blend scarf

Instructions: With the tolerably hot water in the bowl, submerge the lemon under the water. Take a knife and cut the lemon into ¼ inch wide wheels while the lemon is submerged. This enables the water to capture all of the etheric oils from the skin of the lemon as you cut. Take the cotton linen and soak it in the lemon water, then wring it out just so that it doesn't drip. Quickly, so that the linen stays nice and warm, line up the lemon wheels in a row on the open cotton linen and fold it around the wheel to make a narrow band. Wrap this lemon wheel band around the upper throat leaving the back of the neck open with no lemons. On top of this lemon wrap, cover with the wool scarf for up to 30 minutes to keep it warm. The skin may turn red, this is normal.

Appendix D

Iodine Stain Test

This simple test is almost too simple, it costs next to nothing, and it will help you to know when your body is in need of Iodine. I really like how this test demonstrates that just because you give the body a nutrient, it doesn't mean the body will utilize it. In this test, if the iodine stain that you paint on your skin remains on the skin for 24 hours, your body apparently doesn't need it and therefore leaves it on the skin. If your body does need the iodine, often it will be slurped up almost immediately, and the iodine stain will disappear within a few hours. So in one simple test, you can determine if you need more iodine, and you can provide iodine all at the same time.

Instructions:
- Get a 1 ounce bottle of 2% Iodine tincture. (Available for topical use only from any pharmacy.)
- Using the tincture, paint a spot about the size of a silver dollar. Paint the spot in an inconspicuous place -- belly, thigh, or the inside of the arm. Be sure it is dry before putting on clothes to prevent staining the clothing. Do this when you know you will not be taking a shower or bath, since it may wash off.

- If your body level of Iodine is normal, the spot will remain on the skin for 24 hours.
- If the spot disappears in less than 24 hours, this means your body needed Iodine and took it in. (I find it awesome that our body will take in what it needs and leave on the skin what it doesn't need!) This works transdermally much like the now-popular Nicoderm and Estrogen Patches, by soaking into the blood stream via the skin.
- Keep applying the tincture of Iodine every 24 hours, at different places on your body, until the spot stays there for the full 24 hours.

*** Important: If you are presently on thyroid medicine, you may need to cut back on your medicine's dose, or ultimately stop it all together, now that your body has the iodine to manufacture the thyroid hormones it needs.

Purpose:

Iodine is needed by the thyroid to produce thyroxin. This test will let you know if you need more iodine, and it will also supply the iodine your body needs. Once iodine levels are normal in your body (meaning the spot lasts 24 hours), then you can stop applying it for a while and re-check periodically.

Iodine is one of America's most common deficiencies; even though the salt most of us consume has been iodized, this form of iodine seems to not function efficiently in the body. According to a study by the CDC (Center for Disease Control) the number of Americans with low iodine has quadrupled in the last 25 years.[190] Dr. Bernard Jenson, D.C., Ph.D., found that the iodized table salt, which is superheated so that it can pour more easily, is a poor form of iodine for the body. I recommend sun-evaporated sea salt with supplemental iodine. Sun-evaporated sea salt is loaded with trace minerals and does not come with the health risks of regular iodized salt. Sea salt will actually help normalize the fluid-regulating abilities of the body and has been known to normalize edema and high blood pressure.[191]   Once again, just giving your body iodine does not ensure your body can use it. Chlorinated and fluorinated water, which most Americans drink, inhibits the absorption of iodine, and perchlorate, a metabolic form of chlorine, inhibits transportation of iodine in the body.[192] This is one more reason to get a whole-house water purification system. The body will absorb two cups of the water in a 20 minute bath! I know my local municipal water is as blue as any swimming pool and smells just like a pool from all of the chlorine. If our goal is to eliminate anything that is interfering with the body functioning normally, eliminating your consumption of chlorine and supplementing with organic iodine will go a long way towards healing.

Iodine deficiencies may show up as weight gain, lethargy, fatigue, enlarged thyroid, hair loss, fibrous cysts, and mental retardation. In fact, experts say that iodine deficiencies are the world's leading cause of preventable mental retardation.

Replacing the missing iodine in your body may restore normal thyroid function; however, if you find that your spot never seems to last 24 hours, you need to alert your doctor and he can determine what you need to do from there. Many times when this happens, the hypothalamus and adrenal glands are fatigued and need support before the iodine will be efficiently used. Also, a special form of liquid potassium iodide can be taken sublingually while using this skin stain test to determine when you have adequate iodine.

Dietary Sources of Iodine: Dulse, Kelp, or Potassium Iodide or Atomadine™ from a health food store.

[188] Garro, J. et al. The effect of chronic ethanolconsumption on carcinogen metabolism and on *O*-methyl guanine transferase mediated repairs of alkylated DNA. *Alcohol Clin. Exp. Res.* 10: 735. 1986.

[189] Nielsen, Forrest H. Ultratrace Elements of Possible Importance for Human Health: An Update Essential and Toxic Tace Elements in Human Health: An Update, pages 355-376, 1993.

[190] Joseph, G., Hollowell, Norman W., Staehling, J., Staehling, N. *Iodine Nutrition in the United States. Trends and Public Health Implications: Iodine Excretion Data from National Health and Nutrition Examination Surveys I and III (1971–1974 and 1988–1994.* The Journal of Clinical Endocrinology & Metabolism Vol. 83, No. 10 3401-3408. 1998

[191] De Langre, Jacques. *Seasalts Hidden Powers.* Happiness Press, December 1987.

[192] Connett, Paul. *50 Reasons to Oppose Fluoridation, www.slweb.org/50reasons.*

Appendix E

Recommended Reading

The Swiss Secret to Optimal Health:
Dr. Rau's Diet for Whole Body Healing
Thomas Rau, M.D., 2007.

Nourishing Traditions
Sally Fallon, 1999.

Energy Medicine, The Scientific Basis
James Oschman, Ph.D., 2000.

Reference Guide for Essential Oils
Connie and Alan Higley, 2006.

Eat Right for Your Type
Dr. Peter J. D'Adamo, N.M.D., 1996.

Excitotoxins: The taste that kills
Russell L. Blaylock, M.D., 1996

What Your Doctor May Not Tell You About Menopause
John R. Lee, M.D., 2004

Cell-Wall Deficient Forms: **Stealth Pathogens**
Lida Mattman, Ph.D., 2000.

Prozac; Panacea or Pandora
Dr. Ann Blake Tracy, Ph.D., 1991.

The Game of Life and How to Play It
Florence Scovel Shinn, 1925.

Your Erroneous Zones
Dr. Wayne Dyer, 2001.

Appendix F

Internet Resources

Best Lyme Support Groups:

www.healingwell.com – Lyme Disease
www.healthboards.com – Lyme Disease

Lyme Information Organizations:

Lyme Disease Foundation	www.lyme.org
Lyme Disease Network	www.lymenet.org
American Lyme Disease Foundation	www.aldf.com
Lyme Alliance	www.lymealliance.org
National Center for Homeopathy	www.healthy.net/nch
IGENEX Reference Laboratory	www.igenex.com
HealthWorld Online - Free Medline	www.healthy.net

Center for Disease Control - Lyme Disease Site
www.cdc.gov/ncidod/diseases/lyme

Eat Right For Your Type - Dr. D'Adamo
www.dadamo.com

Alternative Medicine Practitioners Directory
www.altmedweb.com

Appendix G

Research on Borrelogen™

Acute Oral Toxicity Test – ISO

Borrelogen has been found to be essentially non-toxic at 150 times the maximum recommended dosage.

ISO is designed to assess the acute oral toxicity of the test substance, Borrelogen, occurring within 14 days of the oral administration of a single dose or multiple doses of the test substance administered within 24 hours.

The test substance, Borrelogen, was evaluated for its potential to produce death following oral administration at a dose of 2 grams/kilogram of body weight in male and female Sprague-Dawley rats. Based on the absence of mortality and the criteria of the study protocol, *the test substance is defined as nontoxic*. This study was conducted in compliance with the U.S. Food and Drug Administration (FDA) regulations set forth in 21 CFR, Part 58 and OECD GLPs, current version. The sections of the regulations not performed by or under the direction of Toxikon Corp, exempt from this Good Laboratory Practice statement, include characterization and stability of the test and its mixture with carriers, 21 CFR, Part 58.105, and 58.113. The assessment of an LD_{50} was not necessary. No toxicity was observed in post study necropsy of the different organ systems.[193]

Research on the Effectiveness of Borrelogen™

Borrelia burgdorferi antigen release stimulation by nutraceutical formula as determined by Lyme Urine Antigen Testing (LUAT)

(Presented at the 1999 International Tick-Borne Diseases Conference, New York City, New York)

It is understood that antigens are the cause of numerous sensitivities resulting in much of the symptomatology experienced in chronic illness. This clinical study was restricted to determining whether Borrelia burgdorferi specific antigen (Literally the dead pieces of Bb) could be purged from circulation by the use of a nutraceutical formula called Borrelogen. The results are very preliminary as more research is needed to rule out physiological interference. LUAT assay was utilized to determine antigen release after 68 subjects used the nutraceutical for one week. Results revealed 73% of the subjects released specific antigen to the degree of being considered positive or highly positive by LUAT. (Only seventeen of the 68 subjects were tested by Lyme Western Blot IgM/IgG prior to starting Borrelogen. All seventeen subjects were either Equivocal or Positive via this serological assay.) This study in itself cannot be used to make definitive statements about the efficacy of Borrelogen, only that an antigen was released from whatever mechanism. **Note:** IGeneX is not in any way endorsing this nutraceutical, nor is IGeneX associated in any way with Jernigan Nutraceuticals,

Inc. IGeneX was blinded to the use of the nutraceutical and only performed the testing procedure. True research seeks to find the truth in an unbiased manner for the betterment of mankind.

Introduction

Bacteria contain many particulate and soluble antigens that evoke strong, often lasting immune responses, both humoral and cellular.[194] According to Stedman's Medical Dictionary, an antigen (allergen) is any substance that, as a result of coming into contact with appropriate tissues, induces a state of sensitivity.[195] Antigens are understood to cause many of the symptoms experienced by Lyme Disease sufferers. It would stand to reason that decreasing the antigen load on the body would correspondingly decrease the number and severity of symptoms. A proprietary nutraceutical formulation was developed in 1998 to specifically target the functional release of spirochetal antigen from the tissues of the body. The historical and pharmacognostic data of the individual plant-based extracts reveal very low toxicity, while being functionally beneficial in many ways to the body. The research presented here was performed as a clinical study to aid in our understanding of the potential effectiveness of the nutraceutical formula Borrelogen□. Lyme Urine Antigen Testing (LUAT) was chosen as a viable determinant due to its specificity to Borrelia burgdorferi antigens seen as a result of a release of antigen from an appropriately applied therapy. Because the body will, as a natural process, release Lyme specific antigen in about 30% of untreated cases, the nutraceutical formula was tested to see if the body could be stimulated to release a greater amount of antigen, with a higher percentage of positive LUATs. A nutraceutical is defined as a plant-based remedy that is specifically formulated to target specific body dysfunctions.[196]

Methods

Participants in this study were pre-selected based on positive Borrelia burgdorferi screening, using Bio-Resonance Scanning☐ assay. The group consisted of 68 people residing in a non-endemic area of the United States. All were suffering from a range of 3 to 44 chronic problems based on a 55-question Lyme Disease symptom questionnaire. Lyme Urine Antigen Testing (LUAT) was utilized to monitor the release of antigen. LUAT testing is an antigen capture assay specific to detection of low levels of antigen, in spite of the presence of other proteins. The antibody being used in this antigen capture is a unique polyclonal antibody that is specific for the 31 kDa (OpsA), 34 kDa (OpsB), 39 kDa, and 93 kDa antigens of Borrelia burgdorferi. This assay appears to be very specific to these antigens with a reported false positive rate of less than 1% in a study of 408 controls.[197] The reference range of a LUAT is based on P-values or confidence levels. Antigen levels reported as ☐32 ng/ml have a 95% confidence level of being positive and distinguishable from a negative population.[198] A LUAT is a highly controlled and reproducible assay which is used in conjunction with patient history, symptoms and serum panels. The nice thing about LUAT assay is that it is positive throughout all three stages of infection: early, which is said to be <60 days (which is before you normally can get a seropositive result); second stage, which is defined as 60 – 360 days; and the third stage, >360 days.[199]

Results

Reporting only the highest score of the three-day urine collection, the majority of positive LUATs scored over 100 ng/ml. Out of the 68 LUATs, performed 44 were reported as positive or highly positive, while there were 4 borderline, and 18 negative results. The total percentage of positive scores was 73%. When the nutraceutical formula was used instead of

Appendix

prescription antibiotics, the majority of positive LUATs were reported over 100 ng/ml, and as high as >400 ng/ml. Although a score of >400 does not indicate that a patient is more highly infected than a score of >45, it does indicate a high rate of antigen release which can only benefit the patient. An interesting side note: only 17 of these 68 cases were also tested by Lyme Western Blot IgM/IgG prior to taking the Borrelogen. All 17 subjects tested as positive or equivocal by Lyme Western Blot.

Conclusion

Based on this study, it appears that this nutraceutical formula does indeed stimulate the purging of Borrelia burgdorferi antigens from the body. This antigen-detox can only be seen as a good thing as these antigens, when circulating throughout the body, cause a multitude of systemic sensitivities, which in turn causes increased suffering in the patient. An infected person does not release antigens daily or uniformly.[200] It is significant that, 73% of the time, a high release of antigen was stimulated while using this nutraceutical. Further research must be performed to determine if a negative control group on the same protocol would yield a similar effect. However, based on positive patient symptomatic response and clinical observations, we are encouraged that this botanical formula may effectively stimulate and increase the tissue elimination of deleterious antigen via the urine. Further research may also result in increased probability of highly positive Lyme Urine Antigen Test confirmations.

Interference studies performed by IGeneX lab confirmed that Borrelogen does not cause a false positive LUAT when negative patient urines were spiked in various concentrations. This *in vitro* assay does not, however, effectively rule out the possibility of *in vivo* interference.

[193] Glenn T. Shwaery, G. TPh. D., 99G-0905m 1999 Toxikon Corp. Sponsored by International Nutraceutical Research Group.
[194] Coltran, Kumar, Robbins. Robbins Pathological Basis of Disease. 4th Edition; p.335.
[195] Stedman's Medical Dictionary. 25th Ed. Williams & Wilkins.
[196] Journal of Nutraceuticals and Functional Foods, 1994.
[197] Journal of Nutraceuticals and Functional Foods, 1994.
[198] Journal of Nutraceuticals and Functional Foods, 1994.
[199] Calllister SM, Schell RF. Laboratory Serodiagnosis of Lyme Borreliosis. J Spirochetal Tick-borne Inf 1998; 1:21.
[200] Harris NS. IGeneX Reference Laboratory Guide, 1998; 4.

Appendix H

Other Jernigan Nutraceuticals™ Products

Many products made by Jernigan Nutraceuticals have already been discussed in this book in detail. This section provides information on others that may be mentioned but have not received as much attention in the Perfect-7 protocol.

Virogen

Of all of the remedies I have created, I enjoy using Virogen the most. I originally created it in order to help restore the damaged crystalline matrix of the Gulf War Veterans suffering from a genetically engineered or "designer microbe" called Mycoplasma fermentans incognitus. Once again, none of the 5000 remedies we had on hand could effectively provide the body with the information and energy needed to deal with this microbe that many experts agree has genetic material spliced into it from some of the world's worst viruses, parasites, and bacteria. Virogen was the result of this research and has resulted in **one of my favorite remedies to create a super-strong, completely integrated crystalline matrix against virtually any of the standard cold and flu bugs.**

I often have families call to tell me how much they like Virogen. They say if they take the Virogen at the first sign of a cold or flu, by the next day they are feeling great again. Virogen has be tested by many doctors that do various forms of sensitive testing and found to be one of their favorite and most trusted remedies. This is definitely a remedy that should be in every household's first aid kit.

From testing with Bio-Resonance Scanning, Virogen is the best overall remedy to assist the body in dealing with viruses. For any viral condition that does not respond to Virogen, Microbojen also has demonstrated phenomenal benefits.

Again, like virtually all of the Jernigan Nutraceutical formulas, Virogen works to restore the proper integrity of the crystalline matrix of the body so that the body can resolve viral invasion.

Molybdenum

Molybdenum is a trace mineral that can dramatically aid in the detoxification of the toxins caused by the dysfunction of multiple tissues in chronic illness. Molybdenum is very useful for detoxifying the toxin aldehyde from the die-off of Candida-type yeast. This is important to Lyme sufferers due to the fact that **aldehydes are also considered neurotoxins,** or nerve poisons. Aldehydes are also the toxins responsible for the hangover experienced by drinking excessive amounts of alcohol. I know of many Lyme patients who complain of this hung-over feeling without having drunk any alcohol. (However, it is our experience that it will not completely detoxify the specific Bb toxin.) Taking molybdenum will help slow the degeneration of tissues and related symptoms from the toxic overload.

Instead of taking a pain killer for a headache, Molybdenum can be taken for a toxic headache instead.

One can also take it before consuming any alcohol. The Molybdenum will bind the alcohol and will help prevent any buzz or hang over.

Yeast Ease

Yeast Ease ™ was the first product we developed that I decided was good enough to sell. Like almost all of the Jernigan Nutraceutical line, its ingredients are unique on the market. We were the first to identify and research the anti-yeast actions of the plants in this formula.

I found these anti-yeast actions using Bio-Resonance Scanning™ and tested Yeast Ease against the best anti-yeast products on the market. According to our tests, Yeast Ease out-performed all of the other products. Our tests also showed it to be very hypoallergenic and low toxicity.

I will never forget the day I arranged for an independent lab to run tests of Yeast Ease™ against five of the most common strains of candida-type yeast. The lead microbiologist confidently informed me that no one product kills all five. I smiled on the inside, knowing from the Bio-Resonance Scanning™ that Yeast Ease™ would be effective against all five strains. When the test results came in, sure enough -- it was very effective against every type of candida.

The lab determined that Yeast Ease™, which is already fairly dilute, would still kill 80% of the candida even when diluted up to 1:3200. This means you could put one gallon of Yeast Ease in 3200 gallons of water, and the Yeast Ease™ would still kill 80% of the candida!

Combine this with the realization that Toxicon Corporation found Yeast Ease is non-toxic up to 150 times the maximum recommended dose. It is so non-toxic that the FDA does not require further testing because it is unlikely that anyone would be drinking gallons of Yeast Ease™.

Yeast Ease™ is a liquid botanical formula; it can be added to your favorite herbal tea, taken directly in the mouth, diluted and added to a douche, applied topically, or added to bath water.

Keep in mind that yeast are a normal body flora – they are supposed to be there, only they are not supposed to grow out of control, so a truly effective treatment program for yeast requires you to change the environment of your body so that yeast cannot continue to grow out of control. Yeast Ease™ and any other product (even the pharmaceuticals) will only assist the body in bringing down the overall population of yeast. There are many other possible causes for yeast infections, such as parasitic infections which alter the pH of the gut, enabling the yeast to thrive, or antibiotic usage, which kills the friendly bacteria, such as acidophilus that normally kill and keep yeast under control, or weakened immune system as seen in AIDS, and in chemotherapy-damaged individuals.

No one product will ever eradicate candida-type yeast because the yeast infection is just a symptom of underlying disturbances in the body. Yeast Ease™ is, however, the best product I know of for a well-rounded treatment program.

Paragen

Parasites should make the news medias' front pages due to their pandemic proportions. The sad thing is that I've heard many people say that their medical doctor says that parasites are only in third-world countries. I'd like to show these doctors the hundreds of round worms and the numerous tapeworms our patients have released in the stool.

Of course, not everyone has tapeworms, but almost everyone that has not been treated, has parasites from microscopic to several inches long. The symptoms are diverse and often get overlooked as being a cold or upset stomach, and they may include any number of symptoms.

As in all of the Jernigan products, we have created what we believe is the best remedy available for restoring the crystalline matrix in regards to its ability to repel and expel a broad spectrum of parasites.

Paragen™ is made from Maclura Pomifera fruit, an inedible fruit from which we make a wonderfully effective extract. There are many anti-parasitic formulas on the market, often just rehashing the same ingredients, most of which are very bitter and next to impossible for children and sensitive adults to take. Paragen has very little flavor and is not bitter.

One of my favorite things to do is to introduce Paragen™ to missionary groups going to third-world countries. Historically speaking, virtually all the people who had gone on missions previously ended up violently sick from parasitic infections. With taking Paragen™ prophylactically, as a preventative, none of the missionaries got sick.

As a parting note, diarrhea, yeast overgrowth, and irritable bowel syndrome are almost always the result of parasites. Try Paragen™ and be amazed.

Pomifetrin

Pomifetrin is frequency-matched to restore and enhance the integrity of the body's crystalline-matrix when abnormal cell-replication is present. A very specific isolate of the Maclura pomifera tree is what gives Pomifetrin its primary action, as summarized here: Abnormal cell-replication is the plague of the century! It is likely viral-induced through various mechanisms. (See Emerging Viruses, Dr. Leonard Horowitz, www.tetrahedron.org.) Pomifetrin is believed to work using a novel method. Based upon Bio-Resonance Scanning™, we have discovered that the Maclura pomifera isolate contains a plant-based viralophage (a virus that attacks viruses, similar to a bacteriophage) that assists the body in eliminating the viruses associated with abnormal cell-replication. Once again, I must stress that all of our formulas are designed for strengthening and restoring the overall performance and integrity of the crystalline-matrix of the body and do not treat disease. Because of Pomifetrin's unique mechanism of action, no antiviral remedies, such as Virogen, Microbojen, or Borrelogen (which has Virogen in it) should be taken at the same time as Pomifetrin.

Abnormal cell replication, no matter where it is found, is not the cause but the end result of a dysregulated and non-reactive global crystalline matrix. The control mechanisms of the human organism lose control, the crystalline integrity is compromised, and the entire organism is affected. Every illness is a loss of the body's ability to morph and adapt in reaction to changes in its internal and external environment. I can tell you this problem always involves both your internal life of the body and the external lifestyle affecting the body. This one remedy, above all of the other top remedies we have tested, addresses this most serious viral fracture of the matrix.

Pomifetrin can be a big part of restoring the quality of life you desire.

Ingredients: Maclura pomifera isolate, Rehmannia root, Dioscorea root, Comus fruit, Mouton root bark, Poria fungus, Alisma rhizome, Ginger root, Schizoneptae. Other ingredients: Energized, distilled water, 20% pharmaceutical-grade ethanol.

Glossary

Allopathic Medicine: The philosophy of conventional medicine which seeks to relieve symptoms as its primary goal.

Applied Kinesiology: a treatment technique used primarily by Doctors of Chiropractic, but also by some Medical Doctors, which uses a patient's neuro-muscular system to identify problem areas in the body to determine the most effective treatment. This type of treatment is very individualized to the patient and helps to eliminate guesswork on the part of the doctor.

Auto-suggestion: a condition where an unconscious reaction to news suggesting that something may happen causes fear, leading to weakening of the body's energetic defenses, setting one up for illness. An example would be the news on television that, "Flu season is here. Reports are coming in that many people are experiencing a scratchy throat and fatigue, with body aches." Upon hearing this report, many start remembering past flus and may "hope" they don't develop this one.

Biological Medicine: The philosophy of medicine which recognizes that any interference with the body, mind, and spirit will cause a disturbance in the interconnectedness of the whole, resulting in disease. The restoration of coherence results in optimum health.

Clinical Kinesiology: the offspring of Applied Kinesiology, which is even more precise in determining not only what the patient's brain thinks is most important, but also uses the patient's brain as a bio-computer to determine the most effective treatments.

Coherence: The state where every aspect of the interconnected and interdependent body, mind, and spirit freely communicates within itself and adapts correctly to any changes in its internal and external environment.

Electro-dermal Testing: this encompasses many different types of machines, which are usually computerized. Through meridian contact points, doctors can determine which systems of the body are being most stressed, what specific problems the body has, and which remedies will correct the problems.

Excitotoxin: a substance added to foods and beverages that literally stimulates neurons to death, causing brain damage of varying degrees. Can be found in, but is not limited to, monosodium glutamate (MSG), aspartame (NutraSweet□), cysteine, hydrolyzed protein, and aspartic acid.

Homeopathy: a form of medicine in which the "electrical signature" of a substance is harnessed and imprinted upon a carrier substance such as distilled water or milk sugar crystals. Most homeopathic remedies contain no molecules of the original substance but only carry the homeopathically modified electrical signature of that substance. *Homeo* means similar, and *pathy* means symptoms. By definition, a homeopathic remedy is a remedy which will create "symptoms" when repeated doses are given to a healthy individual. Conversely, for an unhealthy individual, it may cure the symptoms.

Meridians: Superficial electro-energetic pathways that do not follow nerves. Meridians have been the subject of much controversy in western medicine for hundreds of years, even being called "of the devil" by well-meaning churches. However, the National Institute of Health recently announced that these meridians have been found to be a naturally occurring phenomenon verified by MRI. The controversy was due to the fact that, until recently, no one could physically dissect or see these meridians. A Korean scientist has been reported as having actually dissected these meridians, further documenting their existence. Meridian therapies include low-level lasers, microcurrent therapies, bio-electrical treatments, acupuncture and acupressure. These meridian therapies, as well as Electro-dermal Testing, seek to facilitate healing by stimulating and/or balancing the many meridians of the body.

Mycoplasma: A class of organism which is normally non-pathogenic. Its size is said to be in between that of a virus and a bacteria. Interestingly, the Gulf War Syndrome is causing many of the same symptoms as Lyme Disease and is now said to be caused by Mycoplasma fermentans incognitus.

Number Credulous Medicine: The practice of medicine that focuses on the microscopic view of the blood. This type of medicine reduces the importance of the human as an interdependent, interconnected, fully integrated organism and sees the patient from a strictly numerical basis. Focus is placed primarily upon numbers and percentages on a laboratory blood test and the response of those numbers to the treatments applied.

Nutraceuticals: Complex plant-based medicines.

Pleomorphic: The ability of an organism to change shapes at different stages of its life. *Pleo* means "many," and *morph* means "shapes." A butterfly is said to be pleomorphic in that it starts as a caterpillar and becomes a butterfly.

Preamble: Immediately preceding an event, such as signs and symptoms that come before the actual disease.

Spirochete: A class of pathogenic bacteria typified by its spiral or corkscrew shape. Lyme Disease is caused by a spirochete called Borrelia burgdorferi.

Suppressive Therapies: Medicines and therapies that suppress or weaken the body's natural reactions and mechanisms of bio-regulation. Any time you take a medicine that performs a task that the body should do for itself, the body becomes weak from disuse. Antibiotics are a suppressive treatment in that they weaken the immune system and disturb the normal fluid transportation mechanisms of the body. They also kill the friendly bacteria that help us digest foods correctly and provide us with essential nutrients as a byproduct of their life.

Synergism: Two or more remedies complement the action of the other(s), achieving a greater effect than using either one by itself.

Product Ordering

For products mentioned in this book:

Hansa Center for Optimum Health Retail
316-686-5900
www.hansacenter.com

Jernigan Nutraceuticals Retail or Wholesale
www.jnutra.com

Young Living Essential Oils
800-763-9963
www.youngliving.com
Enroll with sponsor # 497019

BioPro® Products
www.mybiopro.com/hansacenter

Or consult with your healthcare provider for ordering.

Vendors of therapy machines:
(Mention of Dr. Jernigan's name may get you a discount.)

High Tech Health, Infrared Saunas
800-794-5355
www.hightechhealth.com

ELF Labs/Teslar Technology, ST-8 Lymphatic Therapy
618-948-2393
www.elflab.com

A Major Difference, IonCleanse Foot Bath
303-755-0112
www.amajordifference.com

Index

A

Acetaminophen, 264
Acidic pH, 46, 135, 136, 213, 214, 243, 258, 298, 401
Albumen, x
Alkaline, 46, 135
Allopathic Medicine, 54, 74, 154
Aluminum, 144, 188, 262, 264, 325
American Biological Medicine, vi, x, xii, 49, 74, 279
American Dental Association, 260
American Medical Association, 48, 185, 219
Ammonia, 123, 126, 127, 128, 129, 130, 132, 134, 135, 136, 137, 138, 146, 149, 323, 364, 385
Anthocyanidins, 106
Anthrax, 170
Antibiotics, ix, x, 3, 4, 21, 22, 23, 24, 29, 39, 41, 42, 47, 48, 49, 50, 51, 52, 53, 54, 55, 60, 61, 66, 67, 82, 113, 120, 121, 126, 147, 169, 193, 222, 227, 235, 258, 264, 265, 286, 297, 298, 304, 309, 355, 356, 435, 436, 440, 441, 444, 445, 464
Apis, 272
Arginine, 128, 133
Art Therapy, 311
Aspirin, vi, 41, 82, 115, 222, 223, 282, 318, 386
ATP, 365

B

Babesia, 36, 60, 61, 164, 170
Bacterial Biofilms, 8, 157, 158, 220, 227
Bacteriophages, 3, 120
Baking Soda (sodium bicarbonate), 217
Bartonella, 36, 163
Bath, Detox, 8, 146, 196, 207
Bath, Hydrogen peroxide/Epsom Salt, 8, 157, 158
Bath, Mustard Foot, 8, 157, 158, 203, 386
Bath, Strengthening/Nutritive Bath, 8, 157, 158, 204, 207
Beyond Chelation Improved, 383, 390
Biofilms, 227
Bio-hologram, 93
Bio-information, vii, 30, 33, 164, 166, 167, 276
Biological Dentistry, 9, 261, 434, 437
Biological medicine, doctors, 285, 425
Biological Warfare, 60, 169
Biophoton, 34, 90, 91, 96, 109
BioPro® Products, 8, 234, 476
Bio-Resonance Scanning, v, vi, 37, 67, 96, 103, 104, 105, 122, 169, 175, 248, 262, 286, 294, 299, 413, 463, 467, 468, 470
Blood-brain Barrier, 66, 123, 126, 127, 329, 377, 391, 403
Book, Everyday Miracles by God's Design, iv, viii, xi, 69, 148, 292, 294, 335, 348
Book, The Rainbow and the Worm, 95, 108
Borrelia Burgdorferi, 7, 3, 6, 7, 15, 16, 19, 20, 21, 22, 24, 26, 34, 36, 59, 61, 64, 120, 128, 149, 164, 207, 288, 400, 401, 402, 461, 462, 463, 464, 475
Borrelogen
  Ingredients, 165
  Research, 460
  Toxicity Studies, 460
Brain Fog, ii, 116, 141, 440
Breast Cancer, 77, 97, 118
British Medical Journal, 227
Bulls-eye Rash, 5, 15, 16, 22

C

Cancer, 27, 28, 40, 68, 82, 98, 109, 116, 141, 149, 186, 192, 213, 215, 227, 240, 253, 259, 268, 290, 337, 355, 357, 396, 418, 425, 428, 429, 430, 431, 434, *See* Breast Cancer
Candida, 36, 61, 133, 215, 439, 440, 467
Case Studies
   Classic Lyme
     Miss F., 286
   Multiple Sclerosis
     Mrs. L., 288
   Obscure Illness Source
     Mr. M., 294
   Power of the Mind
     Mr. B., 292
     Ms. S., 289
   Scars Interfere
     Mr. W., 296
   Viral Ulcers
     Mrs. P., 297
Cayenne Pepper, 202, 208, 209
Cell-Wall Deficient, 456
Center for Disease Control, 453, 458
Cerebral Allergies, 66, 127, 128
Chelation, 8, 157, 159, 226, 227, 383, 390
Childhood Stress
   Dealing with, 347
   Detecting, 346
   Parental abuse, 344
   School, 345
   Sleep, 345
Chiropractic, 8, 79, 146, 159, 247, 276, 277, 278, 279, 280, 293, 371, 378, 379, 386, 387, 388, 392, 472
Chlorine, inhibition of iodine, 454
Cholera, 29, 34
Cholestyramine, 125
Chronic Fatigue, 19, 59, 61, 127, 128, 187, 246
Cipro, 120
Circiuts of the Body
   Role of Glands, 86
Circuit Healing, 7, v, x, 49, 71, 75, 76, 77, 79, 81, 82, 84, 86, 268, 286, 434

Circuit Healing Chart, 76
Circuits of the Body
   Introduction, 71
   Role of Joints, 79
   Role of Muscles, 84
   Role of Organs, 81
   Role of Symptoms, 82
   Role of Teeth, 77
   Swiss Watch, 75
   Treating, 74
Cleanse, Dr. Joseph's, 8, 157, 158, 189, 190, 192, 210
Cleanse, Master Longevity, 147, 157, 158, 212
Coherence, iii, 26, 38, 46, 54, 68, 90, 91, 93, 96, 102, 105, 108, 109, 119, 154, 156, 382, 472
Colon Cleanse, 157, 158, 189, 190, 192, 210
Colostrum, 16, 17
Colostrums, Fractionated, 17
Computer Tomograms, 337
Computerized Regulation Thermography (CRT), 9, 67, 117, 262, 428
Cookbook Doctoring, 67, 430
Copper Sulfate, 271
Core Warmth, 246, 247, 364, 376
CPK, 5
Cranston, Joe, 48
CT scans, 335

D

Dance, 311, 375
Dental Material, 259
Depression, 9, 47, 312
Detox Cocoa, 7, 157, 158, 177, 178
Detox Coffee, 7, 157, 158, 177, 178, 192
Detox Tea, 7, 157, 158, 177, 192
Detoxification, 116, 122, 123, 126, 133, 136, 141, 145, 146, 157, 158, 166, 168, 175, 176, 177, 185, 192, 193, 204, 213, 214, 215, 226, 245, 259, 262, 263, 264, 272, 323, 388, 416, 417, 420, 422, 467
Diet
   Blood Type Diet, 209

Foods to Avoid, 324
Rotation Diet, 392
Direct Resonance Testing, 129, 136, 137
Dizziness, 174, 387
DNA Imprinting, 403
Drug-induced Illusions, vii, ix, 55, 101
Drugs, high-power, 39
Dry Skin Brushing, 7, 157, 158, 181, 197, 205

E

Echinacea Augustifolia, 178
Edelson, Stephan, 261
Ehrlichia, 36, 61, 164, 170
Eker, T. Harv, v, 319
Electrodermal Screening, 146
Enema, 189, 190, 191, 192, 443
Environmental Protection Agency, 115, 140
Enzymes, viii, 11, 35, 131, 159, 193, 198, 200, 205, 213, 214, 215, 222, 223, 224, 396, 406, 441
Enzymes, Protease, 8, 131, 157, 158, 222, 223, 224, 396, 406
Enzymes, Systemic, 222
EPA, 115, 140, 384, 390, 423
Epidemics, 42
Epsom Salts (magnesium sulfate), 197, 217, 218
Epstein-Barr, 36, 170, 377
Essential Oils, 85, 102, 105, 157, 212, 214, 231, 294, 347, 403, 412, 446
Etheric Field, 270, 271
Excitotoxins, 329, 456

F

F.A.C.T. test, 7, 123, 124, 125, 126, 289, 290, 383
Fasting, 82, 95, 147, 209, 244, 381, 407, 448
Fatigue, ii, 31, 54, 66, 82, 116, 128, 132, 141, 175, 198, 235, 240, 253, 268, 287, 289, 330, 338, 364, 365, 367, 368, 369, 370, 373, 376, 414, 422, 430, 431, 436, 438, 440, 454, 472
Fevers
   Excessive, 393, 395
   Febrile Convulsions in Children, 395
   Gradual Onset, 392
   Sudden Onset, 394
Fiber Optic, 7, 25
Fibromyalgia, 84, 116, 141, 240, 246, 268, 430, 431
Findings, 97, 238, 269, 285, 297, 298, 303, 335, 338, 405, 436
Foods, Cooling, 255
Foods, Warming, 254
Foot Bath, Mustard. *See* Bath, Mustard
Formaldehyde, 140
Free-will, 69
Functional Acuity Contrast Test, 123, 125

G

Germ Theory, xii, 401
German New Medicine, 8, 334, 335, 337, 338, 339, 340, 364, 397
Ginger, 167, 178, 196, 200, 202, 257, 471
Glutamine, 128, 149
Gulf War Syndrome, 59, 61, 474

H

Habits, Changing, 209, 309, 310
Hamer, Ryke Geerd, 335, 337, 338, 339
Hamer, Ryke Geerd Hamer, 334, 337, 364
Hay, Louise, 363
Headache, 41, 82, 245, 282, 318, 387, 468
Health, 8, iii, ix, x, 6, 45, 76, 87, 103, 186, 219, 261, 267, 276, 279, 300, 319, 322, 328, 362, 407, 412, 414, 437, 455, 456, 474, 476
Heart, Electromagnetic Generator, 35, 91, 298, 366

Heart, not a pump, 43, 414
Heavy Metal Detoxification, 262
Heavy metals, sources of, 261
HemiSync, 367, 368
Hepatitis B and C, 170
Herpes, 36, 61, 129, 133, 134, 377
Herxheimer Reaction, 4, 113, 121, 165, 176, 283, 284
Hexagon of Health, 76
High Blood Pressure, 41, 186, 188, 454
HIV, 61, 170, 290
Ho, Mae Wan, 95
Hologram, 92, 93
Homeopathic Remedies, viii, 85, 358, 473
   Aconite, 231, 232, 381, 385, 386, 394, 395
   Belladonna, 392
   Cocculus Comp, 387
   Palladium, 258, 267, 272, 372
   Quartz, 394, 395
   Rescue Remedy, 347, 372
Hormones, 30, 31, 65, 86, 239, 243, 330, 352, 453
Human Herpes Virus-6 (HHV), 36, 377
Hydrogen Peroxide, 197, 200
Hyperbaric Oxygen Therapy, 377, 407

I

Ilio-cecal Valve/Valve of Houston, 424
Illusions of Health, 277
Infrared Sauna, 137, 183, 184, 185, 186
   Illnesses Benefited, 418
Insomnia, 116, 141, 376, 436
Iodine Stain Test, 9, 452
Iscar, 272, 396

J

Jarish-Herxheimer Reaction, 64, 121

L

Leaky Brain Syndrome, 7, 127, 129
Lewis, Ricki, 48
L-Forms, 21
Library of Congress, 95
Light Metabolism, 89, 90, 91, 95, 105, 299
Liquid Crystals, 33, 94
Liver and Gallbladder Flush, 8, 216
Living in the Moment, 303
L-Lysine, 133, 134
Low Body Temperature and
   "Natural" Antibiotics, 265
   Antipsychotics, Fever Reducers, 244
   Contrast Foot Baths, 271
   Death, ii, 52, 77, 137, 149, 239, 240, 242, 252, 347, 366, 404, 460, 473
   Decongestants, 264
   Electromagnetic Pollution, 235, 369
   Fibromyalgia, 19, 59, 61, 128, 187, 241, 248, 376
   Fluid Regulation, 265
   Heavy Metals, 40, 77, 114, 115, 139, 143, 145, 174, 175, 176, 183, 199, 226, 258, 259, 261, 263, 272, 294, 366, 380, 416, 422, 434
   Normal/optimal Range, 364
   Sugar, 36, 204, 209, 212, 214, 244, 324, 330, 369, 381, 439, 473
   Sympathetic Treatments, 264
   Trigger Points, 84, 241, 242
Lyme-related Illnesses
   ALS A, 7, 5, 18, 84, 128, 137, 138, 400
   MS, 5, 18, 19, 84, 128, 400
Lymph Drainage, 117
Lymph System, 117

M

Magnesium, 196, 197, 198, 199, 214, 217, 423

Markolin, Caroline, 8, 336, 337, 364, 397
Master Longevity Cleanse. *See* Cleanse, Master Longevity
Matrix, Crystalline, 30, 31, 32, 33, 36, 37, 38, 40, 41, 46, 60, 64, 90, 91, 92, 93, 94, 95, 96, 98, 99, 101, 102, 104, 106, 134, 155, 239, 289, 294, 296, 299, 466, 467, 470, 471
Mattman, Lida, PhD, 8, 18, 21, 24, 61, 400, 407, 456
McCraty, Rollin, 91
McMakin, Carolyn, 241
Medical Mavericks, 334, 349
Mental Confusion, 244
Mercury Amalgams, 78, 260
Meridian, 40, 96, 296, 412, 473, 474
Miasms, 8, 23, 354, 355
Microbojen, 37, 134, 158, 160, 163, 167, 169, 170, 222, 386, 402, 403, 404, 467, 471
Milk, 13, 16, 17, 132, 146, 193, 204, 255, 256, 257, 330, 331, 473
Mitochondria, 364
Molybdenum, 133, 217, 219, 386, 423, 441, 443, 445, 467, 468
Morphing, 92
Morphogenetic Field, 93
Mosquito, 6, 64, 306
Movie, Under Our Skin, 15
MSG, 324, 329, 473
Multiple Sclerosis, 18, 84, 288, 400, 436
Mustard Foot Bath. *See* Bath, Mustard Foot
Mycoplasma, 59, 170, 466, 474

N

Nanoderm Lotion, 7, 143, 144, 145
National Adipose Tissue Survey, 115, 140
natural, 265
Neural Therapy, 67
Neuro-Antitox II Formulas, 123, 175

Neurotoxins, 4, 34, 119, 120, 121, 124, 125, 126, 133, 158, 175, 193, 289, 364, 376, 405, 467
New England Journal of Medicine, 48
New Scientist, 53, 58
Nicholson, Garth, 60
Ningxia Red Juice, 208, 209, 212, 213
Nitric Oxide, 128, 132, 137, 385
Nitric Oxide Synthetase, 128
Numbness, 65, 174, 232, 244, 246, 296, 297
NutraSweet, 324, 329, 473
Nutrition, 212, 226, 252, 320, 322

O

Oils, Essential, 8, 69, 230, 231, 407, 456
    Forgiveness, 49, 345, 352
    Frankincense, 231, 232, 347
    Harmony, xii, 401
    Joy, viii, 30, 49, 148
    Lavender, 347
    Marjoram, 255, 376, 385
    Peace & Calming, 347
    Primula, 389
    Rosemary, 199, 202, 207, 422
    Solum Uliginosum, 131, 206, 207, 231, 232, 247, 373, 374, 393
    Surrender, 347
    Thieves, 231, 232
    Valor, 231, 232, 347, 371
Olive Oil, Cold Pressed, 217
Optimum Health, x
Oschman, James, 30, 35, 456

P

Painkillers, 282, 283, 386
Paragen, 37, 469, 470
Parasites, 26, 67, 81, 211, 329, 425, 466, 469, 470
Parkinson's, 7, 138, 436
Perfect-7 Protocol, 57, 126, 165, 166, 168, 231, 466
Pesticides, Toxic Effects, 40
Phonons, 36

Phos-Drops, 217, 218
Photons, 30, 32, 89, 90, 94, 95, 104, 105, 107, 299, 417
Plague, 18, 239, 306, 470
Plant Pigments, 89, 106
Pleomorphic, 21, 23, 164, 435, 475
PMS, 188, 328
Polarity, 46, 135, 136, 218, 239, 240, 400, 401, 417
Polarity, Effects of
   Negative, vii, 31, 46, 47, 49, 53, 93, 132, 135, 214, 218, 239, 290, 291, 293, 294, 312, 313, 316, 317, 336, 401, 421, 463, 464
   Positive, ii, 5, 6, 7, 19, 20, 22, 49, 61, 108, 126, 129, 134, 135, 136, 164, 214, 289, 290, 291, 310, 314, 319, 336, 352, 368, 400, 421, 461, 462, 463, 464
Polio, 54
Pomifetrin, 37, 396, 470, 471
Post-graduate Training, 277
Post-Lyme Syndrome, 4, 54, 126, 246
Prayer, 209, 325
Predispositions to Illness, 354
Probiotics, 265, 440, 441
Progesterone, 86, 328, 329, 370, 372
Prozac, 352, 457

Q

Quack, 260

R

Rau, Thomas, 40, 87, 322, 323, 434, 456
Rhythms of the Body, 247
Rife Machines, 166
Riordan, Hugh, 334
Root Canals, 77, 261, 434, 435, 436

S

Scalar Waves, 417
Sea Salt, 324, 453

Silphium, 123, 174, 175, 176, 391, 405
Silver Amalgams, 259, 260
Sleep, 10, 66, 206, 218, 234, 270, 289, 297, 328, 345, 350, 368, 369, 370, 411
Smallpox, 170
Solitons, 36, 90, 91, 102
Strep Throat, 306, 351
Stress
   Adult, 8, 350, 353
   Childhood, 8, 342, 347
   Electromagnetic, vii, 31, 32, 35, 39, 43, 67, 74, 90, 91, 94, 99, 108, 109, 206, 230, 234, 235, 247, 286, 287, 289, 294, 298, 366, 369, 371, 401, 409, 410, 411, 414, 417, 422
   Emotional, 81, 293, 338, 382
   Geopathic, 47, 206
   Mental, 45, 46, 54, 244, 290, 352, 379, 382, 411, 454
   Miasm, 23, 354, 356, 357, 358
   Physical, 37
Sugar Cravings, 244
Sunlight, 311
Supercontinuum Light, 93
Supermarket Toxins, 138
Symptoms, Progression of
   Adrenal fatigue, 373
   Alcohol, worse with, 10, 114, 133, 138, 165, 170, 174, 175, 176, 324, 329, 331, 438, 439, 441, 442, 443, 444, 445, 467, 468
   Asthma, 391
   Auditory, 376
   Auditory/Visual, 376
   Barometric Stress/pain with Weather Change, 374
   Bell's Palsy, 389
   Concentration, Difficult, 382
   Dyslexia, 382
   Ear Noises, 381
   Eyes/vision, 388
   Hair Loss, Unexplained, 13, 454
   Headaches, 386
   Heart Problems, 380
   Hiatal Hernia, 379
   Joint Pain, Swelling, 373
   Memory Problems, 390

Mitochondria Fatigue, 364
Muscle Cramps, Pain, 376
Poor Balance, 387
Sciatica, 385
Sleep Disturbances, Unrefreshing, 368
Stomach Upset, 378
Swollen Glands, 436, 450
Throat Sore, 380
Twitching of Muscles, 384
Vertigo, Dizziness, 387
Weight Loss/gain, 396
Symptonms, Progression of
Fatigue, Tiredness, Poor Stamina, 364
Syphilis, 22

T

Termite Analogy, 23
Therapies
Laser, Low-level, 412
Therapy
Infrared Sauna, 8, 157, 158, 183, 187, 263, 272, 388, 417
IonCleanse, 9, 417, 420, 421, 422, 423, 476
ST-8 Lymphatic Drainage, 263, 386, 388, 416
Suppressive, 355
Thoughts, Extra-low Frequency Waves, 294
Tick, 6, 15, 16, 17, 18, 22, 24, 64, 142, 306, 402, 446, 447, 448, 449
Tick Removal, 9, 446, 447
Toothpaste, 139, 140, 260
Toxicity Symptoms, 116
Toxin
Excito-, 329
Toxin-generating Genes, 3, 120
Toxins
Bacterial, 64, 66, 116, 435
Environmental, 119, 141, 157, 158, 159, 370
Neuro-. *See* Neurotoxins
Skin, 7, 142

Tracy, Ann Blake, 352, 457
Trix® Tick Remover, 447
Trypanosoma Gambiense, 127
Tumor, 40, 82, 109, 212, 214, 337, 338, 430
Tylenol, 82, 147, 245, 386

U

Underwire Bras, 118

V

VCS (Visual Contrast Sensitivity test), 124
Vertigo, 11, 174, 286, 287, 387
Virogen, 37, 134, 466, 467, 471
Vitamins, viii, 41, 42, 67, 212, 214, 215, 250, 265, 266, 294, 308
Voll-testing, 67

W

Water, Municipal, 306
Penta, Young Living, 158, 208, 209, 214, 230, 231, 294, 347, 376, 380, 387, 389, 403, 476
Purified, 133, 176, 325, 379, 424
Tap, 139, 262, 306, 325, 423
Weather, 46, 130, 131, 244, 247, 374, 432
West Nile Virus, 16, 18, 170
Wolf, Otto, 45, 50, 395
Wolfberries, 212, 213

Y

Yeast, 36, 67, 133, 285, 422, 439, 440, 441, 467, 468, 469, 470
Yeast Ease, 37, 440, 441, 442, 468, 469
Young Living Essential Oils, 208, 231, 347, 380, 476